ACSM's
Guidelines for Exercise Testing and Prescription
EIGHTH EDITION

SENIOR EDITOR

Walter R. Thompson, PhD, FACSM
Regents Professor of Kinesiology and
Health (College of Education)
Professor of Nutrition (Division of
Nutrition, School of Health Professions,
College of Health and Human Sciences)
Georgia State University
Atlanta, Georgia

ASSOCIATE EDITORS

**Neil F. Gordon, MD, PhD, MPH,
FACSM**
Chief Medical and Science Officer
Nationwide Better Health
Savannah, Georgia

Linda S. Pescatello, PhD, FACSM
Professor
Department of Kinesiology and Human
Performance Laboratory
Neag School of Education
University of Connecticut
Storrs, Connecticut

ACSM's
Guidelines for
Exercise Testing
and Prescription

EIGHTH EDITION

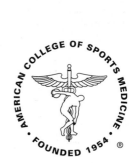

AMERICAN COLLEGE
OF SPORTS MEDICINE

Wolters Kluwer | Lippincott Williams & Wilkins
Health
Philadelphia · Baltimore · New York · London
Buenos Aires · Hong Kong · Sydney · Tokyo

Acquisitions Editor: Emily Lupash
Managing Editor: Andrea M. Klingler
Marketing Manager: Christen Murphy
Production Editor: John Larkin
Creative Director: Doug Smock
Compositor: Aptara, Inc
ACSM *Committee on Certification and Registry Boards Chair*: Dino Costanzo, MA, FACSM
ACSM *Publications Committee Chair*: Jeffrey L. Roitman, EdD
ACSM *Publications Committee Subchair*: Janet P. Wallace, PhD, FACSM
ACSM *Group Publisher*: D. Mark Robertson, Assistant Executive Vice President

Eighth Edition

Copyright © 2010 American College of Sports Medicine

351 West Camden Street   530 Walnut Street
Baltimore, MD 21201   Philadelphia, PA 19106

Printed in China

| First Edition, 1975 | Third Edition, 1986 | Fifth Edition, 1995 | Seventh Edition, 2005 |
| Second Edition, 1980 | Fourth Edition, 1991 | Sixth Edition, 2000 | |

9   8   7   6   5

Library of Congress Cataloging-in-Publication Data

American College of Sports Medicine.
   ACSM's guidelines for exercise testing and prescription / American
College of Sports Medicine ; [senior editor, Walter R. Thompson ;
associate editors, Neil F. Gordon, Linda S. Pescatello ; contributors,
Kelli Allen . . . [et al.]]. — 8th ed.
     p. ; cm.
   Includes bibliographical references and index.
   ISBN 978-0-7817-6903-7 (alk. paper)
  1. Exercise therapy—Standards. 2. Exercise tests—Standards. I.
Thompson, Walter R. II. Gordon, Neil F. III. Pescatello, Linda S. IV.
Title. V. Title: Guidelines for exercise testing and prescription.
   [DNLM: 1. Exertion—Guideline. 2. Exercise
Test—standards—Guideline. 3. Exercise Therapy—standards—Guideline.
WE 103 A514a 2009]
   RM725.A48 2009
   615.8'2—dc22

                             2008033759

DISCLAIMER

To purchase additional copies of this book, call our customer service department at (800) 638-3030 or fax orders to (301) 223-2320. International customers should call (301) 223-2300.

Visit Lippincott Williams & Wilkins on the Internet: http://www.lww.com. Lippincott Williams & Wilkins customer service representatives are available from 8:30 am to 6:00 pm, EST.

For more information concerning American College of Sports Medicine certification and suggested preparatory materials, call (800) 486-5643 or visit the American College of Sports Medicine Website at www.acsm.org

This book is dedicated to the hundreds of volunteer professionals who have, since 1975, contributed thousands of hours developing these internationally adopted Guidelines. Now in its eighth edition, it is the most widely circulated set of guidelines established for both health/fitness and clinical professionals. Specifically, this edition is dedicated to the editors, the writing teams, and the reviewers of this and previous editions who have not only provided their collective expertise, but have also sacrificed precious time with their colleagues, friends, and families to make sure that these Guidelines *met the highest standards in both science and practice.*

In a letter to his friend Robert Hooke on February 5, 1675, English mathematician and physicist Sir Isaac Newton wrote, "If I have seen further, it is by standing on the shoulders of giants." Although Newton lived between 1642 and 1727, this quote could not be truer today, almost 335 years later. The ACSM *Guidelines* had its origins within the ACSM Committee on Certification and Registry Boards (CCRB, formerly known as the Certification and Education Committee and the Preventive and Rehabilitative Exercise Committee). Although the project is still under the auspices of the CCRB, it has become a text that is embraced internationally by ACSM members and nonmembers in health/fitness and clinical practices. Today, it has become *the* resource for anyone conducting exercise programs or exercise testing. It is also the resource for supporting texts produced by ACSM (*ACSM's Resource Manual for Guidelines for Exercise Testing and Prescription, ACSM's Resources for Clinical Exercise Physiology, ACSM's Resources for the Personal Trainer, ACSM's Health-Related Physical Fitness Assessment Manual*, and *ACSM's Exercise Management for Persons with Chronic Diseases and Disabilities*). The author/contributor list is now in the hundreds for this and previous editions, and the following have served in leadership positions and are the "giants" referred to by Newton.

First Edition, 1975

Karl G. Stoedefalke, PhD, FACSM, Co-Chair

John A. Faulkner, PhD, FACSM Co-Chair

Second Edition, 1980

R. Anne Abbott, PhD, FACSM, Chair

Third Edition, 1986

Steven N. Blair, PED, FACSM, Chair

Fourth Edition, 1991

Russell R. Pate, PhD, FACSM, Chair

Fifth Edition, 1995

W. Larry Kenney, PhD, FACSM, Senior Editor

Reed H. Humphrey, PhD, PT, FACSM, Associate Editor Clinical

Cedric X. Bryant, PhD, FACSM, Associate Editor Fitness

Sixth Edition, 2000

Barry A. Franklin, PhD, FACSM, Senior Editor

Mitchell H. Whaley, PhD, FACSM, Associate Editor Clinical

Edward T. Howley, PhD, FACSM, Associate Editor Fitness

Seventh Edition, 2005

Mitchell H. Whaley, PhD, FACSM, Senior Editor

Peter H. Brubaker, PhD, FACSM, Associate Editor Clinical

Robert M. Otto, PhD, FACSM, Associate Editor Fitness

Eighth Edition, 2009

Walter R. Thompson, PhD, FACSM, Senior Editor

Neil F. Gordon, MD, PhD, FACSM, Associate Editor

Linda S. Pescatello, PhD, FACSM, Associate Editor

Preface

The reader of this edition of *ACSM's Guidelines for Exercise Testing and Prescription* will notice four innovations: there is less description; there are fewer references; there are more tables, boxes, and figures; and it is published simultaneously with *ACSM's Resource Manual for Guidelines for Exercise Testing and Prescription, ACSM's Resources for Clinical Exercise Physiology, ACSM's Certification Review Book,* and *ACSM's Exercise Management for Persons with Chronic Diseases and Disabilities.* It is for this last reason that the editors proposed that this edition become more of a *guidelines* book rather than a sole and inclusive *resource.* Going back to the first edition, it was always the intention of this book to be an immediate source of information for health/fitness and clinical professionals. As more scientific and clinical information became available, the *Guidelines* book became thicker and the font smaller between editions 1 and 7. Our goal was to improve the readability of the book so that the reader could easily find a guideline, a brief explanation, and a specific reference or two. We leave expanded explanations and full resourcing to the companion books now that they are published alongside these *Guidelines.* We believe that this edition is in a more usable format for health/fitness and clinical exercise professionals, physicians, nurses, physician assistants, physical and occupational therapists, dietitians, and healthcare administrators.

We also realize that these *Guidelines* are used throughout the world as the definitive text on graded exercise testing and prescription. It is for this reason that we asked international scientists and practitioners from nearly every continent to review and make suggestions about not only the scientific application, but the acceptance of these *Guidelines* in their respective countries. It is our hope that these *Guidelines* will be used throughout the world and, when applicable, translated into numerous languages for local understanding (Note: translation agreements with the publisher need to be in place before engaging in this activity).

INTERNATIONAL REVIEWERS

Jorge E. Franchella, MD, FACSM
Director, Sports Medicine Specialist Course
School of Medicine, Buenos Aires University
Buenos Aires, Argentina

Mark Hargreaves, PhD, FACSM
Professor, Department of Physiology
The University of Melbourne
Melbourne, Australia

Gaston P. Beunen, PhD, FACSM
Department of Biomedical Kinesiology
Faculty of Kinesiology and Rehabilitation Sciences
Katholieke Universiteit
Leuven, Belgium

Victor Matsudo, MD
Scientific Director, São Caetano do Sul
Center of Studies from the Physical Fitness Laboratory
CELAFISCS, Brazil

Constance M. Lebrun, MD, MPE, CCFP, Dip. Sport Med, FACSM
Director, Glen Sather Sports Medicine Clinic
University of Alberta
Edmonton, Alberta

Jürgen Michael Steinacker, MD, FACSM
Professor of Medicine
Sektion Sport- und Rehabilitationsmedizin
Universitätsklinikum Ulm
89070 Ulm
Germany

Stanley Sai-chuen Hui, PhD, FACSM
Professor, Department of Sports Science and Physical Education
The Chinese University of Hong Kong
Shatin, N.T., Hong Kong

Aashish Contractor, MD
Preventive Cardiology and Rehabilitation
Asian Heart Institute
Mumbai, India

Marco Bernardi, MD
Department of Human Physiology and Pharmacology
School of Specialty in Sports Medicine
Faculty of Medicine and Surgery
University of Rome
Rome, Italy

Jasem Ramadan, PhD
Chairman, Department of Physiology
Director, Physical Activity and Exercise Unit
Faculty of Medicine, Kuwait University
Kuwait

Pedro G. Morales Corral, MD
Universidad Autónoma de Nuevo León
Monterrey, Mexico

Wye Mun Low, MBBS, MMed, MSS, FACSM
Sports Physician
The Clinic at Cuppage
Singapore

Rolf Ehrsam, MD, MSc, FACSM
Emeritus Director, Institute for Exercise and Health Sciences
University of Basel
Basel, Switzerland

Sandy S. Hsieh, PhD, FACSM
Graduate Institute of Exercise and Sport Science
National Taiwan Normal University
Taipei, Taiwan

Susan M. Shirreffs, PhD, FACSM
School of Sport and Exercise Sciences
Loughborough University
Loughborough, United Kingdom

It is in this preface that the editors have the opportunity to thank all those who helped make this project a great success. However, in keeping with the theme of this book to remain short, to the point, and without great elaboration, we thank our spouses, friends, and families who ate meals without us, spent weekends, holidays, and vacations without us, and sacrificed a good part of two years enabling us to finish this work. We thank our publisher, and in particular Emily Lupash, acquisitions editor; Andrea Klingler, managing editor; Christen Murphy, marketing manager; and Debra Passan, editorial assistant. We thank former ACSM National Director of Certification Mike Niederpruem, National Director of Certification Richard Cotton, Assistant Director of Certification Hope Wood, Certification Program Coordinator Beth Muhlenkamp, Certification Program Coordinator Kathy Berlin, Certification Assistant Mandy Couch, Administrative Officer for the Committee on Accreditation for the Exercise Sciences Traci Rush, ACSM Assistant Executive Vice President and Group Publisher D. Mark Robertson, and ACSM Publications Committee Chair Dr. Jeff Roitman and his extraordinarily hardworking committee. We thank the ACSM Committee on Certification and Registry Boards, who tirelessly reviewed manuscript drafts and provided great insight. We thank our own students from the University of Connecticut (Amanda Augeri, Bruce Blanchard, Jeffrey Capizzi, Jennifer Klau, Matthew Kostek, and Brian Griffiths) and from Georgia State University (Jessica Lee, Joanna Eure, Caitlin Sales, and Paula Pullen). We are thankful to the senior editors for the companion texts of *Guidelines* (especially Dr. Jon Ehrman, who made it a mission to develop congruency between the *Resource Manual* and the

Guidelines). Finally, we are in great debt to the contributors of these *Guidelines*. It would be impossible for this project to be comprehensive and to include all of the evidence-based best practices without their expertise and devotion to producing this extraordinary text. On a more personal note, I thank my two associate editors, my colleagues, and my friends Dr. Neil Gordon and Dr. Linda Pescatello, who selflessly devoted numerous hours both day and night to this project. Words cannot express my deepest gratitude to you both.

Walter R. Thompson, Ph.D., FACSM
Senior Editor

NOTA BENE

The views and information contained in the eighth edition of *ACSM's Guidelines for Exercise Testing and Prescription* are provided as *guidelines* as opposed to *standards of practice*. This distinction is an important one, because specific legal connotations may be attached to such terminology. The distinction also is critical inasmuch as it gives the exercise professional the freedom to deviate from these guidelines when necessary and appropriate in the course of exercising independent and prudent judgment. *ACSM's Guidelines for Exercise Testing and Prescription* presents a framework whereby the professional may certainly—and in some cases has the obligation to—tailor to individual client or patient needs and alter to meet institutional or legislated requirements.

Contributors

Kelli Allen, PhD
VA Medical Center
Durham, North Carolina

Lawrence E. Armstrong, PhD, FACSM
University of Connecticut
Storrs, Connecticut

Gary J. Balady, MD
Boston University School of Medicine
Boston, Massachusetts

Michael J. Berry, PhD, FACSM
Wake Forest University
Winston-Salem, North Carolina

Craig Broeder, PhD, FACSM
Benedictine University
Lisle, Illinois

John Castellani, PhD, FACSM
U.S. Army Research Institute of
    Environmental Medicine
Natick, Massachusetts

Bernard Clark, MD
St. Francis Hospital and Medical Center
Hartford, Connecticut

Dawn P. Coe, PhD
Grand Valley State University
Allendale, Michigan

Michael Deschenes, PhD, FACSM
College of William and Mary
Willamsburg, Virginia

J. Andrew Doyle, PhD
Georgia State University
Atlanta, Georgia

Barry Franklin, PhD, FACSM
William Beaumont Hospital
Royal Oak, Michigan

Charles S. Fulco, ScD
U.S. Army Research Institute of
    Environmental Medicine
Natick, Massachusetts

Carol Ewing Garber, PhD, FACSM
Columbia University
New York, New York

Paul M. Gordon, PhD, FACSM
University of Michigan
Ann Arbor, Michigan

Sam Headley, PhD, FACSM
Springfield College
Springfield, Massachusetts

John E. Hodgkin, MD
St. Helena Hospital
St. Helena, California

John M. Jakicic, PhD, FACSM
University of Pittsburgh
Pittsburgh, Pennsylvania

Wendy Kohrt, PhD, FACSM
University of Colorado—Denver
Aurora, Colorado

Timothy R. McConnell, PhD, FACSM
Bloomsburg University
Bloomsburg, Pennsylvania

Kyle McInnis, ScD, FACSM
University of Massachusetts
Boston, Massachusetts

Miriam C. Morey, PhD
VA and Duke Medical Centers
Durham, North Carolina

Stephen Muza, PhD
U.S. Army Research Institute of
Environmental Medicine
Natick, Massachusetts

Jonathan Myers, PhD, FACSM
VA Palo Alto Health Care
System/Stanford University
Palo Alto, California

Patricia A. Nixon, PhD, FACSM
Wake Forest University
Winston-Salem, North Carolina

Jeff Rupp, PhD
Georgia State University
Atlanta, Georgia

Ray Squires, PhD, FACSM
Mayo Clinic
Rochester, Minnesota

Clare Stevinson, PhD
University of Alberta
Edmonton, Canada

Scott Thomas, PhD
University of Toronto
Toronto, Canada

Yves Vanlandewijck, PhD
Katholieke Universiteit Leuven
Leuven, Belgium

Contents

SECTION IV: APPENDICES

Abbreviations

AACVPR	American Association of Cardiovascular and Pulmonary Rehabilitation	CAD	coronary artery disease
		CDC	U.S. Centers for Disease Control and Prevention
ABI	ankle/brachial systolic pressure index	CES	ACSM Certified Clinical Exercise Specialist
ACE	angiotensin-converting enzyme	CHF	congestive heart failure
		CHO	carbohydrate
ACGIH	American Conference of Governmental Industrial Hygienists	CI	cardiac index
		COPD	chronic obstructive pulmonary disease
ACOG	American College of Obstetricians and Gynecologists	CPAP	continuous positive airway pressure
		CPK	creatine phosphokinase
ACP	American College of Physicians	CPR	cardiopulmonary resuscitation
ACS	Acute coronary syndromes	CRQ	Chronic Respiratory Questionnaire
ACSM	American College of Sports Medicine	CVD	atherosclerotic cardiovascular disease
ADL	activities of daily living		
AHA	American Heart Association	DBP	diastolic blood pressure
		DOMS	delayed onset muscle soreness
AICD	automatic implantable cardioverter defibrillator	ECG	electrocardiogram (electrocardiographic)
AIHA	American Industrial Hygiene Association	EF	ejection fraction
AMA	American Medical Association	EIB	exercise-induced bronchoconstriction
AMS	acute mountain sickness	EIH	exercise-induced hypotension
AST	aspartate aminotransferase	ERV	expiratory reserve volume
AV	atrioventricular	ES	ACSM Exercise Specialist
BIA	bioelectrical impedance analysis	ETT	ACSM Exercise Test Technologist®
BLS	basic life support	FC	functional capacity
BMI	body mass index	$FEV_{1.0}$	forced expiratory volume in one second
BP	blood pressure		
BR	breathing reserve	FFM	fat-free mass
BUN	blood urea nitrogen	$FICO_2$	fraction of inspired carbon dioxide
CABG(S)	coronary artery bypass graft (surgery)	FIO_2	fraction of inspired oxygen

FN	false negative
FP	false positive
FRV	functional residual volume
FVC	forced vital capacity
GEL	ACSM Group Exercise Leader®
GXT	graded exercise test
HAPE	high-altitude pulmonary edema
HDL	high-density lipoprotein
HFD	ACSM Health/Fitness Director®
HFI	ACSM Health/Fitness Instructor®
HFS	ACSM Certified Health Fitness Specialist
HR	heart rate
HR_{max}	maximal heart rate
HRR	heart rate reserve
HR_{rest}	resting heart rate
IC	inspiratory capacity
ICD	implantable cardioverter defibrillator
IDDM	insulin-dependent diabetes mellitus
JCC	Jewish Community Center
KSAs	knowledge, skills, and abilities
LAD	left axis deviation
LBBB	left bundle-branch block
LDH	lactate dehydrogenase
LDL	low-density lipoprotein
L-G-L	Lown-Ganong-Levine
LLN	lower limit of normal
LV	left ventricle (left ventricular)
MCHC	mean corpuscular hemoglobin concentration
MET	metabolic equivalent
MI	myocardial infarction
MUGA	multigated acquisition (scan)
MVC	maximal voluntary contraction
MVV	maximal voluntary ventilation
NCEP	National Cholesterol Education Program

NIDDM	non–insulin-dependent diabetes mellitus
NIH	National Institutes of Health
NIOSH	National Institute for Occupational Safety and Health
NYHA	New York Heart Association
PAC	premature atrial contraction
P_aO_2	partial pressure of arterial oxygen
PAR-Q	Physical Activity Readiness Questionnaire
PD	ACSM Program Director^{SM}
PE_{max}	maximal expiratory pressure
PI_{max}	maximal inspiratory pressure
PNF	proprioceptive neuromuscular facilitation
PO_2	partial pressure of oxygen
PTCA	percutaneous transluminal coronary angioplasty
PVC	premature ventricular contraction
PVD	peripheral vascular disease
$\dot{Q}$	cardiac output
RAD	right axis deviation
RAL	recommended alert limit
RBBB	right bundle-branch block
RCEP	ACSM Registered Clinical Exercise Physiologist®
rep	repetition
RER	respiratory exchange ratio
RIMT	resistive inspiratory muscle training
1-RM	one-repetition maximum
RPE	rating of perceived exertion
RQ	respiratory quotient
RV	residual volume
RVG	radionuclide ventriculography

RVH	right ventricular hypertrophy	$\dot{V}I$	inspired ventilation per minute VMT
S_aO_2	percent saturation of arterial oxygen		ventilatory muscle training
SBP	systolic blood pressure	$\dot{V}O_2$	volume of oxygen consumed per minute
SEE	standard error of estimate	$\dot{V}O_{2max}$	maximal volume of oxygen
SPECT	single-photon emission computed tomography		consumed per minute (maximal oxygen uptake, maximal oxygen
SVT	supraventricular tachycardia		consumption)
THR	target heart rate	$\dot{V}O_{2peak}$	peak oxygen uptake
TLC	total lung capacity	$\dot{V}O_2R$	oxygen uptake reserve
TN	true negative	$\%\dot{V}O_2R$	percentage of oxygen
TP	true positive		uptake reserve
TPR	total peripheral resistance	VT	ventilatory threshold
TV	tidal volume	WBGT	wet-bulb globe
VC	vital capacity		temperature
$\dot{V}CO_2$	volume of carbon dioxide per minute	WHR	waist-to-hip ratio
		W-P-W	Wolff-Parkinson-White
$\dot{V}E$	expired ventilation per minute	YMCA	Young Men's Christian Association
$\dot{V}E_{max}$	maximal expired ventilation	YWCA	Young Women's Christian Association

Health Appraisal
and Risk Assessment

CHAPTER 1

Benefits and Risks Associated with Physical Activity

The purpose of this chapter is to provide current information concerning the benefits as well as the risks of physical activity and/or exercise. For clarification purposes, key terms used throughout this text related to physical activity and fitness are defined in the beginning of this chapter. Additional definitions specific to a condition or situation are explained within the context of the chapter in which it occurs. Also, given the increasingly important role of physical activity in the prevention and treatment of hypokinetic diseases, the public health perspective that forms the basis of the current physical activity recommendations is presented. At the end of this chapter, there are recommendations for reducing the incidence and severity of exercise-related complications for both primary and secondary prevention programs.

PHYSICAL ACTIVITY AND FITNESS TERMINOLOGY

Physical activity and exercise are often used interchangeably, but these terms are not synonymous. *Physical activity* is defined as any bodily movement produced by the contraction of skeletal muscles that result in a substantial increase over resting energy expenditure (5,36). *Exercise* is a type of physical activity consisting of planned, structured, and repetitive bodily movement done to improve or maintain one or more components of physical fitness (5). *Physical fitness* has typically been defined as a set of attributes or characteristics that people have or achieve that relates to the ability to perform physical activity (5). These characteristics are usually separated into either health-related or skill-related components (Box 1.1).

In addition to defining physical activity, exercise, and physical fitness, it is important to clearly define the wide range of intensities associated with physical activity. This has been accomplished using several methods, including percentages of maximal oxygen consumption ($\dot{V}O_{2max}$), oxygen consumption reserve ($\dot{V}O_2R$), heart rate reserve (HRR), maximal heart rate (HR_{max}), or metabolic equivalents (METs). Each of these methods for describing the intensity of physical activity has benefits and limitations. Although determining the most appropriate method is left to the exercise professional, Chapter 7 provides the methodology and guidelines for selecting a suitable method.

BOX 1.1	Health-Related and Skill-Related Physical Fitness Components

HEALTH-RELATED PHYSICAL FITNESS COMPONENTS
- Cardiovascular endurance: The ability of the circulatory and respiratory system to supply oxygen during sustained physical activity.
- Body composition: The relative amounts of muscle, fat, bone, and other vital parts of the body.
- Muscular strength: The ability of muscle to exert force.
- Muscular endurance: The ability of muscle to continue to perform without fatigue.
- Flexibility: The range of motion available at a joint.

SKILL-RELATED PHYSICAL FITNESS COMPONENTS
- Agility: The ability to change the position of the body in space with speed and accuracy.
- Coordination: The ability to use the senses, such as sight and hearing, together with body parts in performing tasks smoothly and accurately.
- Balance: The maintenance of equilibrium while stationary or moving.
- Power: The ability or rate at which one can perform work.
- Reaction time: The time elapsed between stimulation and the beginning of the reaction to it.
- Speed: The ability to perform a movement within a short period of time.

Adapted from U.S. Department of Health and Human Services. *Physical activity and health: a Report of the Surgeon General*. Atlanta, GA: Centers for Disease Control and Prevention; 1996. President's Council on Physical Fitness. Definitions: health, fitness, and physical activity. [Internet]. 2000. Available from http://www.fitness.gov/digest_mar2000.htm

METs are a useful and convenient way to describe the intensity of a variety of physical activities. In a recent update to a joint American College of Sports Medicine (ACSM) and Centers for Disease Control and Prevention (CDC) publication, light physical activity was defined as requiring <3 METs, moderate activities 3–6 METs, and vigorous activities >6 METs (19). Table 1.1 gives specific examples of activities in each of these areas. A fairly complete list of activities and their associated estimates of energy expenditure can be found in the companion book of these Guidelines (*ACSM's Resource Manual for Guidelines for Exercise Testing and Prescription*).

Because maximal aerobic capacity usually declines with age (1), the exercise professional should understand that when older and younger individuals work at the same MET level, the relative exercise intensity (%$\dot{V}O_{2max}$) will usually be different. In other words, the older individual will be working at a greater relative percentage of $\dot{V}O_{2max}$. Table 1.2 shows the approximate relationships between relative and absolute exercise intensities and various aerobic capacities (6–12 METs). It should also be noted that physically active older adults may have

TABLE 1.1. MET VALUES OF COMMON PHYSICAL ACTIVITIES CLASSIFIED AS LIGHT, MODERATE, OR VIGOROUS INTENSITY

LIGHT (<3 METs)	MODERATE (3–6 METs)	VIGOROUS (>6 METs)
Walking	**Walking**	**Walking, jogging, and running**
Walking slowly around home, store or office = 2.0^a	Walking 3.0 mph = 3.0^a Walking at very brisk pace (4 mph) = 5.0^a	Walking at very, very brisk pace (4.5 mph) = 6.3^a Walking/hiking at moderate pace and grade with no or light pack (<10 pounds) = 7.0
Household and occupation	**Household and occupation**	Hiking at steep grades and pack 10–42 pounds = 7.5–9.0
Sitting—using computer, work at desk, using light hand tools = 1.5 Standing performing light work, such as making bed, washing dishes, ironing, preparing food or store clerk = 2.0–2.5	Cleaning, heavy—washing windows, car, clean garage = 3.0 Sweeping floors or carpet, vacuuming, mopping = 3.0–3.5 Carpentry—general = 3.6 Carrying and stacking wood = 5.5 Mowing lawn—walk power mower = 5.5	Jogging at 5 mph = 8.0^a Jogging at 6 mph = 10.0^a Running at 7 mph = 11.5^a **Household and occupation** Shoveling sand, coal, etc. = 7.0 Carrying heavy loads, such as bricks = 7.5 Heavy farming, such as bailing hay = 8.0 Shoveling, digging ditches = 8.5
Leisure time and sports	**Leisure time and sports**	
Arts and crafts, playing cards = 1.5 Billiards = 2.5 Boating—power = 2.5 Croquet = 2.5 Darts = 2.5 Fishing—sitting = 2.5 Playing most musical instruments = 2.0–2.5	Badminton—recreational = 4.5 Basketball—shooting a round = 4.5 Bicycling on flat—light effort (10–12 mph) = 6.0 Dancing—ballroom slow = 3.0; ballroom fast = 4.5 Fishing from riverbank and walking = 4.0 Golf—walking pulling clubs = 4.3 Sailing boat, wind surfing = 3.0 Swimming leisurely = 6.0^b Table tennis = 4.0 Tennis doubles = 5.0 Volleyball—noncompetitive = 3.0–4.0	**Leisure time and sports** Basketball game = 8.0 Bicycling on flat—moderate effort (12–14 mph) = 8 fast (14–16 mph) = 10 Skiing cross country—slow (2.5 mph = 7.0; fast (5.0–7.9 mph) = 9.0 Soccer—casual = 7.0; competitive = 10.0 Swimming—moderate/hard = $8–11^b$ Tennis singles = 8.0 Volleyball—competitive at gym or beach = 8.0

MET, metabolic equivalent; mph, miles per hour.

^{a}On flat, hard surface.

^{b}MET values can vary substantially from person to person during swimming as a result of different strokes and skill levels.

Adapted and modified from Ainsworth B, Haskell WL, White MC, et al. Compendium of physical activities: an update of activity codes and MET intensities. *Med Sci Sports Exerc.* 2000;32(suppl):S498–S504.

TABLE 1.2. CLASSIFICATION OF PHYSICAL ACTIVITY INTENSITY

	RELATIVE INTENSITY		ABSOLUTE INTENSITY RANGES (METs) ACROSS FITNESS LEVELS			
INTENSITY	$\dot{V}O_2R$ (%) HRR (%)	MAXIMAL HR (%)	12 MET $\dot{V}O_{2max}$	10 MET $\dot{V}O_{2max}$	8 MET $\dot{V}O_{2max}$	6 MET $\dot{V}O_{2max}$
Very light	<20	<50	<3.2	<2.8	<2.4	<2.0
Light	20–39	50–63	3.2–5.3	2.8–4.5	2.4–3.7	2.0–3.0
Moderate	40–59	64–76	5.4–7.5	4.6–6.3	3.8–5.1	3.1–4.0
Hard (vigorous)	60–84	77–93	7.6–10.2	6.4–8.6	5.2–6.9	4.1–5.2
Very hard	≥85	≥94	≥10.3	≥8.7	≥7.0	≥5.3
Maximal	100	100	12	10	8	6

METs, metabolic equivalent units (1 MET − 3.5 mL · kg^{-1} · min^{-1}); $\dot{V}O_2R$, oxygen uptake reserve; HRR, heart rate reserve; HR, heart rate.

Adapted from U.S. Department of Health and Human Services. *Physical activity and health: a Report of the Surgeon General*. Washington (DC): Atlanta, GA: Centers for Disease Control and Prevention; 1996. American College of Sports Medicine. The recommended quantity and quality of exercise for developing and maintaining cardiorespiratory and muscular fitness, and flexibility in healthy adults. *Med Sci Sports Exerc*. 1998;30:975–91. Howley ET. Type of activity: resistance, aerobic and leisure versus occupational physical activity. *Med Sci Sports Exerc*. 2001;33:S364–9.

aerobic capacities comparable to or greater than those of sedentary younger adults.

PUBLIC HEALTH PERSPECTIVE FOR CURRENT RECOMMENDATIONS

More than ten years ago, the U.S. Surgeon General (45), the National Institutes of Health (30), and the American College of Sports Medicine, in conjunction with CDC (34), issued landmark publications on physical activity and health. These publications called attention to the health-related benefits of regular physical activity that did not meet traditional criteria for improving fitness levels (e.g., <20 minutes per session and <50% of aerobic capacity).

An important goal of these reports was to clarify for the public and exercise professionals the amounts and intensities of physical activity needed for improved health, lowered susceptibility to disease (morbidity), and decreased mortality (30,34,45). In addition, these reports documented the dose-response relationship between physical activity and health (i.e., some activity is better than none, and more activity, up to a point, is better than less). Although this dose–response relationship was not particularly emphasized in these reports, it is clear that physical activity meeting these minimal recommendations results in improved health. More recently, a meta-analysis of 23 sex-specific cohorts of physical activity or fitness representing 1,325,004 person-years of follow-up clearly showed the dose-response relationship between physical activity, physical fitness, and the risks of coronary artery disease and cardiovascular disease (Fig. 1.1) (54). It is clear that additional amounts of physical activity or increased physical fitness levels provide additional health benefits. There is also evidence for an inverse dose-response relationship between physical activity and all-cause

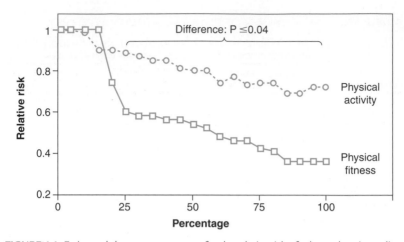

FIGURE 1.1. Estimated dose-response curve for the relative risk of atherosclerotic cardio-vascular disease (CVD) by sample percentages of fitness and physical activity. Studies weighted by person-years of experience. Used with permission from Williams PT. Physical fitness and activity as separate heart disease risk factors: a meta-analysis. *Med Sci Sports Exerc.* 2001;33(5):754–61.

mortality, overweight, obesity and fat distribution, type 2 diabetes, colon cancer, quality of life, and independent living in older adults (22). Table 1.3 illustrates these relationships and the type of evidence available to support the relationship.

Two important conclusions from the U.S. Surgeon General's Report (45) that have affected the development of the guidelines appearing in this book are:

- Important health benefits can be obtained by including a moderate amount of physical activity on most, if not all, days of the week.
- Additional health benefits result from greater amounts of physical activity. People who maintain a regular program of physical activity that is longer in duration or is more vigorous in intensity are likely to derive greater benefit.

In 1995, the CDC and the ACSM issued the recommendation that "every U.S. adult should accumulate 30 minutes or more of moderate physical activity on most, preferably all, days of the week" (34). The intent of this statement was to increase public awareness of the importance and health-related benefits of moderate physical activity. Unfortunately, although there is some evidence that leisure-time physical inactivity has decreased (6), sedentary behavior is still a major public health concern. Specifically, only 49.1% of U.S. adults met the CDC-ACSM physical activity recommendation as reported in a recent survey (7).

As indicated earlier, the inverse relationship between physical activity and chronic disease and premature mortality has been well established. Since the release of the U.S. Surgeon General's Report in 1996 (45), several reports have been published advocating physical activity levels above the minimum recommendations (12,21,39,46). These guidelines and recommendations refer to the

TABLE 1.3. EVIDENCE FOR DOSE-RESPONSE RELATIONSHIP BETWEEN PHYSICAL ACTIVITY AND HEALTH OUTCOME

VARIABLE	EVIDENCE FOR INVERSE DOSE-RESPONSE RELATIONSHIP	CATEGORY OF EVIDENCE
All-cause mortality	Yes	C
Cardiovascular and coronary heart disease	Yes	C
Blood pressure and hypertension	No[a]	B
Blood lipids and lipoproteins	Insufficient data	
Coagulation and hemostatic factors	Insufficient data	
Overweight, obesity, and fat distribution	Yes	C
Type 2 diabetes mellitus	Yes[b]	C
Colon cancer	Yes	C
Low back pain, osteoarthritis, and osteoporosis	Insufficient data	
Quality of life and independent living in older persons	Yes	C
Depression and anxiety	No[a]	B

Category A: Evidence is from endpoints of well-designed randomized clinical trials (RCTs) (or trials that depart only minimally from randomization) that provide a consistent pattern of findings in the population for which the recommendation is made. It requires substantial numbers of studies involving substantial number of participants. *Category B:* Evidence is from endpoints of intervention studies that include only a limited number of RCTs, post hoc or subgroup analysis of RCT, or meta-analysis of RCTs. In general, Category B pertains when few randomized trials exist, they are small in size, and the trial results are somewhat inconsistent, or the trials were undertaken in a population that differs from the target population of the recommendation. *Category C:* Evidence is from outcomes of uncontrolled or nonrandomized trials or observational studies. *Category D:* Expert judgment is based on the panel's synthesis of evidence from experimental research described in the literature and/or derived from the consensus of panel members based on clinical experience or knowledge that does not meet the listed criteria. This category is used only in cases in which the provision of some guidance was deemed valuable, but an adequately compelling clinical literature addressing the subject of the recommendation was deemed insufficient to justify placement in one of the other categories (A through C).

[a]*No* indicates a lack of evidence for a "dose response" for the relationship between the health outcome and physical activity; it does not indicate the absence of a favorable relationship.

[b]Inverse dose response for primary prevention, but not for improvement in blood glucose control in patients with diabetes.

Used with permission from Kesaniemi YK, Danforth Jr E, Jensen MD, et al. Dose-response issues concerning physical activity and health: an evidence-based symposium. *Med Sci Sports Exerc.* 2001;33:S351–8.

volume of physical activity required to prevent weight gain and/or obesity and should not be viewed as contradictory. The physical activity guidelines and relevant updates illustrate the dose-response relationship independent of obesity (19). In other words, physical activity beyond the minimum recommendations is likely to manage and/or prevent the additional problems of weight gain and obesity.

As a result of this continuing sedentary behavior and because of some confusion and misinterpretation of the original physical activity recommendations, the ACSM and the American Heart Association (AHA) issued updated recommendations for physical activity and health in 2007 (19). Since the original 1995 recommendation, several large-scale epidemiologic studies have been performed that further document the dose-response relationship between physical activity and cardiovascular disease and premature mortality (24,26,33,38,42,56). The primary recommendations from this ACSM-AHA update include (19):

- All healthy adults aged 18 to 65 need moderate-intensity aerobic physical activity for a minimum of 30 minutes five days per week, or vigorous activity for a minimum of 20 minutes three days per week.
- Combinations of moderate and vigorous intensity exercise can be performed to meet this recommendation.
- Moderate-intensity aerobic activity can be accumulated toward the 30-minute minimum by performing bouts each lasting 10 or more minutes.
- Every adult should perform activities that maintain or increase muscular strength and endurance a minimum of two days each week.
- Because of the dose-response relation between physical activity and health, persons who wish to further improve their personal fitness, reduce their risk for chronic diseases and disabilities, or prevent unhealthy weight gain may benefit by exceeding the minimum recommended amounts of physical activity.

BENEFITS OF REGULAR PHYSICAL ACTIVITY AND/OR EXERCISE

Evidence to support the inverse relationship between physical activity and cardiovascular disease, hypertension, stroke, osteoporosis, type 2 diabetes, obesity, colon cancer, breast cancer, anxiety, and depression continues to accumulate (Table 1.3). This evidence has resulted from laboratory-based studies, as well as large-scale, population-based observational studies (11,19,22,25,45,51). Since the last edition of this text, additional evidence has strengthened this relationship. As stated in the recent ACSM-AHA Updated Recommendation on Physical Activity and Health (19), "since the 1995 recommendation, several large-scale observational epidemiologic studies, enrolling thousands to tens of thousands of people, have clearly documented a dose-response relation between physical activity and risk of cardiovascular disease and premature mortality in men and women, and in ethnically diverse participants" (24,26,32,38,42,56). Box 1.2 summarizes the benefits of regular physical activity and/or exercise.

Recently, the ACSM and the AHA released a statement on Physical Activity and Public Health in Older Adults (31). In general, these recommendations are similar to the updated guidelines for adults (19), but the recommended intensity of aerobic activity is related to the older adult's aerobic fitness level. In addition, age-specific recommendations are made concerning the importance of flexibility, balance, and muscle-strengthening activities, as well as the importance of developing an activity plan that integrates therapeutic and preventive measures (31).

RISKS ASSOCIATED WITH EXERCISE

In general, exercise does not provoke cardiovascular events in healthy individuals with normal cardiovascular systems. The risk of sudden cardiac arrest or myocardial infarction is very low in healthy individuals performing moderate-intensity activities (50,53). However, there is an acute and transient increase in

BOX 1.2	Benefits of Regular Physical Activity and/or Exercise

IMPROVEMENT IN CARDIOVASCULAR AND RESPIRATORY FUNCTION

- Increased maximal oxygen uptake resulting from both central and peripheral adaptations
- Decreased minute ventilation at a given absolute submaximal intensity
- Decreased myocardial oxygen cost for a given absolute submaximal intensity
- Decreased heart rate and blood pressure at a given submaximal intensity
- Increased capillary density in skeletal muscle
- Increased exercise threshold for the accumulation of lactate in the blood
- Increased exercise threshold for the onset of disease signs or symptoms (e.g., angina pectoris, ischemic ST-segment depression, claudication)

REDUCTION IN CORONARY ARTERY DISEASE RISK FACTORS

- Reduced resting systolic/diastolic pressures
- Increased serum high-density lipoprotein cholesterol and decreased serum triglycerides
- Reduced total body fat, reduced intra-abdominal fat
- Reduced insulin needs, improved glucose tolerance
- Reduced blood platelet adhesiveness and aggregation

DECREASED MORBIDITY AND MORTALITY

- Primary prevention (i.e., interventions to prevent the initial occurrence)
  - Higher activity and/or fitness levels are associated with lower death rates from coronary artery disease
  - Higher activity and/or fitness levels are associated with lower incidence rates for combined cardiovascular diseases, coronary artery disease, stroke, type 2 diabetes, osteoporotic fractures, cancer of the colon and breast, and gallbladder disease
- Secondary prevention (i.e., interventions after a cardiac event [to prevent another])
  - Based on meta-analyses (pooled data across studies), cardiovascular and all-cause mortality are reduced in postmyocardial infarction patients who participate in cardiac rehabilitation exercise training, especially as a component of multifactorial risk factor reduction
  - Randomized controlled trials of cardiac rehabilitation exercise training involving postmyocardial infarction patients do not support a reduction in the rate of nonfatal reinfarction >

> Box 1.2. continued

OTHER BENEFITS
- Decreased anxiety and depression
- Enhanced physical function and independent living in older persons
- Enhanced feelings of well-being
- Enhanced performance of work, recreational, and sport activities
- Reduced risk of falls and injuries from falls in older persons
- Prevention or mitigation of functional limitations in older adults
- Effective therapy for many chronic diseases in older adults

Adapted from references 3, 22, 26: U.S. Department of Health and Human Services. *Physical activity and health: a Report of the Surgeon General*, Atlanta, GA: Centers for Disease Control and Prevention; 1996. Kesaniemi YK, Danforth Jr E, Jensen MD, et al. Dose-response issues concerning physical activity and health: an evidence-based symposium. *Med Sci Sports Exerc.* 2001; 33:S351–8. Nelson M, Rajeski JW, Blair SN, et al. Physical activity and public health in older adults: recommendation from the American College of Sports Medicine and the American Heart Association. *Med Sci Sports Exerc.* 2007;39(8):1435–45.

the risk of sudden cardiac death and/or myocardial infarction in individuals performing vigorous exercise with either diagnosed or occult cardiovascular disease (16,29,40,43,50,55). Therefore, the risk of these events during exercise increases with the prevalence of cardiac disease in the population. Chapter 2 includes guidelines for risk stratification of individuals who wish to increase their physical activity levels.

SUDDEN CARDIAC DEATH AMONG YOUNG INDIVIDUALS

The risk of sudden cardiac death in individuals younger than 30 to 40 years of age is very low because of the low prevalence of cardiovascular disease in this population. In 2007, the AHA released a scientific statement on Exercise and Acute Cardiovascular Events: Placing the Risks into Perspective (2). Table 1.4 (taken from this publication) shows the cardiovascular causes of exercise-related sudden death in young athletes. It is clear from these data that the most common causes of death in young individuals are congenital and hereditary abnormalities, including hypertrophic cardiomyopathy, coronary artery abnormalities, and aortic stenosis. The absolute risk of exercise-related death among high school and college athletes is one per 133,000 men and 769,000 women (47). It should be noted that these rates, although low, include all sports-related nontraumatic deaths. Of the 136 total identifiable causes of death, 100 were caused by cardiac disease.

In a population-based study from Italy, the death rate was reported as one per 33,000 young athletes per year (9). It is not clear why this rate is higher, but it may be related to reporting all deaths, not just those related to exercise. In addition, the intensity of activity may have been higher than reported in other studies.

TABLE 1.4. CARDIOVASCULAR CAUSES OF EXERCISE-RELATED SUDDEN DEATH IN YOUNG ATHLETES[a]

	VAN CAMP (n = 100)[b] (47)	MARON (n = 134) (27)	CORRADO (n = 55)[c] (9)
Hypertrophic CM	51	36	1
Probable hypertrophic CM	5	10	0
Coronary anomalies	18	23	9
Valvular and subvalvular aortic stenosis	8	4	0
Possible myocarditis	7	3	5
Dilated and nonspecific CM	7	3	1
Atherosclerotic CVD	3	2	10
Aortic dissection/rupture	2	5	1
Arrhythmogenic right ventricular CM	1	3	11
Myocardial scarring	0	3	0
Mitral valve prolapse	1	2	6
Other congenital abnormalities	0	1.5	0
Long QT syndrome	0	0.5	0
Wolff-Parkinson-White syndrome	1	0	1
Cardiac conduction disease	0	0	3
Cardiac Sarcoidosis	0	0.5	0
Coronary artery aneurysm	1	0	0
Normal heart at necropsy	7	2	1
Pulmonary thromboembolism	0	0	1

CM, cardiomyopathy; CVD, atherosclerotic cardiovascular disease.

[a]Ages ranged from 13 to 24 (44), 12 to 40 (25), and 12 to 35 (9) years. References 44 and 25 used the same database and include many of the same athletes. All (47), 90% (27), and 89% (9) had symptom onset during or within an hour of training or competition.

[b]Total exceeds 100% because several athletes had multiple abnormalities.

[c]Includes some athletes whose deaths were not associated with recent exertion. Includes aberrant artery origin and course, tunneled arteries, and other abnormalities.

Used with permission from American Heart Association. Exercise and acute cardiovascular events: placing the risks into perspective. A Scientific Statement from the American Heart Association Council on Nutrition, Physical Activity, and Metabolism and the Council on Clinical Cardiology. *Circulation.* 2007;115:1643-55.

EXERCISE-RELATED CARDIAC EVENTS IN ADULTS

The risk of sudden cardiac death or acute myocardial infarction is higher in adults than in younger individuals. This is due to the higher prevalence of cardiovascular disease in the older population. The absolute risk of sudden cardiac death during vigorous physical activity has been estimated at one per year for every 15,000–18,000 people (40,44). Another study reported a risk estimate of 0.3 to 2.7 events per 10,000 person-hours for men and 0.6 to 6.0 events for women (15). Although these rates are low and since these studies were published, additional research has confirmed the increased rate of sudden cardiac death and acute myocardial infarction in adults performing vigorous exercise when compared with their younger counterparts (16,29,40,44,55). In addition, the rates of sudden cardiac death and acute myocardial infarction are disproportionately higher in the most sedentary individuals when they perform unaccustomed or infrequent exercise (2).

Exercise professionals should understand that although there is an increased risk of sudden cardiac death and acute myocardial infarction with vigorous exercise, the physically active adult has between one fourth to one half the risk of developing cardiovascular disease (35,54). The exact mechanism of sudden cardiac death during vigorous exercise with asymptomatic adults is not completely understood. However, evidence exists that the increased frequency of cardiac contraction and the increased excursion of the coronary arteries produces bending and flexing of the coronary arteries. This may cause cracking of the atherosclerotic plaque with resulting platelet aggregation and possible acute thrombosis. This process has been documented angiographically in individuals with exercise-induced cardiac events (4,8,17).

EXERCISE TESTING AND THE RISK OF CARDIAC EVENTS

As with vigorous exercise, the risk of cardiac events during exercise testing varies directly with the incidence of cardiovascular disease. Several studies have looked at the risks of exercise testing (3,14,20,23,28,37,41). Table 1.5 summarizes the risks of various cardiac events, including acute myocardial infarction, ventricular fibrillation, hospitalization, and death. These data indicate that in a mixed population, the risk of exercise testing is low, with approximately six cardiac events per 10,000 tests. One of these studies includes data for which the exercise testing was supervised by nonphysicians (23). In addition, the majority of these studies used symptom-limited exercise tests. Therefore, it would be expected that the risk of submaximal testing in a similar population would be lower.

RISKS OF CARDIAC EVENTS DURING CARDIAC REHABILITATION

It is clear that the highest risk of cardiovascular events occurs in those individuals with diagnosed coronary artery disease. In one survey, there was one nonfatal complication per 34,673 hours and one fatal cardiovascular complication per 116,402 hours of cardiac rehabilitation (18). More recent studies have found a lower rate, one cardiac arrest per 116,906 patient-hours, one myocardial infarction per 219,970 patient-hours, one fatality per 752,365 patient-hours, and one major complication per 81,670 patient-hours (10,13,48,49). These studies are presented in Table 1.6 (2). Although these complication rates are low, it should be noted that patients were screened and exercised in medically supervised settings equipped to handle emergencies. The mortality rate appears to be six times higher when patients exercised in facilities without the ability to successfully manage cardiac arrest (2,10,13,48,49). Interestingly, however, a review of home-based cardiac rehabilitation programs found no increase in cardiovascular complications versus formal center-based exercise programs (52).

PREVENTION OF EXERCISE-RELATED CARDIAC EVENTS

Because of the low incidence of cardiac events related to vigorous exercise, it is very difficult to test the effectiveness of strategies to reduce the occurrence of these events. According to a recent statement by the AHA, "Physicians should not overestimate the risks of exercise because the benefits of habitual physical

TABLE 1.5. CARDIAC COMPLICATIONS DURING EXERCISE TESTING[a]

REFERENCE	YEAR	SITE	NO. TESTS	MI	VF	DEATH	HOSPITALIZATION	COMMENT
Rochmis (37)	1971	73 U.S. centers	170,000	NA	NA	1	3	34% of tests were symptom limited; 50% of deaths in 8 hr; 50% over next 4 days
Irving (20)	1977	15 Seattle facilities	10,700	NA	4.67	0	NR	
McHenry (28)	1977	Hospital	12,000	0	0	0	0	
Atterhog (3)	1979	20 Swedish centers	50,000	0.8	0.8	6.4	5.2	
Stuart (41)	1980	1,375 U.S. centers	518,448	3.58	4.78	0.5	NR	VF includes other dysrhythmias requiring treatment
Gibbons (14)	1989	Cooper Clinic	71,914	0.56	0.29	0	NR	Only 4% of men and 2% of women had CVD
Knight (23)	1995	Geisinger Cardiology Service	28,133	1.42	1.77	0	NR	25% were inpatient tests supervised by non-MDs

MI, myocardial infarction; VF, ventricular fibrillation; CVD, atherosclerotic cardiovascular disease; MD, medical doctor; NA, not applicable; NR, not reported.

[a]Events are per 10,000 tests.

13

TABLE 1.6. SUMMARY OF CONTEMPORARY EXERCISE-BASED CARDIAC REHABILITATION PROGRAM COMPLICATION RATES

INVESTIGATOR	YEAR	PATIENT EXERCISE HOURS	CARDIAC ARREST	MYOCARDIAL INFARCTION	FATAL EVENTS	MAJOR COMPLICATIONS[a]
Van Camp (48)	1980–1984	2,351,916	1/111,996[b]	1/293,990	1/783,972	1/81,101
Digenio (10)	1982–1988	480,000	1/120,000[c]		1/160,000	1/120,000
Vongvanich (49)	1986–1995	268,503	1/89,501[d]	1/268,503[d]	0/268,503	1/67,126
Franklin (13)	1982–1998	292,254	1/146,127[d]	1/97,418[d]	0/292,254	1/58,451
Average			1/116,906	1/219,970	1/752,365	1/81,670

[a]MI and cardiac arrest

[b]Fatal 14%

[c]Fatal 75%

[d]Fatal 0%

Used with permission from American Heart Association. Exercise and acute cardiovascular events: placing the risks into perspective. A Scientific Statement from the American Heart Association Council on Nutrition, Physical Activity, and Metabolism and the Council on Clinical Cardiology. *Circulation*; 2007;1643–55.

activity substantially outweigh the risks." This report also recommends several strategies to reduce these cardiac events during vigorous exercise (2):

- Healthcare professionals should know the pathologic conditions associated with exercise-related events so that physically active children and adults can be appropriately evaluated.
- Active individuals should know the nature of cardiac prodromal symptoms and seek prompt medical care if such symptoms develop (see Table 2.2).
- High school and college athletes should undergo preparticipation screening by qualified professionals.
- Athletes with known cardiac conditions should be evaluated for competition using published guidelines.
- Healthcare facilities should ensure that their staffs are trained in managing cardiac emergencies and have a specified plan and appropriate resuscitation equipment (Appendix B).
- Active individuals should modify their exercise program in response to variations in their exercise capacity, habitual activity level, and the environment.

Although strategies for reducing the number of cardiovascular events during vigorous exercise have not been systematically studied, it is incumbent on the exercise professional to take reasonable precautions when working with individuals who wish to increase their physical activity and/or fitness levels. This is particularly true when the exercise program will be vigorous in nature. Although many sedentary individuals can safely begin a light- to moderate-intensity physical activity program, individuals of all ages should be risk stratified according to need for further medical evaluation and/or clearance; need for and type of exercise testing (maximal or submaximal); and need for medical supervision during testing (Fig. 2.4). Sedentary individuals or those who exercise infrequently should begin their programs at lower intensities and progress at a slower rate because a disproportionate number of cardiac events occur in this population. Individuals with known or suspected cardiovascular, pulmonary, or metabolic disease should obtain medical clearance before beginning a vigorous exercise program. Exercise professionals who supervise vigorous exercise programs should have current training in cardiac life support and emergency procedures. These procedures should be reviewed and practiced at regular intervals (Appendix B). Finally, individuals should be educated on the signs and symptoms of cardiovascular disease and should be referred to a physician for further evaluation should these symptoms occur.

REFERENCES

1. American College of Sports Medicine. The recommended quantity and quality of exercise for developing and maintaining cardiorespiratory and muscular fitness, and flexibility in healthy adults. *Med Sci Sports Exerc.* 1998;30(6):975–91.
2. American College of Sports Medicine, American Heart Association. Exercise and acute cardiovascular events: placing the risks into perspective. *Med Sci Sports Exerc.* 2007;39(5):886–97.
3. Atterhog JH, Jonsson B, Samuelsson R. Exercise testing: a prospective study of complication rates. *Am Heart J.* 1979;98(5):572–9.
4. Black A, Black MM, Gensini G. Exertion and acute coronary artery injury. *Angiology.* 1975;26(11):759–83.

5. Caspersen CJ, Powell KE, Christenson GM. Physical activity, exercise, and physical fitness: definitions and distinctions for health-related research. *Public Health Rep.* 1985;100(2):126–31.

6. Centers for Disease Control and Prevention. Adult participation in recommended levels of physical activity: United States, 2001 and 2003. *MMWR Morb Mortal Wkly Rep.* 2005;54:1208–12.

7. Centers for Disease Control and Prevention. Trends in leisure time physical inactivity by age, sex, and race/ethnicity: United States—1994–2004. *MMWR Morb Mortal Wkly Rep.* 2005;54:991–4.

8. Ciampricotti R, Deckers JW, Taverne R, El GM, Relik-Van WL, Pool J. Characteristics of conditioned and sedentary men with acute coronary syndromes. *Am J Cardiol.* 1994;73(4):219–22.

9. Corrado D, Basso C, Rizzoli G, Schiavon M, Thiene G. Does sports activity enhance the risk of sudden death in adolescents and young adults? *J Am Coll Cardiol.* 2003;42(11):1959–63.

10. Digenio AG, Sim JG, Dowdeswell RJ, Morris R. Exercise-related cardiac arrest in cardiac rehabilitation: the Johannesburg experience. *S Afr Med J.* 1991;79(4):188–91.

11. Feskanich D, Willett W, Colditz G. Walking and leisure-time activity and risk of hip fracture in postmenopausal women. *JAMA.* 2002;288(18):2300–06.

12. Food and Nutrition Board, Institute of Medicine. *Dietary reference intakes for energy, carbohydrates, fiber, fat, protein and amino acids (macronutrients).* Washington (DC): National Academy Press, 2002.

13. Franklin BA, Bonzheim K, Gordon S, Timmis GC. Safety of medically supervised outpatient cardiac rehabilitation exercise therapy: a 16-year follow-up. *Chest.* 1998;114(3):902–6.

14. Gibbons L, Blair SN, Kohl HW, Cooper K. The safety of maximal exercise testing. *Circulation.* 1989;80(4):846–52.

15. Gibbons LW, Cooper KH, Meyer BM, Ellison RC. The acute cardiac risk of strenuous exercise. *JAMA.* 1980;244(16):1799–1801.

16. Giri S, Thompson PD, Kiernan FJ, et al. Clinical and angiographic characteristics of exertion-related acute myocardial infarction. *JAMA.* 1999;282(18):1731–6.

17. Hammoudeh AJ, Haft JI. Coronary-plaque rupture in acute coronary syndromes triggered by snow shoveling. *N Engl J Med.* 1996;335(26):2001.

18. Haskell WL. Cardiovascular complications during exercise training of cardiac patients. *Circulation.* 1978;57(5):920–4.

19. Haskell WL, Lee IM, Pate RR, et al. Physical activity and public health: updated recommendation from the American College of Sports Medicine and the American Heart Association. *Med Sci Sports Exerc.* 2007;39(8):1423–34.

20. Irving JB, Bruce RA, DeRouen TA. Variations in and significance of systolic pressure during maximal exercise (treadmill) testing. *Am J Cardiol.* 1977;39(6):841–8.

21. Jakicic JM, Clark K, Coleman E, et al. American College of Sports Medicine position stand. Appropriate intervention strategies for weight loss and prevention of weight regain for adults. *Med Sci Sports Exerc.* 2001;33(12):2145–56.

22. Kesaniemi YK, Danforth E, Jr Jensen MD, Kopelman PG, Lefebvre P, Reeder BA. Dose-response issues concerning physical activity and health: an evidence-based symposium. *Med Sci Sports Exerc.* 2001;33(6 Suppl):S351–8.

23. Knight JA, Laubach CA, Jr Butcher RJ, Menapace FJ. Supervision of clinical exercise testing by exercise physiologists. *Am J Cardiol.* 1995;75(5):390–1.

24. Lee IM, Rexrode KM, Cook NR, Manson JE, Buring JE. Physical activity and coronary heart disease in women: is "no pain, no gain" passe? *JAMA.* 2001;285(11):1447–54.

25. Leitzmann MF, Rimm EB, Willett WC, et al. Recreational physical activity and the risk of cholecystectomy in women. *N Engl J Med.* 1999;341(11):777–84.

26. Manson JE, Greenland P, LaCroix AZ, et al. Walking compared with vigorous exercise for the prevention of cardiovascular events in women. *N Engl J Med.* 2002;347(10):716–25.

27. Maron BJ, Shirani J, Poliac LC, Mathenge R, Roberts WC, Mueller FO. Sudden death in young competitive athletes: clinical, demographic, and pathological profiles. *JAMA* 1996;276(3):199–204.

28. McHenry PL. Risks of graded exercise testing. *Am J Cardiol.* 1977;39(6):935–7.

29. Mittleman MA, Maclure M, Tofler GH, Sherwood JB, Goldberg RJ, Muller JE. Triggering of acute myocardial infarction by heavy physical exertion: protection against triggering by regular exertion. Determinants of Myocardial Infarction Onset Study Investigators. *N Engl J Med.* 1993;329(23):1677–83.

30. National Institutes of Health. Physical activity and cardiovascular health. NIH Consensus Development Panel on Physical Activity and Cardiovascular Health. *JAMA* 1996;276(3):241–6.

31. Nelson M, Rajeski W, Blair SN, et al. Physical activity and public health in older adults: recommendation from the American College of Sports Medicine and the American Heart Association. *Med Sci Sports Exer.* 2007;39(8):1435–45.
32. Paffenbarger RS, Hyde RT, Wing AL, Lee IM, Jung DL, Kampert JB. The association of changes in physical-activity level and other lifestyle characteristics with mortality among men. *N Engl J Med.* 1993;328(8):538–45.
33. Paffenbarger RS, Lee IM. Smoking, physical activity, and active life expectancy. *Clin J Sport Med.* 1999;9(4):244.
34. Pate RR, Pratt M, Blair SN, et al. Physical activity and public health: a recommendation from the Centers for Disease Control and Prevention and the American College of Sports Medicine. *JAMA.* 1995;273(5):402–7.
35. Powell KE, Thompson PD, Caspersen CJ, Kendrick JS. Physical activity and the incidence of coronary heart disease. *Annu Rev Public Health.* 1987;8:253–87.
36. President's Council on Physical Fitness. *Definitions: health, fitness, and physical activity.* [Internet]. 2000. Available from http://www.fitness.gov/digest_mar2000.htm
37. Rochmis P, Blackburn H. Exercise tests: a survey of procedures, safety, and litigation experience in approximately 170,000 tests. *JAMA.* 1971;217(8):1061–6.
38. Rockhill B, Willett WC, Manson JE, Leitzmann MF, Stampfer MJ, Hunter DJ, Colditz GA. Physical activity and mortality: a prospective study among women. *Am J Public Health.* 2001;91(4):578–83.
39. Saris WH, Blair SN, Van Baak MA, et al. How much physical activity is enough to prevent unhealthy weight gain? Outcome of the IASO 1st Stock Conference and consensus statement. *Obes Rev.* 2003;4(2):101–14.
40. Siscovick DS, Weiss NS, Fletcher RH, Lasky T. The incidence of primary cardiac arrest during vigorous exercise. *N Engl J Med.* 1984;311(14):874–7.
41. Stuart RJ, Ellestad MH. National survey of exercise stress testing facilities. *Chest.* 1980;77(1):94–7.
42. Tanasescu M, Leitzmann MF, Rimm EB, Willett WC, Stampfer MJ, Hu FB. Exercise type and intensity in relation to coronary heart disease in men. *JAMA.* 2002;288(16):1994–2000.
43. Thompson PD, Funk EJ, Carleton RA, Sturner WQ. Incidence of death during jogging in Rhode Island from 1975 through 1980. *JAMA.* 1982;247(18):2535–8.
44. Thompson PD, Stern MP, Williams P, Duncan K, Haskell WL, Wood PD. Death during jogging or running: a study of 18 cases. *JAMA.* 1979;242(12):1265–7.
45. U.S. Department of Health and Human Services. *Physical activity and health: a Report of the Surgeon General,* Atlanta, GA: Centers for Disease Control and Prevention; 1996.
46. U.S. Department of Health and Human Services. *Dietary guidelines for Americans.* Washington, DC: Department of Agriculture and Department of Health and Human Services; 2005.
47. Van Camp SP, Bloor CM, Mueller FO, Cantu RC, Olson HG. Nontraumatic sports death in high school and college athletes. *Med Sci Sports Exerc.* 1995;27(5):641–7.
48. Van Camp SP, Peterson RA. Cardiovascular complications of outpatient cardiac rehabilitation programs. *JAMA.* 1986;256(9):1160–3.
49. Vongvanich P, Paul-Labrador MJ, Merz CN. Safety of medically supervised exercise in a cardiac rehabilitation center. *Am J Cardiol.* 1996;77(15):1383–5.
50. Vuori I. The cardiovascular risks of physical activity. *Acta Med Scand Suppl.* 1986;711:205–14.
51. Wenger NK, Froelicher ES, Smith LK, et al. Cardiac rehabilitation as secondary prevention. Agency for Health Care Policy and Research and National Heart, Lung, and Blood Institute. *Clin Pract Guidel Quick Ref Guide Clin.* 1995;Oct(17):1–23.
52. Wenger NK, Froelicher ES, Smith LK, et al. Cardiac rehabilitation. Clinical practice guideline no. 17. Washington (DC): U.S. Department of Health and Human Services, Public Health, Agency for Health Care Policy and Research and National Heart, Lung and Blood Institute; 1995.
53. Whang W, Manson JE, Hu FB, et al. Physical exertion, exercise, and sudden cardiac death in women. *JAMA.* 2006;295(12):1399–1403.
54. Williams PT. Physical fitness and activity as separate heart disease risk factors: a meta-analysis. *Med Sci Sports Exerc.* 2001;33(5):754–61.
55. Willich SN, Lewis M, Lowel H, Arntz HR, Schubert F, Schroder R. Physical exertion as a trigger of acute myocardial infarction. Triggers and Mechanisms of Myocardial Infarction Study Group. *N Engl J Med.* 1993;329(23):1684–90.
56. Yu S, Yarnell JW, Sweetnam PM, Murray L. What level of physical activity protects against premature cardiovascular death? The Caerphilly study. *Heart.* 2003;89(5):502–6.

CHAPTER 2

Preparticipation Health Screening and Risk Stratification

Numerous physiologic, psychologic, and metabolic health/fitness benefits result from participation in regular physical activity. As illustrated in Chapter 1, however, there are documented risks associated with physical activity. Although there is risk of acute musculoskeletal injury during exercise, the major concern is the increased risk of sudden cardiac death and myocardial infarction that is sometimes associated with vigorous physical exertion. A major public health goal is to increase individual participation in regular, moderate-to-vigorous physical activity. Pursuit of this goal must include a process for identifying individuals at increased risk for adverse exercise-related events. At the same time, the risk stratification process should not present a significant barrier to participation. This chapter presents guidelines for (a) evaluating an individual's risk for adverse exercise-related events and (b) making appropriate recommendations regarding the initiation, continuation, or progression of an individual's physical activity program to reduce the potential occurrence of these types of catastrophic events.

Potential participants should be screened for the presence, signs, symptoms, and/or risk factors of various cardiovascular, pulmonary, and metabolic diseases as well as other conditions (e.g., pregnancy, orthopedic injury) that require special attention (16,18,19) to (a) optimize safety during exercise testing and (b) aid in the development of a safe and effective exercise prescription. The purposes of the preparticipation health screening include the following:

- Identification of individuals with medical contraindications for exclusion from exercise programs until those conditions have been abated or are under control
- Recognition of persons with clinically significant disease(s) or conditions who should participate in a medically supervised exercise program
- Detection of individuals at increased risk for disease because of age, symptoms, and/or risk factors who should undergo a medical evaluation and exercise testing before initiating an exercise program or increasing the frequency, intensity, or duration of their current program
- Recognition of special needs of individuals that may affect exercise testing and programming

Risk stratification procedures initially take into consideration whether individuals are guiding themselves through the process or are consulting a healthcare or fitness professional. The self-guided individual will most likely need a relatively simple tool and decision-making process to determine if his or her risk is elevated to the extent that a physician should be consulted before initiating a physical activity program, particularly if the intended exercise intensity is vigorous (1,6,7). A healthcare or fitness professional should have a logical and practical sequence for gathering and evaluating an individual's health information, assessing risk, and providing appropriate recommendations about additional screening procedures and physical activity recommendations (e.g., the Frequency, Intensity, Time, and Type or FITT framework; see Chapter 7). The American College of Sports Medicine (ACSM) provides guidelines for risk stratification in this chapter, but recognizes guidelines for risk stratification published by other organizations such as the American Heart Association (AHA) (1,12,18,19) and the American Association of Cardiovascular and Pulmonary Rehabilitation (AACVPR) (4). Exercise and health/fitness professionals should also be familiar with these other guidelines when establishing individual and program-specific policies for preparticipation health screening and medical clearance, particularly for populations with known cardiovascular disease.

PREPARTICIPATION SCREENING

Preparticipation screening procedures and tools must be valid, providing relevant and accurate information about the individual's health history, current medical conditions, risk factors, signs/symptoms, current physical activity/exercise habits, and medications. Another consideration is the literacy level of the instrument used to obtain this information (i.e., participant education level and language).

SELF-GUIDED SCREENING FOR PHYSICAL ACTIVITY

A self-guided screening for physical activity program is initiated and guided by the individual with little or no input or supervision from an exercise or health/fitness professional. Individuals seeking to start a physical activity program on their own may have questions about whether it is appropriate and safe to do so. Therefore, they need an easy-to-use screening tool to guide them through the process. At the most basic level, participants may follow the recommendation of the Surgeon Generals' Report on Physical Activity and Health (1996) (23): "previously inactive men over age 40 and women over age 50, and people at high risk for cardiovascular disease (CVD) should first consult a physician before embarking on a program of vigorous physical activity to which they are unaccustomed." The participant may also use a self-guided questionnaire or instrument such as the Physical Activity Readiness Questionnaire (PAR-Q; Fig. 2.1) (9) or the AHA/ACSM Health/Fitness Facility Preparticipation Screening Questionnaire (Fig. 2.2), which serves to alert those with elevated risk to consult a physician (or other appropriate healthcare provider) before participation (6,7).

Other types of *self-administered* surveys that may be incorporated into the exercise screening process include (a) routine paperwork completed within the scope of a physician office visit, (b) entry procedures at health/fitness or clinical

Physical Activity Readiness
Questionnaire - PAR-Q
(revised 2002)

PAR-Q & YOU

(A Questionnaire for People Aged 15 to 69)

Regular physical activity is fun and healthy, and increasingly more people are starting to become more active every day. Being more active is very safe for most people. However, some people should check with their doctor before they start becoming much more physically active.

If you are planning to become much more physically active than you are now, start by answering the seven questions in the box below. If you are between the ages of 15 and 69, the PAR-Q will tell you if you should check with your doctor before you start. If you are over 69 years of age, and you are not used to being very active, check with your doctor.

Common sense is your best guide when you answer these questions. Please read the questions carefully and answer each one honestly: check YES or NO.

YES	NO		
☐	☐	1.	Has your doctor ever said that you have a heart condition **and** that you should only do physical activity recommended by a doctor?
☐	☐	2.	Do you feel pain in your chest when you do physical activity?
☐	☐	3.	In the past month, have you had chest pain when you were not doing physical activity?
☐	☐	4.	Do you lose your balance because of dizziness or do you ever lose consciousness?
☐	☐	5.	Do you have a bone or joint problem (for example, back, knee or hip) that could be made worse by a change in your physical activity?
☐	☐	6.	Is your doctor currently prescribing drugs (for example, water pills) for your blood pressure or heart condition?
☐	☐	7.	Do you know of **any other reason** why you should not do physical activity?

If you answered

YES to one or more questions

Talk with your doctor by phone or in person BEFORE you start becoming much more physically active or BEFORE you have a fitness appraisal. Tell your doctor about the PAR-Q and which questions you answered YES.

• You may be able to do any activity you want — as long as you start slowly and build up gradually. Or, you may need to restrict your activities to those which are safe for you. Talk with your doctor about the kinds of activities you wish to participate in and follow his/her advice.
• Find out which community programs are safe and helpful for you.

NO to all questions

If you answered NO honestly to all PAR-Q questions, you can be reasonably sure that you can:
• start becoming much more physically active — begin slowly and build up gradually. This is the safest and easiest way to go.
• take part in a fitness appraisal — this is an excellent way to determine your basic fitness so that you can plan the best way for you to live actively. It is also highly recommended that you have your blood pressure evaluated. If your reading is over 144/94, talk with your doctor before you start becoming much more physically active.

DELAY BECOMING MUCH MORE ACTIVE:
• if you are not feeling well because of a temporary illness such as a cold or a fever — wait until you feel better; or
• if you are or may be pregnant — talk to your doctor before you start becoming more active.

PLEASE NOTE: If your health changes so that you then answer YES to any of the above questions, tell your fitness or health professional. Ask whether you should change your physical activity plan.

Informed Use of the PAR-Q: The Canadian Society for Exercise Physiology, Health Canada, and their agents assume no liability for persons who undertake physical activity, and if in doubt after completing this questionnaire, consult your doctor prior to physical activity.

No changes permitted. You are encouraged to photocopy the PAR-Q but only if you use the entire form.

NOTE: If the PAR-Q is being given to a person before he or she participates in a physical activity program or a fitness appraisal, this section may be used for legal or administrative purposes.

"I have read, understood and completed this questionnaire. Any questions I had were answered to my full satisfaction."

NAME _____

SIGNATURE _____   DATE _____

SIGNATURE OF PARENT _____   WITNESS _____
or GUARDIAN (for participants under the age of majority)

Note: This physical activity clearance is valid for a maximum of 12 months from the date it is completed and becomes invalid if your condition changes so that you would answer YES to any of the seven questions.

CSEP SCPE © Canadian Society for Exercise Physiology   Supported by: 🍁 Health Canada   Santé Canada

continued on other side...

FIGURE 2.1. Physical Activity Readiness (PAR-Q) Form. (Source: Physical Activity Readiness Questionnaire [PAR-Q], Public Health Agency of Canada and the Canadian Society for Exercise Physiology, reproduced with the permission of the Minister of Public Works and Government Services Canada, 2007).

exercise program facilities, and (c) physical activity promotional materials designed for and distributed to the general public. When a participant completes a self-guided instrument and medical clearance is recommended from the questionnaire results, participants should consult their physician and obtain clearance before participation in a physical activity/exercise program. For self-guided physical

Assess your health status by marking all *true* statements

History
You have had:
_____ a heart attack
_____ heart surgery
_____ cardiac catheterization
_____ coronary angioplasty (PTCA)
_____ pacemaker/implantable cardiac
         defibrillator/rhythm disturbance
_____ heart valve disease
_____ heart failure
_____ heart transplantation
_____ congenital heart disease

If you marked any of these statements in this section, consult your physician or other appropriate health care provider before engaging in exercise. You may need to use a facility with a **medically qualified staff.**

Symptoms
_____ You experience chest discomfort with exertion
_____ You experience unreasonable breathlessness
_____ You experience dizziness, fainting, or blackouts
_____ You take heart medications.

Other health issues
_____ You have diabetes
_____ You have asthma or other lung disease
_____ You have burning or cramping sensation in your
         lower legs when walking short distances
_____ You have musculoskeletal problems that limit
         your physical activity
_____ You have concerns about the safety of exercise
_____ You take prescription medications
_____ You are pregnant

Cardiovascular risk factors
_____ You are a man older than 45 years
_____ You are a woman older than 55 years, have had a
         hysterectomy, or are postmenopausal
_____ You smoke, or quit smoking within the previous 6 months
_____ Your blood pressure is >140/90 mm Hg
_____ You do not know your blood pressure
_____ You take blood pressure medication
_____ Your blood cholesterol level is >200 mg/dL
_____ You do not know your cholesterol level
_____ You have a close blood relative who had a
         heart attack or heart surgery before age
         55 (father or brother) or age
         65 (mother or sister)
_____ You are physically inactive (i.e., you get
         <30 minutes of physical activity on at
         least 3 days per week)
_____ You are >20 pounds overweight

If you marked two or more of the statements in this section you should consult your physician or other appropriate health care provider before engaging in exercise. You might benefit from using a facility with a **professionally qualified exercise staff**[a] *to guide your exercise program.*

_____ None of the above

You should be able to exercise safely without consulting your physician or other appropriate health care provider in a self-guided program or almost any facility that meets your exercise program needs.

[a]Professionally qualified exercise staff refers to appropriately trained individuals who possess academic training, practical and clinical knowledge, skills, and abilities commensurate with the credentials defined in Appendix D.

FIGURE 2.2. AHA/ACSM Health/Fitness Facility Preparticipation Screening Questionnaire (Modified from American College of Sports Medicine Position Stand and American Heart Association. Recommendations for cardiovascular screening, staffing, and emergency policies at health/fitness facilities. *Med Sci Sports Exerc.* 1998;30(6):1009–18.)

activity regimens conducted at low (<40% oxygen update reserve $\dot{V}O_2R$) to moderate (40%–60% $\dot{V}O_2R$) exercise intensity, little additional assessment is needed beyond the ACSM/AHA Questionnaires (1), provided that one adheres to all medical clearance recommendations contained within the form. Such regimens should incorporate the physical activity recommendations from the U.S. Surgeon General (6,23). A specific self-guided exercise regimen suitable for previously sedentary individuals may be found in the *ACSM Fitness Book* (6).

PROFESSIONALLY GUIDED SCREENING FOR PHYSICAL ACTIVITY

Professionally guided implies that the health fitness/clinical assessment is conducted by—and the exercise program is designed and supervised by—appropriately trained personnel who possess academic training and practical/clinical knowledge, skills, and abilities commensurate with the credentials defined in Appendix D.

Self-guided surveys are effective in identifying individuals who would benefit from medical consultation before participation in an exercise program (1). A more advanced process administered by professionally trained personnel provides greater detail regarding CVD risk factors and signs/symptoms and identifies a broader scope of chronic diseases and/or conditions that need special consideration before engaging in an exercise program. The professionally guided preparticipation screening process involves (a) the review of more detailed health/medical history information and specific risk stratification, and (b) detailed recommendations for physical activity/exercise, medical examination, exercise testing, and physician supervision.

Many health/fitness and clinical exercise program facilities use a more elaborate health/medical history questionnaire designed to provide additional details regarding selected health/fitness habits and medical history, such as the AHA/ACSM Questionnaire (1) (Fig. 2.2). This questionnaire may be used as a basic instrument for this process, but additional information needs to be obtained related to specific CVD risk factors.

RISK STRATIFICATION

Appropriate recommendations for medical examination, physical activity/exercise, exercise testing, and physician supervision are made based on a risk stratification process that assigns participants into one of three risk categories: (a) low, (b) moderate, or (c) high risk (Table 2.1). The process by which individuals are assigned to one of these risk categories is called risk stratification and is based on:

- The presence or absence of known cardiovascular, pulmonary, and/or metabolic disease
- The presence or absence of signs or symptoms suggestive of cardiovascular, pulmonary, and/or metabolic disease
- The presence or absence of CVD risk factors

   Low risk: Individuals classified as low risk are those who do not have signs/symptoms of or have diagnosed cardiovascular, pulmonary, and/or metabolic disease and have no more than one (i.e., ≤1) CVD risk factor. The risk of an acute cardiovascular event in this population is low, and a physical

TABLE 2.1. ACSM RISK STRATIFICATION CATEGORIES FOR ATHEROSCLEROTIC CARDIOVASCULAR DISEASE

Low risk	Asymptomatic men and women who have ≤1 CVD risk factor from Table 2.3
Moderate risk	Asymptomatic men and women who have ≥2 risk factors from Table 2.3
High risk	Individuals who have known cardiovascular,[a] pulmonary,[b] or metabolic[c] disease *or* one or more signs and symptoms listed in Table 2.2

ACSM, American College of Sports Medicine; CVD, cardiovascular disease.

[a]Cardiac, peripheral vascular, or cerebrovascular disease.

[b]Chronic obstructive pulmonary disease, asthma, interstitial lung disease, or cystic fibrosis.

[c]Diabetes mellitus (type 1, type 2), thyroid disorders, renal, or liver disease.

activity/exercise program may be pursued safely without the necessity for medical examination and clearance (1,20,22,23).

Moderate risk: Individuals classified as moderate risk do not have signs/symptoms of or diagnosed cardiovascular, pulmonary, and/or metabolic disease, but have two or more (i.e., >2) CVD risk factors. The risk of an acute cardiovascular event in this population is increased, although in most cases, individuals at moderate risk may safely engage in low- to moderate-intensity physical activities without the necessity for medical examination and clearance. However, it is advisable to have a medical examination and an exercise test before participation in vigorous intensity exercise (i.e., >60% $\dot{V}O_2R$) (14,15).

High risk: Individuals classified as high risk are those who have one or more signs/symptoms of or diagnosed cardiovascular, pulmonary, and/or metabolic disease. The risk of an acute cardiovascular event in this population is increased to the degree that a thorough medical examination should take place and clearance given before initiating physical activity or exercise at any intensity.

The exercise or health/fitness professional may evaluate the individual's medical/health history information and follow a logical sequence considering this risk-stratification process to determine into which appropriate risk category an individual should be placed. Exercise or health/fitness professionals should have a thorough knowledge of (a) the criteria for known cardiovascular, pulmonary, and metabolic diseases; (b) the descriptions of signs and symptoms for these diseases; (c) the specific criteria that determine the CVD risk-factor schemes; and (d) the criteria for each risk category. The flow chart in Figure 2.3 may be used to move sequentially through the process to determine the risk-category placement for each individual.

UNDISCLOSED OR UNAVAILABLE CARDIOVASCULAR DISEASE RISK-FACTOR INFORMATION

Health/fitness and exercise professionals and clinicians are encouraged to adopt a conservative approach to CVD risk-factor identification for the purposes of risk stratification, especially when (a) risk-factor information is missing and/or (b) the criteria for identifying the presence or absence of a specific risk factor

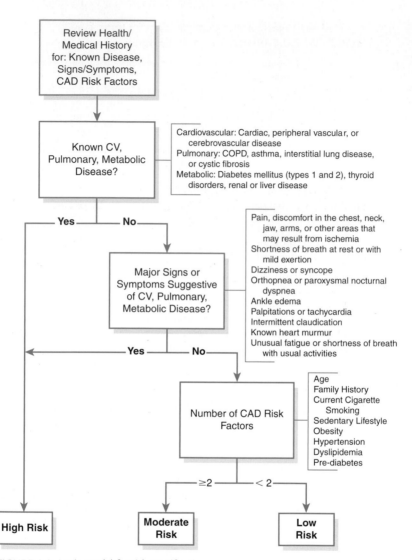

FIGURE 2.3. Logic model for risk stratification.

cannot be determined or is not available. If the presence or absence of a specific risk factor is not disclosed or is unavailable, the risk factor should be counted as a risk factor, except for prediabetes (8) (see Table 10.2 for diagnostic criteria for prediabetes). Missing or unknown criteria for prediabetes should be counted as a risk factor in the presence of age (≥45 years), particularly for those with a body mass index ≥25 kg·m^{-2}, and for those who are younger, have a body mass index ≥25 kg·m^{-2}, and have additional risk factors for prediabetes (8).

See Box 2.1 for case studies that involve undisclosed or unavailable CVD risk-factor information.

KNOWN CARDIOVASCULAR, PULMONARY, AND METABOLIC DISEASE

An individual has known cardiovascular, pulmonary, and/or metabolic disease if a physician has diagnosed one of the following conditions:

- Cardiovascular disease (CVD): cardiac, peripheral artery (PAD), or cerebrovascular disease
- Pulmonary disease: chronic obstructive pulmonary disease (COPD), asthma, interstitial lung disease, or cystic fibrosis (5)
- Metabolic disease: diabetes mellitus (type 1 or type 2), thyroid disorders, and renal or liver disease

MAJOR SIGNS/SYMPTOMS SUGGESTIVE OF CARDIOVASCULAR, PULMONARY, AND METABOLIC DISEASE

Table 2.2 presents a listing of major signs or symptoms suggestive of cardiovascular, pulmonary and/or metabolic disease in addition to information aiding the clinician in the clarification and significance of each sign or symptom. The presence of most of these signs/symptoms may be identified using the AHA/ACSM Questionnaire (1) (Fig. 2.2); however, a few signs/symptoms (i.e., orthopnea, ankle edema, and heart murmur) require a more thorough medical history and/or examination. These signs/symptoms must be interpreted within the clinical context in which they appear because they are not necessarily specific for cardiovascular, pulmonary, or metabolic disease.

ATHEROSCLEROTIC CARDIOVASCULAR DISEASE RISK FACTORS

ACSM risk stratification is based, in part, on the presence or absence of the CVD risk factors listed in Table 2.3 (2,3,8,10,23). The health/medical history should be reviewed to determine if the individual meets any of the criteria for positive risk factors shown in Table 2.3. The number of positive risk factors is then summed. Because of the cardioprotective effect of high-density lipoprotein cholesterol (HDL-C), HDL-C is considered a negative risk factor. For individuals having HDL-C $\geq$60 mg$\cdot$dL^{-1} (1.55 mmol$\cdot$L^{-1}), one positive risk factor is subtracted from the sum of positive risk factors.

The risk factors in Table 2.3 should not be viewed as an all-inclusive list of factors associated with elevated risk for CVD. Rather, Table 2.3 contains *clinically relevant established CVD risk factor* criteria that should be considered collectively when making decisions about (a) the level of medical clearance, (b) the need for exercise testing before initiating participation, and (c) the level of supervision for both exercise testing and exercise program participation. The intended use for the CVD risk factor list in Table 2.3 is to aid in the identification of occult coronary

(*text continues on page 28*)

TABLE 2.2. MAJOR SIGNS OR SYMPTOMS SUGGESTIVE OF CARDIOVASCULAR, PULMONARY, OR METABOLIC DISEASE[a]

SIGN OR SYMPTOM	CLARIFICATION/SIGNIFICANCE
Pain, discomfort (or other anginal equivalent) in the chest, neck, jaw, arms, or other areas that may result from ischemia	One of the cardinal manifestations of cardiac disease, in particular coronary artery disease Key features *favoring an ischemic origin* include: • *Character:* Constricting, squeezing, burning, "heaviness" or "heavy feeling" • *Location:* Substernal, across midthorax, anteriorly; in one or both arms, shoulders; in neck, cheeks, teeth; in forearms, fingers in interscapular region • *Provoking factors:* Exercise or exertion, excitement, other forms of stress, cold weather, occurrence after meals Key features *against an ischemic origin* include: • *Character:* Dull ache; "knifelike," sharp, stabbing; "jabs" aggravated by respiration • *Location:* In left submammary area; in left hemithorax • *Provoking factors:* After completion of exercise, provoked by a specific body motion
Shortness of breath at rest or with mild exertion	Dyspnea (defined as an abnormally uncomfortable awareness of breathing) is one of the principal symptoms of cardiac and pulmonary disease. It commonly occurs during strenuous exertion in healthy, well-trained persons and during moderate exertion in healthy, untrained persons. However, it should be regarded as abnormal when it occurs at a level of exertion that is not expected to evoke this symptom in a given individual. Abnormal exertional dyspnea suggests the presence of cardiopulmonary disorders, in particular left ventricular dysfunction or chronic obstructive pulmonary disease.
Dizziness or syncope	Syncope (defined as a loss of consciousness) is most commonly caused by a reduced perfusion of the brain. Dizziness and, in particular, syncope *during* exercise may result from cardiac disorders that prevent the normal rise (or an actual fall) in cardiac output. Such cardiac disorders are potentially life-threatening and include severe coronary artery disease, hypertrophic cardiomyopathy, aortic stenosis, and malignant ventricular dysrhythmias. Although dizziness or syncope shortly *after* cessation of exercise should not be ignored, these symptoms may occur even in healthy persons as a result of a reduction in venous return to the heart.
Orthopnea or paroxysmal nocturnal dyspnea	Orthopnea refers to dyspnea occurring at rest in the recumbent position that is relieved promptly by sitting upright or standing. Paroxysmal nocturnal dyspnea refers to dyspnea, beginning usually 2–5 h after the onset of sleep, which may be relieved by sitting on the side of the bed or getting out of bed. Both are symptoms of left ventricular dysfunction. Although nocturnal dyspnea may occur in persons with chronic obstructive pulmonary *(continued)*

TABLE 2.2. MAJOR SIGNS OR SYMPTOMS SUGGESTIVE OF CARDIOVASCULAR, PULMONARY, OR METABOLIC DISEASE[a] (*Continued*)

SIGN OR SYMPTOM	CLARIFICATION/SIGNIFICANCE
	disease, it differs in that it is usually relieved after the person relieves himself or herself of secretions rather than specifically by sitting up.
Ankle edema	Bilateral ankle edema that is most evident at night is a characteristic sign of heart failure or bilateral chronic venous insufficiency. Unilateral edema of a limb often results from venous thrombosis or lymphatic blockage in the limb. Generalized edema (known as anasarca) occurs in persons with the nephrotic syndrome, severe heart failure, or hepatic cirrhosis.
Palpitations or tachycardia	Palpitations (defined as an unpleasant awareness of the forceful or rapid beating of the heart) may be induced by various disorders of cardiac rhythm. These include tachycardia, bradycardia of sudden onset, ectopic beats, compensatory pauses, and accentuated stroke volume resulting from valvular regurgitation. Palpitations also often result from anxiety states and high cardiac output (or hyperkinetic) states, such as anemia, fever, thyrotoxicosis, arteriovenous fistula, and the so-called idiopathic hyperkinetic heart syndrome.
Intermittent claudication	Intermittent claudication refers to the pain that occurs in a muscle with an inadequate blood supply (usually as a result of atherosclerosis) that is stressed by exercise. The pain does not occur with standing or sitting, is reproducible from day to day, is more severe when walking upstairs or up a hill, and is often described as a cramp, which disappears within 1–2 min after stopping exercise. Coronary artery disease is more prevalent in persons with intermittent claudication. Patients with diabetes are at increased risk for this condition.
Known heart murmur	Although some may be innocent, heart murmurs may indicate valvular or other cardiovascular disease. From an exercise safety standpoint, it is especially important to exclude hypertrophic cardiomyopathy and aortic stenosis as underlying causes because these are among the more common causes of exertion-related sudden cardiac death.
Unusual fatigue or shortness of breath with usual activities	Although there may be benign origins for these symptoms, they also may signal the onset of, or change in the status of cardiovascular, pulmonary, or metabolic disease.

[a]These signs or symptoms must be interpreted within the clinical context in which they appear because they are not all specific for cardiovascular, pulmonary, or metabolic disease.

Modified from Gordon SMBS. Health appraisal in the non-medical setting. In: Durstine JL, King AC, Painter PL. *ACSM's resource manual for guidelines for exercise testing and prescription.* Philadelphia (PA): Lea & Febiger; 1993. p. 219–28.

TABLE 2.3. ATHEROSCLEROTIC CARDIOVASCULAR DISEASE (CVD) RISK FACTOR THRESHOLDS FOR USE WITH ACSM RISK STRATIFICATION

POSITIVE RISK FACTORS	DEFINING CRITERIA
Age	Men ≥45 yr; Women ≥55 yr
Family history	Myocardial infarction, coronary revascularization, or sudden death before 55 yr of age in father or other male first-degree relative, or before 65 yr of age in mother or other female first-degree relative
Cigarette smoking	Current cigarette smoker or those who quit within the previous 6 months or exposure to environmental tobacco smoke
Sedentary lifestyle	Not participating in at least 30 min of moderate intensity (40%–60% $\dot{V}O_2R$) physical activity on at least three days of the week for at least three months (20,23)
Obesity[a]	Body mass index ≥30 kg·m^2 *or* waist girth >102 cm (40 inches) for men and >88 cm (35 inches) for women (2)
Hypertension	Systolic blood pressure ≥140 mm Hg and/or diastolic ≥90 mm Hg, confirmed by measurements on at least two separate occasions, *or* on antihypertensive medication (10)
Dyslipidemia	Low-density lipoprotein (LDL-C) cholesterol ≥130 mg·dL^{-1} (3.37 mmol·L^{-1}) *or* high-density lipoprotein (HDL-C) cholesterol <40 mg·dL^{-1} (1.04 mmol·L^{-1}) *or* on lipid-lowering medication. If total serum cholesterol is all that is available use ≥200 mg·dL^{-1} (5.18 mmol·L^{-1}) (3)
Prediabetes	Impaired fasting glucose (IFG) = fasting plasma glucose ≥100 mg·dL^{-1} (5.50 mmol·L^{-1}) but <126 mg·dL^{-1} (6.93 mmol·L^{-1}) *or* impaired glucose tolerance (IGT) = 2-hour values in oral glucose tolerance test (OGTT) ≥140 mg·dL^{-1} (7.70 mmol·L^{-1}) but <200 mg·dL^{-1} (11.00 mmol·L^{-1}) confirmed by measurements on at least two separate occasions (8)
NEGATIVE RISK FACTOR	DEFINING CRITERIA
High-serum HDL cholesterol[†]	≥60 mg·dL^{-1} (1.55 mmol·L^{-1})

Note: It is common to sum risk factors in making clinical judgments. If HDL is high, subtract one risk factor from the sum of positive risk factors, because high HDL decreases CVD risk.

[a]Professional opinions vary regarding the most appropriate markers and thresholds for obesity; therefore, allied health professionals should use clinical judgment when evaluating this risk factor.

artery disease. The *scope* of the list and the *threshold* for each risk factor are not inconsistent with other risk-factor lists established by other health organizations that are intended for use in predicting coronary events prospectively during long-term follow up (24). Furthermore, other risk factors, such as the inflammatory markers C-reactive protein and fibrinogen, also have been suggested as positive and emerging CVD risk factors (11,13), but are not included in this list. Refer to Case Studies in Box 2.1 for further explanation.

BOX 2.1	Case Studies to be Used to Establish Risk Stratification

CASE STUDY I

Female, age 21 years, smokes socially on weekends ($\sim$10–20 cigarettes). Drinks alcohol one or two nights a week, usually on weekends. Height = 63 in (160 cm), weight = 124 lb (56.4 kg), BMI = 22 kg·m^{-2}. RHR = 76 beats·min^{-1}, systolic/diastolic BP = 118/72 mm Hg. Total cholesterol = 178 mg·dL^{-1} (4.61 mmol·L^{-1}), LDL-C = 98 mg·dL^{-1} (2.54 mmol·L^{-1}), HDL-C = 57 mg·dL^{-1} (1.48 mmol·L^{-1}), FBG unknown. Currently taking oral contraceptives. Attends group exercise class two to three times a week. Reports no symptoms. Both parents living and in good health.

CASE STUDY II

Male, age 54 years, nonsmoker. Height = 72 inches (182.9 cm), weight = 168 pounds (76.4 kg), BMI = 22.8 kg·m^{-2}. RHR = 64 bpm, RBP = 124/78 mm Hg. Total cholesterol = 187 mg·dL^{-1} (4.84 mmol·L^{-1}), LDL = 103 mg·dL^{-1} (2.67 mmol·L^{-1}), HDL = 52 mg·dL^{-1} (1.35 mmol·L^{-1}), FBG = 88 mg·dL^{-1} (4.84 mmol·L^{-1}). Recreationally competitive runner, runs four to seven days per week, completes one to two marathons and numerous other road races every year. No medications other than OTC ibuprofen as needed. Reports no symptoms. Father died at age 77 years of a heart attack, mother died at age 81 years of cancer.

CASE STUDY III

Male, age 44 years, nonsmoker. Height = 70 inches (177.8 cm), weight = 216 pounds (98.2 kg), BMI = 31.0 kg·m^{-2}. RHR = 62 bpm, RBP = 128/84 mm Hg. Total serum cholesterol = 184 mg·dL^{-1} (4.77 mmol·L^{-1}), LDL = 106 mg·dL^{-1} (2.75 mmol·L^{-1}), HDL = 44 mg · dL^{-1} (1.14 mmol·L^{-1}), FBG unknown. Walks two to three miles two to three times a week. Father had type 2 diabetes and died at age 67 of a heart attack; mother living, no CVD. No medications; reports no symptoms.

CASE STUDY IV

Female, age 36 years, nonsmoker. Height = 64 inches (162.6 cm), weight = 108 pounds (49.1 kg), BMI = 18.5 kg·m^{-2}. RHR = 61 bpm, RBP = 114/62 mm Hg. Total cholesterol = 174 mg·dL^{-1} (4.51 mmol·L^{-1}), blood glucose normal with insulin injections. Type 1 diabetes diagnosed at age 7. Teaches dance aerobic classes three times a week, walks approximately 45 minutes four times a week. Reports no symptoms. Both parents in good health with no history of cardiovascular disease. >

> Box 2.1. continued

	CASE STUDY I	CASE STUDY II	CASE STUDY III	CASE STUDY IV
Known CV, Pulmonary, and/or Metabolic Disease?	No	No	No	Yes—diagnosed Type 1 diabetes
Major Signs or Symptoms?	No	No	No	No
CVD Risk Factors:				
Age?	No	Yes	No	No
Family History?	No	No	No	No
Current Cigarette Smoking?	Yes	No	No	No
Sedentary Lifestyle?	No	No	No	No
Obesity?	No	No	Yes—BMI >30 kg·m^{-2}	No
Hypertension?	No	No	No	No
Hypercholesterolemia?	No	No	No	No
Pre-diabetes?	Unknown—count as No in absence of Age or Obesity as risk factors	No	Unknown—count as Yes in presence of Obesity	Diagnosed Type 1 diabetes
Risk Stratification Category:	Low Risk—no known disease, no major signs or symptoms, 1 CVD risk factor	Low Risk—no known disease, no major signs or symptoms, 1 CVD risk factor	Moderate Risk—no known disease, no major signs or symptoms, 2 CVD risk factors	High Risk—diagnosed metabolic disease

BMI = body mass index, RHR = resting heart rate, FBG = fasting blood glucose, BP = blood pressure, LDL-C = low density lipoprotein cholesterol, HDL-C = high density lipoprotein cholesterol

EXERCISE TESTING AND PARTICIPATION RECOMMENDATIONS BASED ON RISK CATEGORY

Once the risk category has been established for an individual as low, medium, or high, appropriate recommendations may be made regarding:

- The necessity for medical examination and clearance before initiating a physical activity/exercise program or substantially changing the FITT framework of an existing physical activity/exercise program
- The necessity for an exercise test before initiating a physical activity/exercise program or substantially changing the FITT framework of an existing activity program
- The necessity for physician supervision when participating in a maximal or submaximal exercise test

EXERCISE TESTING AND TESTING SUPERVISION RECOMMENDATIONS BASED ON RISK CATEGORY

No set of guidelines for exercise testing and participation covers all situations. Local circumstances and policies vary, and specific program procedures also are properly diverse. To provide guidance on the need for a medical examination and exercise test before participation in a moderate to vigorous intensity exercise program, ACSM suggests the recommendations presented in Figure 2.4 for determining when a medical examination and diagnostic exercise test are appropriate and when physician supervision is recommended. Although it is recommended that exercise testing for those individuals classified as low risk is not a necessity, the information gathered from an exercise test may be useful in establishing a safe and effective exercise prescription for these individuals. Recommending an exercise test for low-risk individuals should not be viewed as inappropriate if the purpose of the test is to design an effective exercise program. The exercise testing recommendations found in Figure 2.4 reflect the notion that the risk of cardiovascular events increases as a direct function of exercise intensity (i.e., vigorous > moderate > low exercise intensity) and the presence of risk factors. Although Figure 2.4 provides both absolute and relative thresholds for moderate and vigorous exercise intensity, health/fitness and exercise professionals should choose the most applicable definition (i.e., relative or absolute) for their setting and population when making decisions about the level of screening necessary before exercise training and for physician supervision during exercise testing. It should be noted that the recommendations for medical examination and exercise testing for individuals at moderate risk desiring to participate in vigorous-intensity exercise (Fig. 2.4) are consistent with those found within recent AHA Guidelines (1) (Box 2.2).

The degree of medical supervision of exercise testing varies appropriately from physician-supervised tests to situations in which there may be no physician present (12). The degree of physician supervision may differ with local policies

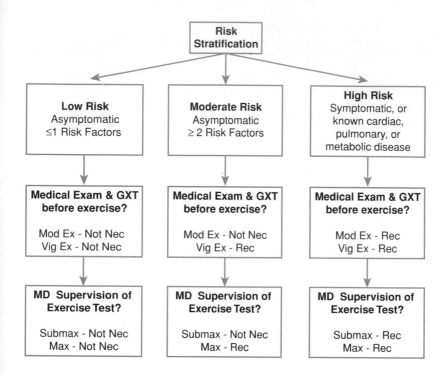

Mod Ex: Moderate intensity exercise; 40-60% of $\dot{V}O_{2max}$; 3-6 METs; "an intensity well within the individual's capacity, one which can be comfortably sustained for a prolonged period of time (~45 minutes)"

Vig Ex: Vigorous intensity exercise; > 60% of $\dot{V}O_{2max}$; > 6 METs; "exercise intense enough to represent a substantial cardiorespiratory challenge"

Not Nec: Not Necessary; reflects the notion that a medical examination, exercise test, and physician supervision of exercise testing would not be essential in the preparticipation screening, however, they should not be viewed as inappropriate

Rec: Recommended; when MD supervision of exercise testing is "Recommended," the MD shonld be in close proximity and readily available should there be an emergent need

FIGURE 2.4. Exercise Testing and Testing Supervision Recommendations Based on Risk Stratification.

and circumstances, the health status of the patient, and the training and experience of the laboratory staff. Physicians responsible for supervising exercise testing should meet or exceed the minimal competencies for supervision and interpretation of results as established by the AHA (21). In all situations in which exercise testing is performed, site personnel should at least be certified at a level

BOX 2.2 American Heart Association (AHA) Risk Stratification Criteria

CLASS A: APPARENTLY HEALTHY INDIVIDUALS

- Includes the following individuals
  1. Children, adolescents, men <45 years, and women <55 years who have no symptoms of or known presence of heart disease or major atherosclerotic cardiovascular disease (CVD) risk factors
  2. Men ≥45 years and women ≥55 years who have no symptoms or known presence of heart disease and with less than two major CVD risk factors
  3. Men ≥45 years and women ≥55 years who have no symptoms or known presence of heart disease and with two or more CVD risk factors
- Activity guidelines: No restrictions other than basic guidelines
- Electrocardiogram (ECG) and blood pressure monitoring: Not required
- Supervision required: None, although it is suggested that persons classified as Class A-2 and particularly Class A-3 undergo a medical examination and possibly a medically supervised exercise test before engaging in vigorous exercise (12)

CLASS B: PRESENCE OF KNOWN, STABLE CARDIOVASCULAR DISEASE WITH LOW RISK FOR COMPLICATIONS WITH VIGOROUS EXERCISE, BUT SLIGHTLY GREATER THAN FOR APPARENTLY HEALTHY INDIVIDUALS

- Includes individuals with any of the following diagnoses:
  1. Coronary artery disease (myocardial infarction, coronary artery bypass graft surgery, percutaneous transluminal coronary angioplasty, angina pectoris, abnormal exercise test, and abnormal coronary angiograms) whose condition is stable and who have the clinical characteristics outlined below
  2. Valvular heart disease, excluding severe valvular stenosis or regurgitation with the clinical characteristics outlined below
  3. Congenital heart disease
  4. Cardiomyopathy; ejection fraction ≤30%; includes stable patients with heart failure with any of the clinical characteristics as outlined below but not hypertrophic cardiomyopathy or recent myocarditis
  5. Exercise test abnormalities that do not meet the criteria outlined in Class C
- *Clinical characteristics*:
  1. New York Heart Association Class 1 or 2
  2. Exercise capacity ≤6 METs
  3. No evidence of congestive heart failure
  4. No evidence of myocardial ischemia or angina at rest or on the exercise test at or below 6 METs >

> **Box 2.2. continued**

---

5. Appropriate rise in systolic blood pressure during exercise
6. Absence of sustained or nonsustained ventricular tachycardia at rest or with exercise
7. Ability to satisfactorily self-monitor intensity of activity
- *Activity guidelines*: Activity should be individualized, with exercise prescription by qualified individuals and approved by primary health-care provider
- *Supervision required*: Medical supervision during initial prescription session is beneficial. Supervision by appropriate trained nonmedical personnel for other exercise sessions should occur until the individual understands how to monitor his or her activity. Medical personnel should be trained and certified in advanced cardiac life support. Nonmedical personnel should be trained and certified in basic life support (which includes CPR).
- *ECG and blood pressure monitoring*: Useful during the early prescription phase of training, usually 6 to 12 sessions

CLASS C: THOSE AT MODERATE TO HIGH RISK FOR CARDIAC COMPLICATIONS DURING EXERCISE AND/OR UNABLE TO SELF-REGULATE ACTIVITY OR UNDERSTAND RECOMMENDED ACTIVITY LEVEL

- Includes individuals with any of the following diagnoses:
  1. CVD with the clinical characteristics outlined below
  2. Valvular heart disease, excluding severe valvular stenosis or regurgitation with the clinical characteristics outlined below
  3. Congenital heart disease; risk stratification should be guided by the 27th Bethesda Conference recommendations[a]
  4. Cardiomyopathy; ejection fraction ≤30%; includes stable patients with heart failure with any of the clinical characteristics as outlined below but not hypertrophic cardiomyopathy or recent myocarditis
  5. Complex ventricular arrhythmias not well controlled
- *Clinical characteristics*:
  1. NYHA class 3 or 4
  2. Exercise test results:
     - Exercise capacity <6 METs
     - Angina or ischemia ST depression at workload <6METs
     - Fall in systolic blood pressure below resting levels with exercise
     - Nonsustained ventricular tachycardia with exercise
  3. Previous episode of primary cardiac arrest (17) (i.e., cardiac arrest that did not occur in the presence of an acute myocardial infarction or during a cardiac procedure)
  4. A medical problem that the physician believes may be life threatening
     - *Activity guidelines*: Activity should be individualized, with exercise prescription provided by qualified individuals and approved by primary healthcare provider >

> **Box 2.2. continued**

- *Supervision*: Medical supervision during all exercise sessions until safety is established
- *ECG and blood pressure monitoring*: Continuous during exercise sessions until safety is established, usually ≥12 sessions

CLASS D: UNSTABLE DISEASE WITH ACTIVITY RESTRICTION[b]
- Includes individuals with
  1. Unstable ischemia
  2. Severe and symptomatic valvular stenosis or regurgitation
  3. Congenital heart disease; criteria for risk that would prohibit exercise conditioning should be guided by the 27th Bethesda Conference recommendations[a]
  4. Heart failure that is not compensated
  5. Uncontrolled arrhythmias
  6. Other medical conditions that could be aggravated by exercise
- *Activity guidelines*: No activity is recommended for conditioning purposes. Attention should be directed to treating the patient and restoring the patient to class C or better. Daily activities must be prescribed on the basis of individual assessment by the patient's personal physician.

[a]Fuster V, Gotto AM, Libby P. 27th Bethesda Conference: Matching the intensity of risk factor management with the hazard for coronary disease events. *J Am Coll Cardiol*. 1996;27:964–76.

[b]Exercise for conditioning purposes is not recommended.

Adapted from Fletcher GF, Balady GJ, Amsterdam EA, et al. Exercise standards for testing and training. A statement for health care professionals from the American Heart Association. *Circulation*. 2001;104:1694–1740.

---

of basic life support (CPR, cardiopulmonary resuscitation) and have automated external defibrillator (AED) training. Preferably, one or more staff members should also be certified in first aid and advanced cardiac life support (ACLS) (17).

Hypertension represents a unique risk factor in that it may be aggravated by acute exercise. Therefore, although it appears within Table 2.3, special consideration should be given to patients with hypertension when screening for exercise testing or training (see Chapter 10 for the special considerations in exercise testing for individuals with hypertension). Because hypertension is commonly clustered with other risk factors associated with CVD (i.e., dyslipidemia, obesity, diabetes mellitus, and the metabolic syndrome), most patients with hypertension presenting for exercise testing or training fall into the *moderate* or *high* risk category as defined in Table 2.1. For such individuals, the requisite medical examination in Table 2.3 is consistent with the screening recommendations for patients with hypertension outlined in JNC7

(10) and Chapter 10. However, in cases when hypertension is the only presenting risk factor from those listed in Table 2.3, prudent recommendations for preparticipation screening should be based on the severity of the hypertension (see Table 3.1 for JNC7 classifications) and the desired intensity of exercise.

RISK STRATIFICATION FOR CARDIAC PATIENTS

Cardiac patients may be further stratified regarding safety during exercise using published guidelines (4). Risk stratification criteria from the AACVPR are presented in Box 2.3 (4). The AHA has developed a more extensive risk-classification system for medical clearance of cardiac patients (Box 2.2) (12). The AHA guidelines provide recommendations for participant and/or patient monitoring and supervision and for activity restriction. Exercise program professionals should recognize that the AHA guidelines do not consider comorbidities (e.g., type 2 diabetes mellitus, morbid obesity, severe pulmonary disease, and debilitating neurologic or orthopedic conditions) that could result in modification of the recommendations for monitoring and supervision during exercise training.

BOX 2.3	American Association of Cardiovascular and Pulmonary Rehabilitation Risk Stratification Criteria for Cardiac Patients

LOWEST RISK

Characteristics of patients at lowest risk for exercise participation (all characteristics listed must be present for patients to remain at lowest risk)

- Absence of complex ventricular dysrhythmias during exercise testing and recovery
- Absence of angina or other significant symptoms (e.g., unusual shortness of breath, light-headedness, or dizziness, during exercise testing and recovery)
- Presence of normal hemodynamics during exercise testing and recovery (i.e., appropriate increases and decreases in heart rate and systolic blood pressure with increasing workloads and recovery)
- Functional capacity ≥ 7 METs

Nonexercise Testing Findings

- Resting ejection fraction $\geq 50\%$
- Uncomplicated myocardial infarction or revascularization procedure
- Absence of complicated ventricular dysrhythmias at rest >

> **Box 2.3. continued**

- Absence of congestive heart failure
- Absence of signs or symptoms of postevent/postprocedure ischemia
- Absence of clinical depression

MODERATE RISK

Characteristics of patients at moderate risk for exercise participation (any one or combination of these findings places a patient at moderate risk)

- Presence of angina or other significant symptoms (e.g., unusual shortness of breath, light-headedness, or dizziness occurring only at high levels of exertion [≥7 METs])
- Mild to moderate level of silent ischemia during exercise testing or recovery (ST-segment depression <2 mm from baseline)
- Functional capacity <5 METs

Nonexercise Testing Findings

- Rest ejection fraction = 40%–49%

HIGHEST RISK

Characteristics of patients at high risk for exercise participation (any one or combination of these findings places a patient at high risk)

- Presence of complex ventricular dysrhythmias during exercise testing or recovery
- Presence of angina or other significant symptoms (e.g., unusual shortness of breath, light-headedness, or dizziness at low levels of exertion [<5 METs] or during recovery)
- High level of silent ischemia (ST-segment depression ≥2 mm from baseline) during exercise testing or recovery
- Presence of abnormal hemodynamics with exercise testing (i.e., chronotropic incompetence or flat or decreasing systolic BP with increasing workloads) or recovery (i.e., severe postexercise hypotension)

Nonexercise Testing Findings

- Rest ejection fraction <40%
- History of cardiac arrest or sudden death
- Complex dysrhythmias at rest
- Complicated myocardial infarction or revascularization procedure
- Presence of congestive heart failure
- Presence of signs or symptoms of postevent/postprocedure ischemia
- Presence of clinical depression

Reprinted from Williams MA. Exercise testing in cardiac rehabilitation: exercise prescription and beyond. *Cardiol Clin.* 2001;19:415–431, with permission from Elsevier.

REFERENCES

1. American College of Sports Medicine Position Stand and American Heart Association. Recommendations for cardiovascular screening, staffing, and emergency policies at health/fitness facilities. *Med Sci Sports Exerc.* 1998;30(6):1009–18.
2. Executive summary of the clinical guidelines on the identification, evaluation, and treatment of overweight and obesity in adults. *Arch Intern Med.* 1998;158(17):1855–67.
3. Third Report of the National Cholesterol Education Program (NCEP) Expert Panel on Detection, Evaluation, and Treatment of High Blood Cholesterol in Adults (Adult Treatment Panel III) final report. *Circulation.* 2002;106(25):3143–421.
4. American Association of Cardiovascular and Pulmonary Rehabilitation. *Guidelines for Cardiac Rehabilitation and Secondary Prevention Programs.* 4th ed. Champaign (IL): Human Kinetics; 2004.
5. American Association of Cardiovascular and Pulmonary Rehabilitation. *Guidelines for Pulmonary Rehabilitation Programs.* Champaign (IL): Human Kinetics; 2004.
6. American College of Sports Medicine. *ACSM Fitness Book.* 3rd ed. Champaign (IL): Human Kinetics; 2003.
7. American College of Sports Medicine. *ACSM's Health/Fitness Facility Standards and Guidelines.* 3rd ed. Champaign (IL): Human Kinetics; 2007.
8. American Diabetes Association. Diagnosis and Classification of Diabetes Mellitus. *Diabetes Care.* 2007;30(suppl 1):S42–7.
9. Canada's Physical Activity Guide to Healthy Active Living. *Health Canada 1998* [Internet]. 2002. [cited 2007 June 15] Available from: http://www.hc-sc.gc.ca/hppb/paguide/pdf/guideEng.pdf
10. Chobanian AV, Bakris GL, Black HR, et al. The Seventh Report of the Joint National Committee on Prevention, Detection, Evaluation, and Treatment of High Blood Pressure: the JNC 7 report. *JAMA.* 2003; 289(19):2560–72.
11. Ferketich AK, Schwartzbaum JA, Frid DJ, Moeschberger ML. Depression as an antecedent to heart disease among women and men in the NHANES I study. National Health and Nutrition Examination Survey. *Arch Intern Med.* 2000;160(9):1261–8.
12. Fletcher GF, Balady GJ, Amsterdam EA, et al. Exercise standards for testing and training: a statement for healthcare professionals from the American Heart Association. *Circulation.* 2001;104(14): 1694–1740.
13. Ford DE, Mead LA, Chang PP, Cooper-Patrick L, Wang NY, Klag MJ. Depression is a risk factor for coronary artery disease in men: the precursors study. *Arch Intern Med.* 1998;158(13):1422–6.
14. Gibbons RJ, Balady GJ, Beasley JW, et al. ACC/AHA guidelines for exercise testing. A report of the American College of Cardiology/American Heart Association Task Force on Practice Guidelines (Committee on Exercise Testing). *J Am Coll Cardiol.* 1997;30(1):260–311.
15. Gibbons RJ, Balady GT, Bricker TJ, et al. ACC/AHA 2002 guideline update for exercise testing: summary article. A report of the American college of cardiology/American heart association task force on practice guidelines (committee to update the 1997 exercise testing guidelines). *J Am Coll Cardiol.* 2002;40(8):1531–40.
16. Gordon SMBS. Health appraisal in the non-medical setting. In: Durstine JL, King AC, Painter PL, editors. *ACSM's Resource Manual for Guidelines for Exercise Testing and Prescription.* Philadelphia (PA): Lea & Febiger; 1993. p. 219–28.
17. Kern KB, Halperin HR, Field J. New Guidelines for cardiopulmonary resuscitation and emergency cardiac care: changes in the management of cardiac arrest. *JAMA.* 2001;285(10):1267–9.
18. Maron BJ, Araujo CG, Thompson PD, et al. Recommendations for preparticipation screening and the assessment of cardiovascular disease in masters athletes: an advisory for healthcare professionals from the working groups of the World Heart Federation, the International Federation of Sports Medicine, and the American Heart Association Committee on Exercise, Cardiac Rehabilitation, and Prevention. *Circulation.* 2001;103(2):327–34.
19. Maron BJ, Thompson PD, Puffer JC, et al. Cardiovascular preparticipation screening of competitive athletes. A statement for health professionals from the Sudden Death Committee (clinical cardiology) and Congenital Cardiac Defects Committee (cardiovascular disease in the young), American Heart Association. *Circulation.* 1996;94(4):850–6.
20. Pate RR, Pratt M, Blair SN, et al. Physical activity and public health. A recommendation from the Centers for Disease Control and Prevention and the American College of Sports Medicine. *JAMA.* 1995;273(5):402–7.

21. Rodgers GP, Ayanian JZ, Balady G, et al. American College of Cardiology/American Heart Association Clinical Competence Statement on Stress Testing. A Report of the American College of Cardiology/American Heart Association/American College of Physicians–American Society of Internal Medicine Task Force on Clinical Competence. *Circulation*. 2000;102(14):1726–38.
22. Thompson PD, Buchner D, Pina IL, et al. Exercise and physical activity in the prevention and treatment of atherosclerotic cardiovascular disease: a statement from the Council on Clinical Cardiology (Subcommittee on Exercise, Rehabilitation, and Prevention) and the Council on Nutrition, Physical Activity, and Metabolism (Subcommittee on Physical Activity). *Circulation*. 2003;107(24): 3109–16.
23. U.S. Department of Health and Human Services. *Physical activity and health: a report of the Surgeon General*. Washington (DC): U.S. Department of Health and Human Services, Office of Surgeon General; 1996.
24. Wilson PW, D'Agostino RB, Levy D, Belanger AM, Silbershatz H, Kannel WB. Prediction of coronary heart disease using risk factor categories. *Circulation*. 1998;97(18):1837–47.

II

Exercise Testing

> > > > > > > > > > > > >

CHAPTER 3

Pre-Exercise Evaluations

This chapter contains information related to pre-exercise testing procedures and serves as a bridge between the risk stratification concepts presented in Chapter 2, the fitness assessment (Chapter 4), and/or clinical exercise testing concepts (Chapters 5 and 6). Although each of the chapter elements (e.g., medical history, physical examination, identification of exercise contraindications, informed-consent procedures) relate to health/fitness and clinical exercise settings, the lower-risk population typically encountered in the health and fitness setting generally justifies a less sophisticated approach to the pre-exercise test procedures. Therefore, abbreviated versions of the medical history and physical examination procedures described within this chapter are reasonable within the health and fitness setting.

The extent of medical evaluation necessary before exercise testing depends on the assessment of risk as determined from the procedures outlined in Chapters 1 and 2. For many persons, especially those with atherosclerotic cardiovascular disease (CVD) and other cardiovascular disorders, the exercise test and accompanying physical examination are critical to the development of a safe and effective exercise program. In today's healthcare environment, not all persons warrant extensive testing; however, it is important to work with healthcare providers in understanding the importance of the baseline exercise evaluation. This evaluation provides greater assurance of exercise safety by identifying residual myocardial ischemia, significant dysrhythmias, and the effect of certain medical therapies.

A comprehensive pre-exercise test evaluation in the clinical setting generally includes a medical history, physical examination, and laboratory tests. The goal of this chapter is not to be totally inclusive or to supplant more specific references on each subject, but rather to provide a concise set of guidelines for the pre-exercise test participant assessment.

MEDICAL HISTORY, PHYSICAL EXAMINATION, AND LABORATORY TESTS

The pre-exercise test medical history should be thorough and include both past and current information. Appropriate components of the medical history are presented in Box 3.1. A preliminary physical examination should be performed by a physician or other qualified personnel before exercise testing moderate- and

BOX 3.1 Components of the Medical History

Appropriate components of the medical history may include the following:

- Medical diagnosis. Cardiovascular disease, including myocardial infarction and other acute coronary syndromes; percutaneous coronary artery procedures, including angioplasty and coronary stent(s); coronary artery bypass surgery; valvular surgery(s) and valvular dysfunction (e.g., aortic stenosis/mitral valve disease); other cardiac surgeries, such as left ventricular aneurysmectomy and cardiac transplantation; pacemaker and/or implantable cardioverter defibrillator; presence of aortic aneurysm; ablation procedures for dysrhythmias; symptoms of angina pectoris; heart failure; peripheral vascular disease; hypertension; diabetes; metabolic syndrome; obesity; pulmonary disease, including asthma, emphysema, and bronchitis; cerebrovascular disease, including stroke and transient ischemic attacks; anemia and other blood dyscrasias (e.g., lupus erythematosus); phlebitis, deep vein thrombosis or emboli; cancer; pregnancy; osteoporosis; musculoskeletal disorders; emotional disorders; eating disorders.
- Previous physical examination findings. Murmurs, clicks, gallop rhythms, other abnormal heart sounds, and other unusual cardiac and vascular findings; abnormal pulmonary findings (e.g., wheezes, rales, crackles); plasma glucose, hemoglobin A1c, serum lipids and lipoproteins, or other significant laboratory abnormalities; high blood pressure; edema.
- History of symptoms. Discomfort (e.g., pressure, tingling, pain, heaviness, burning, tightness, squeezing, numbness) in the chest, jaw, neck, back, or arms; light-headedness, dizziness, or fainting; temporary loss of visual acuity or speech, transient unilateral numbness or weakness; shortness of breath; rapid heart beats or palpitations, especially if associated with physical activity, eating a large meal, emotional upset, or exposure to cold (or any combination of these activities).
- Recent illness, hospitalization, new medical diagnoses, or surgical procedures.
- Orthopedic problems, including arthritis, joint swelling, and any condition that would make ambulation or use of certain test modalities difficult.
- Medication use, drug allergies.
- Other habits, including caffeine, alcohol, tobacco, or recreational (illicit) drug use.
- Exercise history. Information on readiness for change and habitual level of activity: type of exercise, frequency, duration, and intensity.
- Work history with emphasis on current or expected physical demands, noting upper- and lower-extremity requirements.
- Family history of cardiac, pulmonary, or metabolic disease, stroke, or sudden death.

Adapted from Bickley LS. *Bates' Pocket Guide to Physical Examination and History Taking.* 4th ed. Philadelphia (PA): Lippincott Williams & Wilkins; 2003.

BOX 3.2	Components of the Pre-exercise Test Physical Examination

Appropriate components of the physical examination may include the following:

- Body weight; in many instances, determination of body mass index (BMI), waist girth, and/or body composition (percent body fat) is desirable
- Apical pulse rate and rhythm
- Resting blood pressure, seated, supine, and standing
- Auscultation of the lungs with specific attention to uniformity of breath sounds in all areas (absence of rales, wheezes, and other breathing sounds)
- Palpation of the cardiac apical impulse, point of maximal impulse (PMI)
- Auscultation of the heart with specific attention to murmurs, gallops, clicks, and rubs
- Palpation and auscultation of carotid, abdominal, and femoral arteries
- Evaluation of the abdomen for bowel sounds, masses, visceromegaly, and tenderness
- Palpation and inspection of lower extremities for edema and presence of arterial pulses
- Absence or presence of tendon xanthoma and skin xanthelasma
- Follow-up examination related to orthopedic or other medical conditions that would limit exercise testing
- Tests of neurologic function, including reflexes and cognition (as indicated)
- Inspection of the skin, especially of the lower extremities in known diabetes patients

Adapted from Bickley LS. *Bate's Pocket Guide to Physical Examination and History Taking.* 4th ed. Philadelphia (PA): Lippincott Williams & Wilkins; 2003.

high-risk subjects (see Fig. 2.4). Appropriate components of the physical examination specific to subsequent exercise testing are presented in Box 3.2. An expanded discussion and alternatives can be found in *ACSM'S Resource Manual for Guidelines for Exercise Testing and Prescription.*

Identification and risk stratification of persons with CVD and those at high risk of developing CVD are facilitated by review of previous test results, such as coronary angiography or exercise nuclear or echocardiography studies (6). Additional testing may include ambulatory electrocardiogram (ECG) (Holter) monitoring and pharmacologic stress testing to further clarify the need for and extent of intervention, assess response to treatment such as medical therapies and revascularization procedures, or determine the need for additional assessment. As outlined in Box 3.3, other laboratory tests may be warranted based on the level of risk and clinical status of the patient. These laboratory tests may include, but are

BOX 3.3	Recommended Laboratory Tests by Level of Risk and Clinical Assessment

Apparently healthy (low risk) or individuals at increased risk, but without known disease (moderate risk)

- Fasting serum total cholesterol, LDL cholesterol, HDL cholesterol, and triglycerides
- Fasting plasma glucose, especially in individuals ≥45 years old and younger individuals who are overweight (BMI ≥25 kg·m^{-2}) and have one or more of the following risk factors for type 2 diabetes: a first-degree relative with diabetes, member of a high-risk ethnic population (e.g., African American, Latino, Native American, Asian American, and Pacific Islander), delivered a baby weighing >9 lbs (4.08 kg) or history of gestational diabetes, hypertension (BP ≥140/90 mm Hg in adults), HDL cholesterol of <40 mg·dL^{-1} (<1.04 mmol·L^{-1}) and/or triglyceride level ≥150 mg·dL^{-1} (≥1.69 mmol·L^{-1}), previously identified impaired glucose tolerance or impaired fasting glucose (fasting glucose ≥100 mg·dL^{-1}; ≥5.55 mmol·L^{-1}), habitual physical inactivity, polycystic ovary disease, and history of vascular disease
- Thyroid function, as a screening evaluation especially if dyslipidemia is present

Patients with known or suspected cardiovascular disease (high risk)

- Preceding tests plus pertinent previous cardiovascular laboratory tests (e.g., resting 12-lead ECG, Holter monitoring, coronary angiography, radionuclide or echocardiography studies, previous exercise tests)
- Carotid ultrasound and other peripheral vascular studies
- Consider measures of Lp(a), high-sensitivity C-reactive protein, LDL particle size and number, and HDL subspecies (especially in young persons with a strong family history of premature CVD and in those persons without traditional coronary risk factors)
- Chest radiograph, if heart failure is present or suspected
- Comprehensive blood chemistry panel and complete blood count as indicated by history and physical examination (Table 3.3)

Patients with pulmonary disease

- Chest radiograph
- Pulmonary function tests (Table 3.4)
- Other specialized pulmonary studies (e.g., oximetry or blood gas analysis)

not limited to, serum chemistries, complete blood count, serum lipids and lipoproteins, fasting plasma glucose, and pulmonary function. Detailed guidelines for several chronic diseases can be found in other chapters within this text.

Although a detailed description of all the physical examination procedures listed in Box 3.2 and the recommended laboratory tests listed in Box 3.3 are beyond the scope of this text, additional basic information related to assessment of blood pressure, lipids and lipoproteins, other blood chemistries, and pulmonary function are provided in the following section. For more detailed descriptions of these assessments, the reader is referred to the work of Bickley (3).

BLOOD PRESSURE

Measurement of resting blood pressure (BP) is an integral component of the pre-exercise test evaluation. Subsequent decisions should be based on the average of two or more properly measured, seated BP readings recorded during each of two or more office visits (11,14). Specific techniques for measuring BP are critical to accuracy and detection of high BP and are presented in Box 3.4. In addition to high BP readings, unusually low readings also should be evaluated for clinical significance. The Seventh Report of the Joint National Committee on Prevention, Detection, Evaluation, and Treatment of High Blood Pressure (JNC7) provides guidelines for

---

BOX 3.4   Procedures for Assessment of Resting Blood Pressure

1. Patients should be seated quietly for at least 5 minutes in a chair with back support (rather than on an examination table) with their feet on the floor and their arm supported at heart level. Patients should refrain from smoking cigarettes or ingesting caffeine during the 30 minutes preceding the measurement.
2. Measuring supine and standing values may be indicated under special circumstances.
3. Wrap cuff firmly around upper arm at heart level; align cuff with brachial artery.
4. The appropriate cuff size must be used to ensure accurate measurement. The bladder within the cuff should encircle at least 80% of the upper arm. Many adults require a large adult cuff.
5. Place stethoscope bell below the antecubital space over the brachial artery.
6. Quickly inflate cuff pressure to 20 mm Hg above first Korotkoff sound.
7. Slowly release pressure at rate equal to 2 to 5 mm Hg per second.
8. Systolic BP is the point at which the first of two or more Korotkoff sounds is heard (phase 1) and diastolic BP is the point before the disappearance of Korotkoff sounds (phase 5).
9. At least two measurements should be made (minimum of 1 minute apart).
10. Provide to patients, verbally and in writing, their specific BP numbers and BP goals.

Modified from National High Blood Pressure Education Program. *The Seventh Report of the Joint National Committee on Prevention, Detection, Evaluation, and Treatment of High Blood Pressure (JNC7).* Washington, DC: 2003; 03-5233. For additional, more detailed recommendations, see Pickering TG, Hall JE, Appel LJ, et al. Recommendations for blood pressure measurement in humans and experimental animals. *Hypertension.* 2005;45:142–61.

TABLE 3.1. CLASSIFICATION AND MANAGEMENT OF BLOOD PRESSURE FOR ADULTS[a]

| | | | | INITIAL DRUG THERAPY | |
BP CLASSI-FICATION	SBP mm Hg	DBP mm Hg	LIFESTYLE MODIFICA-TION	WITHOUT COMPELLING INDICATION	WITH COMPELLING INDICATIONS
Normal	<120	And <80	Encourage		
Prehypertension	120–139	Or 80–89	Yes	No antihypertensive drug indicated	Drug(s) for compelling indications[b]
Stage 1 hypertension	140–159	Or 90–99	Yes	Antihypertensive drug(s) indicated	Drug(s) for compelling indications[b] Other antihyper-tensive drugs, as needed
Stage 2 hypertension	≥160	Or ≥100	Yes	Antihypertensive drug(s) indicated Two-drug combination for most[c]	

BP, blood pressure; DBP, diastolic blood pressure; SBP, systolic blood pressure.

Adapted from National High Blood Pressure Education Program. *The Seventh Report of the Joint National Committee on Prevention, Detection, Evaluation, and Treatment of High Blood Pressure (JNC7).* 2003; 3:5233.

[a]Treatment determined by highest BP category.

[b]Compelling indications include heart failure, post–myocardial infarction, high coronary heart disease risk, diabetes, chronic kidney disease, and recurrent stroke prevention. Treat patients with chronic kidney disease or diabetes to BP goal of <130/80 mm Hg.

[c]Initial combined therapy should be used cautiously in those at risk for orthostatic hypotension.

Adapted from National High Blood Pressure Education Program. *The Seventh Report of the Joint National Committee on Prevention, Detection, Evaluation, and Treatment of High Blood Pressure (JNC7).* 2003;3:5233.

hypertension detection and management (11). Table 3.1 summarizes the JNC7 recommendations for the classification and management of BP for adults.

The relationship between BP and risk for cardiovascular events is continuous, consistent, and independent of other risk factors. For individuals 40 to 70 years of age, each increment of 20 mm Hg in systolic BP or 10 mm Hg in diastolic BP doubles the risk of cardiovascular disease across the entire BP range from 115/75 to 185/115 mm Hg. According to JNC7, persons with a systolic BP of 120 to 139 mm Hg or a diastolic BP of 80 to 89 mm Hg should be considered as *prehypertensive* and require health-promoting lifestyle modifications to prevent cardiovascular disease (2,11).

Lifestyle modification—including physical activity, weight reduction (if needed), a DASH eating plan (i.e., a diet rich in fruits, vegetables, and low-fat dairy products with a reduced content of saturated and total fat), dietary sodium reduction (no more than 100 mmol or 2.4 g sodium/day), and moderation of alcohol consumption—remains the cornerstone of antihypertensive therapy (2,11). However, JNC7 emphasizes that most patients with hypertension who require drug therapy in addition to lifestyle modification require two or more antihypertensive medications to achieve the goal BP (i.e., <140/90 mm Hg, or <130/80 mm Hg for patients with diabetes or chronic kidney disease) (11).

LIPIDS AND LIPOPROTEINS

The Third Report of the Expert Panel on Detection, Evaluation, and Treatment of High Blood Cholesterol in Adults (Adult Treatment Panel III, or ATP III) outlines the National Cholesterol Education Program's (NCEP's) recommendations for cholesterol testing and management (Table 3.2) (10). ATP III and subsequent updates by the National Heart, Lung, and Blood Institute, American Heart Association, and American College of Cardiology identify low-density lipoprotein (LDL) cholesterol as the primary target for cholesterol-lowering therapy (8,10,15). This designation is based on a wide variety of evidence indicating that elevated LDL cholesterol is a

TABLE 3.2. ATP III CLASSIFICATION OF LDL, TOTAL, AND HDL CHOLESTEROL (mg · dL^{-1})

LDL CHOLESTEROL	
<100^a	Optimal
100–129	Near optimal/above optimal
130–159	Borderline high
160–189	High
≥190	Very high

TOTAL CHOLESTEROL	
<200	Desirable
200–239	Borderline high
≥240	High

HDL CHOLESTEROL	
<40	Low
≥60	High

TRIGLYCERIDES	
<150	Normal
150–199	Borderline high
200–499	High
≥500	Very high

LDL, low-density lipoprotein; HDL, high-density lipoprotein.

^{a}According to the American Heart Association/American College of Cardiology 2006 update (endorsed by the National Heart, Lung, and Blood Institute), it is reasonable to treat LDL cholesterol to <70 mg · dL^{-1} (<1.81 mmol · L^{-1}) in patients with coronary and other atherosclerotic vascular disease (15).

NOTE: To convert LDL cholesterol, total cholesterol, and HDL cholesterol from mg · dL^{-1} to mmol · L^{-1}, multiply by 0.0259. To convert triglycerides from mg · dL^{-1} to mmol · L^{-1}, multiply by 0.0113.

Adapted from National Cholesterol Education Program. *Third Report of the National Cholesterol Education Program (NCEP) Expert Panel on Detection, Evaluation, and Treatment of High Blood Cholesterol in Adults (Adult Treatment Panel III).* Washington, DC:2002. NIH Publication No. 02–5215.

powerful risk factor for CVD and that lowering of LDL cholesterol results in a striking reduction in the incidence of CVD. Table 3.2 summarizes the ATP III classifications of LDL, total, and high-density lipoprotein (HDL) cholesterol and triglycerides.

According to ATP III, a low HDL cholesterol level is strongly and inversely associated with the risk for CVD. Clinical trials provide suggestive evidence that raising HDL cholesterol levels reduces the risk for CVD. However, it is now known that the serum HDL cholesterol level does not assess HDL's functional properties and it remains uncertain whether raising HDL cholesterol levels per se, independent of other changes in lipid and/or nonlipid risk factors, always reduces the risk for CVD. In view of this, ATP III does not identify a specific HDL cholesterol goal level to reach with therapy. Rather, nondrug and drug therapies that raise HDL cholesterol that also are part of the management of other lipid and nonlipid risk factors are encouraged by ATP III.

There is growing evidence for a strong association between elevated triglyceride levels and CVD risk. Recent studies suggest that some species of triglyceride-rich lipoproteins, notably, cholesterol-enriched remnant lipoproteins, promote atherosclerosis and predispose to CVD. Because these remnant lipoproteins appear to have atherogenic potential similar to that of LDL cholesterol, ATP III recommends that they be added to LDL cholesterol to become a secondary target of therapy for persons with elevated triglycerides. To accomplish this, non-HDL cholesterol is calculated by subtracting HDL cholesterol from the total cholesterol level.

The metabolic syndrome is characterized by a constellation of metabolic risk factors in one individual. Abdominal obesity, atherogenic dyslipidemia (i.e., elevated triglycerides, small LDL cholesterol particles, and reduced HDL cholesterol), elevated blood pressure, insulin resistance, prothrombotic state, and proinflammatory state generally are accepted as being characteristic of the metabolic syndrome. The root causes of the metabolic syndrome are overweight and obesity, physical inactivity, and genetic factors. Because the metabolic syndrome has emerged as an important contributor to CVD, ATP III places emphasis on the metabolic syndrome as a risk enhancer.

ATP III designates hypertension, cigarette smoking, diabetes, overweight and obesity, physical inactivity, and an atherogenic diet as modifiable nonlipid risk factors, whereas age, male sex, and family history of premature CVD are nonmodifiable nonlipid risk factors for CVD. Triglycerides, lipoprotein remnants, lipoprotein (a), small LDL particles, HDL subspecies, apolipoproteins B and A-1, and total cholesterol-to-HDL cholesterol ratio are designated by ATP III as emerging lipid risk factors. Thrombogenic and hemostatic factors, inflammatory markers (e.g., high-sensitivity C-reactive protein), impaired fasting glucose, and homocysteine are designated by ATP III as emerging nonlipid risk factors. Regarding the latter, recent studies suggest that homocysteine-lowering therapy does not result in a reduction in CVD risk.

The guiding principle of ATP III and subsequent updates by the National Heart, Lung, and Blood Institute, American Heart Association, and American College of Cardiology is that the intensity of LDL-lowering therapy should be adjusted to the individual's absolute risk for CVD (8,10,15). The ATP III treatment guidelines and subsequent updates by the National Heart, Lung, and Blood Institute, American Heart Association, and American College of Cardiology are summarized in the ACSM Resource Manual.

BLOOD PROFILE ANALYSES

Multiple analyses of blood profiles are commonly evaluated in clinical exercise programs. Such profiles may provide useful information about an individual's overall health status and ability to exercise and may help to explain certain ECG abnormalities. Because of varied methods of assaying blood samples, some caution is advised when comparing blood chemistries from different laboratories. Table 3.3 gives normal ranges for selected blood chemistries, derived from a variety of sources. For many patients with CVD, medications for dyslipidemia and hypertension are common. Many of these medications act in the liver to lower blood

TABLE 3.3. TYPICAL RANGES OF NORMAL VALUES FOR SELECTED BLOOD VARIABLES IN ADULTS[a]

VARIABLE	MEN	NEUTRAL	WOMEN
Hemoglobin $(g \cdot dL^{-1})$	13.5–17.5		11.5–15.5
Hematocrit (%)	40–52		36–48
Red cell count $(\times 10^{12}/L)$	4.5–6.5		3.9–5.6
Mean cell hemoglobin concentration (MCHC)		30–35 $(g \cdot dL^{-1})$	
White blood cell count		4–11 $(\times 10^9/L)$	
Platelet count		150–450 $(\times 10^9/L)$	
Fasting glucose[b]		60–99 $mg \cdot dL^{-1}$	
Blood urea nitrogen (BUN)		4–24 $mg \cdot dL^{-1}$	
Creatinine		0.3–1.4 $mg \cdot dL^{-1}$	
BUN/creatinine ratio		7–27	
Uric acid $(mg \cdot dL^{-1})$	4.0–8.9	2.3–7.8	
Sodium		135–150 $mEq \cdot dL^{-1}$	
Potassium		3.5–5.5 $mEq \cdot dL^{-1}$	
Chloride		98–110 $mEq \cdot dL^{-1}$	
Osmolality		278–302 mOsm/kg	
Calcium		8.5–10.5 $mg \cdot dL^{-1}$	
Calcium, ion		4.0–5.2 $mg \cdot dL^{-1}$	
Phosphorus		2.5–4.5 $mg \cdot dL^{-1}$	
Protein, total		6.0–8.5 $g \cdot dL^{-1}$	
Albumin		3.0–5.5 $g \cdot dL^{-1}$	
Globulin		2.0–4.0 $g \cdot dL^{-1}$	
A/G ratio		1.0–2.2	
Iron, total $(mcg \cdot dL^{-1})$	40–190		35–180
Liver Function Tests			
Bilirubin		<1.5 $mg \cdot dL^{-1}$	
SGOT (AST)	8–46 $U \cdot L^{-1}$		7–34 $U \cdot L^{-1}$
SGPT (ALT)	7–46 $U \cdot L^{-1}$		4–35 $U \cdot L^{-1}$

SGOT, serum glutamic-oxaloacetic transaminase; AST, aspartate transaminase (formerly SGOT); SGPT, serum glutamic-pyruvic transaminase; ALT, alanine transaminase (formerly SGPT).

[a]Certain variables must be interpreted in relation to the normal range of the issuing laboratory.

[b]Fasting blood glucose 100–125 $mg \cdot dL^{-1}$ is considered impaired fasting glucose or prediabetes.

NOTE: For a complete list of Système International (SI) conversion factors, please see http://jama.ama-assn.org/content/vol295/issue1/images/data/103/DC6/ JAMA_auinst_si.dtl cholesterol and in the kidneys to lower blood pressure. One should pay particular attention to liver function tests such as alanine transaminase (ALT), aspartate transaminase (AST), and bilirubin as well as to renal (kidney) function tests such as creatinine, glomerular filtration rate, blood urea nitrogen (BUN), and BUN/creatinine ratio in patients on such medications. Indication of volume depletion and potassium abnormalities can be seen in the sodium and potassium measurements. These tests should be applied judiciously and not used as finite ranges of normal.

PULMONARY FUNCTION

Pulmonary function testing with spirometry is recommended for all smokers older than age 45 years and in any person presenting with dyspnea (shortness of breath), chronic cough, wheezing, or excessive mucus production (5). Spirometry is a simple and noninvasive test that can be performed easily. Indications for spirometry are listed in Table 3.4. When performing spirometry, standards for the performance of the test should be followed (9).

Although many measurements can be made from a spirometric test, the most commonly used include the forced vital capacity (FVC), the forced expiratory volume in one second (FEV$_1$), and the FEV$_1$/FVC ratio. Results from these measurements can help to identify the presence of restrictive or obstructive respiratory abnormalities, sometimes before symptoms or signs of disease are present. The FEV$_1$/FVC is diminished with obstructive airway diseases [e.g., asthma, chronic bronchitis, emphysema, and chronic obstructive pulmonary disease (COPD)], but remains normal with restrictive disorders (e.g., kyphoscoliosis, neuromuscular disease, pulmonary fibrosis, and other interstitial lung diseases).

The Global Initiative for Chronic Obstructive Lung Disease has classified the presence and severity of COPD as seen in Table 3.4 (12). The term COPD can be used when chronic bronchitis, emphysema, or both are present, and the spirometry documents an obstructive defect. A different approach for classifying the severity of obstructive and restrictive defects has been taken by the American Thoracic Society (ATS) and European Respiratory Society (ERS) Task Force on Standardization of Lung Function Testing, as presented in Table 3.4 (13). This ATS/ERS Task Force prefers to use the largest available vital capacity (VC), whether it is obtained on inspiration (IVC), slow expiration (SVC), or forced expiration (FVC). An obstructive defect is defined by a reduced FEV$_1$/VC ratio below the fifth percentile of the predicted value. In contrast with using a fixed value for FEV$_1$/VC or FEV$_1$/FVC of 0.7 as the dividing line between normal and abnormal, the use of the fifth percentile of the predicted value as the lower limit of normal does not lead to an overestimation of the presence of an obstructive defect in older people. A restrictive defect is characterized by a reduction in the total lung capacity (TLC), as measured on a lung volume study, below the fifth percentile of the predicted value, and a normal FEV$_1$/VC.

The spirometric classification of lung disease has been useful in predicting health status, use of health resources, and mortality. Abnormal spirometry can also be indicative of an increased risk for lung cancer, heart attack, and stroke and can be used to identify patients in which interventions, such as smoking cessation and use of pharmacologic agents, would be most beneficial.

TABLE 3.4. INDICATIONS FOR SPIROMETRY

A. INDICATIONS FOR SPIROMETRY

Diagnosis
To evaluate symptoms, signs, or abnormal laboratory tests
To measure the effect of disease on pulmonary function
To screen individuals at risk of having pulmonary disease
To assess preoperative risk
To assess prognosis
To assess health status before beginning strenuous physical activity programs

Monitoring
To assess therapeutic intervention
To describe the course of diseases that affect lung function
To monitor people exposed to injurious agents
To monitor for adverse reactions to drugs with known pulmonary toxicity

Disability/Impairment Evaluations
To assess patients as part of a rehabilitation program
To assess risks as part of an insurance evaluation
To assess individuals for legal reasons

Public Health
Epidemiologic surveys
Derivation of reference equations
Clinical research

B. THE GLOBAL INITIATIVE FOR CHRONIC OBSTRUCTIVE LUNG DISEASE SPIROMETRIC CLASSIFICATION OF COPD SEVERITY BASED ON POSTBRONCHODILATOR FEV_1

Stage I	Mild	FEV_1/FVC <0.70
		FEV_1 ≥80% of predicted
Stage II	Moderate	FEV_1/FVC <0.70
		50% ≤FEV_1 <80% predicted
Stage III	Severe	FEV_1/FVC <0.70
		30% ≤FEV_1 <50% predicted
Stage IV	Very severe	FEV_1/FVC <0.70
		FEV_1 <30% predicted or FEV_1 <50% predicted plus chronic respiratory failure

C. THE AMERICAN THORACIC SOCIETY AND EUROPEAN RESPIRATORY SOCIETY CLASSIFICATION OF SEVERITY OF ANY SPIROMETRIC ABNORMALITY BASED ON FEV_1

Degree of Severity	FEV_1 % Predicted
Mild	Less than the LLN but ≥70
Moderate	60–69
Moderately severe	50–59
Severe	35–49
Very severe	< 35

COPD, chronic obstructive pulmonary disease; FEV_1, forced expiratory volume in one second; FVC, forced vital capacity; respiratory failure, arterial partial pressure of oxygen (PaO_2) <8.0 kPa (60 mm Hg) with or without arterial partial pressure of CO_2 (PaO_2) >6.7 kPa (50 mm Hg) while breathing air at sea level; LLN, lower limit of normal.

Modified from Pauwels RA, Buist AS, Calverly PM, et al. Global strategy for the diagnosis, management, and prevention of chronic obstructive pulmonary disease. NHLBI/WHO Global Initiative for Chronic Obstructive Lung Disease (GOLD) Workshop summary. *Am J Respir Crit Care Med*. 2001;163:1256–76. Available from: http//www.goldcopd.com (last major revision, November 2006); Pellegrino R, Viegi G, Enright P, et al. Interpretive strategies for lung function tests. ATS/ERS Task Force: standardisation of lung function testing. *Eur Respir J*. 2005;26:948–68.

The determination of the maximal voluntary ventilation (MVV) should also be obtained during routine spirometric testing (9,13). This measurement can be used to estimate breathing reserve during maximal exercise. The MVV should be measured rather than estimated by multiplying the FEV_1 by a constant value, as is often done in practice (13).

CONTRAINDICATIONS TO EXERCISE TESTING

For certain individuals the risks of exercise testing outweigh the potential benefits. For these patients it is important to carefully assess risk versus benefit when deciding whether the exercise test should be performed. Box 3.5 outlines both absolute and relative contraindications to exercise testing (7). Performing the pre-exercise test evaluation and the careful review of prior medical history, as described earlier in this chapter, helps identify potential contraindications and increases the safety of the exercise test. Patients with absolute contraindications should not perform exercise tests until such conditions are stabilized or adequately treated. Patients with relative contraindications may be tested only after careful evaluation of the risk/benefit ratio. However, it should be emphasized that contraindications might not apply in certain specific clinical situations, such as soon after acute myocardial infarction, revascularization procedure, or bypass surgery or to determine the need for, or benefit of, drug therapy. Finally, conditions exist that preclude reliable diagnostic ECG information from exercise testing (e.g., left bundle-branch block, digitalis therapy). The exercise test may still provide useful information on exercise capacity, dysrhythmias, and hemodynamic responses to exercise. In these conditions, additional evaluative techniques such as respiratory gas exchange analyses, echocardiography or nuclear imaging can be added to the exercise test to improve sensitivity, specificity, and diagnostic capabilities.

Emergency departments may perform an exercise test on low-risk patients who present with chest pain (i.e., within 4 to 8 hours) to rule out myocardial infarction (4,7). Generally, these patients include those who are no longer symptomatic and who have unremarkable ECGs and no change in serial cardiac enzymes. However, exercise testing in this setting should be performed only as part of a carefully constructed patient management protocol and only after patients have been screened for high-risk features or other indicators for hospital admission. Table 3.5 is a quick reference source for the time-course of changes in serum cardiac biomarkers for myocardial damage or necrosis (1).

INFORMED CONSENT

Obtaining adequate informed consent from participants before exercise testing and participation in an exercise program is an important ethical and legal consideration. Although the content and extent of consent forms may vary, enough information must be present in the informed-consent process to ensure that the participant knows and understands the purposes and risks associated with the

BOX 3.5   Contraindications to Exercise Testing

Absolute
- A recent significant change in the resting ECG suggesting significant ischemia, recent myocardial infarction (within 2 days), or other acute cardiac event
- Unstable angina
- Uncontrolled cardiac dysrhythmias causing symptoms or hemodynamic compromise
- Symptomatic severe aortic stenosis
- Uncontrolled symptomatic heart failure
- Acute pulmonary embolus or pulmonary infarction
- Acute myocarditis or pericarditis
- Suspected or known dissecting aneurysm
- Acute systemic infection, accompanied by fever, body aches, or swollen lymph glands

Relative[a]
- Left main coronary stenosis
- Moderate stenotic valvular heart disease
- Electrolyte abnormalities (e.g., hypokalemia, hypomagnesemia)
- Severe arterial hypertension (i.e., systolic BP of >200 mm Hg and/or a diastolic BP of >110 mm Hg) at rest
- Tachydysrhythmia or bradydysrhythmia
- Hypertrophic cardiomyopathy and other forms of outflow tract obstruction
- Neuromuscular, musculoskeletal, or rheumatoid disorders that are exacerbated by exercise
- High-degree atrioventricular block
- Ventricular aneurysm
- Uncontrolled metabolic disease (e.g., diabetes, thyrotoxicosis, or myxedema)
- Chronic infectious disease (e.g., mononucleosis, hepatitis, AIDS)
- Mental or physical impairment leading to inability to exercise adequately

[a]Relative contraindications can be superseded if benefits outweigh risks of exercise. In some instances, these individuals can be exercised with caution and/or using low-level end points, especially if they are asymptomatic at rest.

Modified from Gibbons RJ, Balady GJ, Bricker J, et al. ACC/AHA 2002 guideline update for exercise testing: a report of the American College of Cardiology/American Heart Association Task Force on Practice Guidelines (Committee on Exercise Testing) [Internet]. 2002. cited 2007 June 15]. Available from: www.acc.org/clinical/guidelines/exercise/dirIndex.htm

TABLE 3.5. TIME-COURSE OF CHANGES IN SERUM CARDIAC BIOMARKERS FOR MYOCARDIAL DAMAGE

BIOMARKER	RANGE OF TIMES TO INITIAL ELEVATION	MEAN TIME TO PEAK ELEVATIONS (NON-REPERFUSED)	TIME TO RETURN TO NORMAL RANGE
CK-MB	3–12 h	24 h	48–72 h
cTnI	3–12 h	24 h	5–10 d
cTnT	3–12 h	12 h–2 d	5–14 d

CK-MB, MB isoenzyme of creatine kinase; cTnI, cardiac troponin I; cTnT, cardiac troponin T.

NOTE: Standard reference ranges are not available for the above cardiac biomarkers. The following are biochemical indicators for detecting myocardial damage: (a) maximal concentration of cTnI or cTnT exceeding the decision limit (ninety-ninth percentile of the values for a reference control group) on at least one occasion during the first 24 hours after the index clinical event; (b) maximal value of CK-MB exceeding the ninety-ninth percentile of the values for a reference control group on two successive samples, or maximal value exceeding twice the upper limit of normal for the specific institution on one occasion during the first hours after the index clinical event. In the absence of availability of a troponin or CK-MB assay, total CK (greater than two times the upper reference limit) or the B fraction of CK may be employed, but these last two biomarkers are considerably less satisfactory than CK-MB.

Adapted from Antman EM, Anbe DT, Armstrong PW, et al. ACC/AHA guidelines for the management of patients with ST-elevation myocardial infarction. *Circulation.* 2004;110:588–636.

test or exercise program. The consent form should be verbally explained and include a statement indicating that the patient has been given an opportunity to ask questions about the procedure and has sufficient information to give informed consent. Note specific questions from the participant on the form along with the responses provided. The consent form must indicate that the participant is free to withdraw from the procedure at any time. If the participant is a minor, a legal guardian or parent must sign the consent form. It is advisable to check with authoritative bodies (e.g., hospital risk management, institutional review boards, facility legal counsel) to determine what is appropriate for an acceptable informed-consent process. Also, all reasonable efforts must be made to protect the privacy of the patient's health information (e.g., medical history, test results) as described in the Health Insurance Portability and Accountability Act (HIPAA) of 1996. A sample consent form for exercise testing is provided in Figure 3.1. No sample form should be adopted for a specific program unless approved by local legal counsel.

When the exercise test is for purposes other than diagnosis or prescription (i.e., for experimental purposes), this should be indicated during the consent process and reflected on the *Informed Consent Form,* and applicable policies for the testing of human subjects must be implemented. A copy of the Policy on Human Subjects for Research is periodically published in ACSM's journal, *Medicine and Science in Sports and Exercise.*

Because most consent forms include a statement that emergency procedures and equipment are available, the program must ensure that available personnel are appropriately trained and authorized to carry out emergency procedures that use such equipment. Written emergency policies and procedures should be in place, and emergency drills should be practiced at least once every 3 months or

Informed Consent for an Exercise Test

1. Purpose and Explanation of the Test

You will perform an exercise test on a cycle ergometer or a motor-driven treadmill. The exercise intensity will begin at a low level and will be advanced in stages depending on your fitness level. We may stop the test at any time because of signs of fatigue or changes in your heart rate, ECG, or blood pressure, or symptoms you may experience. It is important for you to realize that you may stop when you wish because of feelings of fatigue or any other discomfort.

2. Attendant Risks and Discomforts

There exists the possibility of certain changes occurring during the test. These include abnormal blood pressure; fainting; irregular, fast, or slow heart rhythm; and, in rare instances, heart attack, stroke, or death. Every effort will be made to minimize these risks by evaluation of preliminary information relating to your health and fitness and by careful observations during testing. Emergency equipment and trained personnel are available to deal with unusual situations that may arise.

3. Responsibilities of the Participant

Information you possess about your health status or previous experiences of heart-related symptoms (e.g. shortness of breath with low-level activity, pain, pressure, tightness, heaviness in the chest, neck, jaw, back, and/or arms) with physical effort may affect the safety of your exercise test. Your prompt reporting of these and any other unusual feelings with effort during the exercise test itself is very important. You are responsible for fully disclosing your medical history, as well as symptoms that may occur during the test. You are also expected to report all medications (including nonprescription) taken recently and, in particular, those taken today, to the testing staff.

4. Benefits to Be Expected

The results obtained from the exercise test may assist in the diagnosis of your illness, in evaluating the effect of your medications or in evaluating what type of physical activities you might do with low risk.

5. Inquiries

Any questions about the procedures used in the exercise test or the results of your test are encouraged. If you have any concerns or questions, please ask us for further explanations.

6. Use of Medical records

The information that is obtained during exercise testing will be treated as privileged and confidential as described in the Health Insurance Portability and Accountability Act of 1996. It is not to be released or revealed to any person except your referring physician without your written consent. However, the information obtained may be used for statistical analysis or scientific purposes with your right to privacy retained.

FIGURE 3.1. Sample of informed consent form for a symptom-limited exercise test.

7. Freedom of Consent

I hereby consent to voluntarily engage in an exercise test to determine my exercise capacity and state of cardiovascular health. My permission to perform this exercise test is given voluntarily. I understand the I am free to stop the test at any point if I so desire.

I have read this form, and I understand the test procedures that I will perform and the attendant risks and discomforts. Knowing these risks and discomforts, and having had an opportunity to ask questions that have been answered to my satisfaction, I consent to participate in this test.

_____   _____
Date   Signature of Patient

_____   _____
Date   Signature of Witness

_____   _____
Date   Signature of Physician or Authorized Delegate

FIGURE 3.1. (Continued)

more often when there is a change in staff. See Appendix B for more information on emergency management.

PARTICIPANT INSTRUCTIONS

Explicit instructions for participants before exercise testing increase test validity and data accuracy. Whenever possible, written instructions along with a description of the evaluation should be provided well in advance of the appointment so the client or patient can prepare adequately. The following points should be considered for inclusion in such preliminary instructions; however, specific instructions vary with test type and purpose.

- Participants should refrain from ingesting food, alcohol, or caffeine or using tobacco products within 3 hours of testing.
- Participants should be rested for the assessment, avoiding significant exertion or exercise on the day of the assessment.
- Clothing should permit freedom of movement and include walking or running shoes. Women should bring a loose-fitting, short-sleeved blouse that buttons down the front and should avoid restrictive undergarments.
- If the evaluation is on an outpatient basis, participants should be made aware that the evaluation may be fatiguing and that they may wish to have someone accompany them to the assessment to drive home afterward.
- If the test is for diagnostic purposes, it may be helpful for patients to discontinue prescribed cardiovascular medications, but only with physician approval. Currently prescribed antianginal agents alter the hemodynamic

response to exercise and significantly reduce the sensitivity of ECG changes for ischemia. Patients taking intermediate- or high-dose β-blocking agents may be asked to taper their medication over a two- to four-day period to minimize hyperadrenergic withdrawal responses.

- If the test is for functional or exercise prescription purposes, *patients should continue their medication regimen* on their usual schedule so that the exercise responses will be consistent with responses expected during exercise training.
- Participants should bring a list of their medications, including dosage and frequency of administration, to the assessment and should report the last actual dose taken. As an alternative, participants may wish to bring their medications with them for the exercise testing staff to record.
- Drink ample fluids over the 24-hour period preceding the test to ensure normal hydration before testing.

REFERENCES

1. Antman EM, Anbe DT, Armstrong PW, et al. ACC/AHA guidelines for the management of patients with ST-elevation myocardial infarction. *Circulation.* 2004;110:282–92.
2. Appel LJ, Brands MW, Daniels SR, et al. Dietary approaches to prevent and treat hypertension: a scientific statement from the American Heart Association. *Circulation.* 2006;47:296–308.
3. Bickley LS. Bate's pocket guide to physical examination and history taking. 4th ed. Philadelphia (PA): Lippincott Williams & Wilkins; 2003.
4. Braunwald E, Antman EM, Beasley JW, et al. ACC/AHA 2002 guideline update for the management of patients with unstable angina and non-ST-segment elevation myocardial infarction: a report of the American College of Cardiology/American Heart Association task force on practice guidelines [Internet]. 2002 [cited 2007 June 15]. Available from: http://www.acc.org/clinical/guidelines/unstable/unstable.pdf
5. Ferguson GT, Enright PL, Buist AS, et al. Office spirometry for lung health assessment in adults: a consensus statement from the National Lung Health Education Program. *Chest.* 2000;117: 1146–61.
6. Fuster V, Pearson TA. 27th Bethesda Conference: Matching the intensity of risk factor management with the hazard for coronary disease events. September 14–15, 1995. *J Am Coll Cardiol.* 1996;27:957–1047.
7. Gibbons RJ, Balady GJ, Bricker JT, et al. ACC/AHA 2002 Guideline Update for Exercise Testing; a report of the American College of Cardiology/American Heart Association Task Force on Practice Guidelines; Committee on Exercise Testing, 2002. *Circulation.* 2002;106(14):1883–92.
8. Grundy SM, Cleeman JI, Bairey Merz NC, et al. Implications of recent clinical trials for the National Cholesterol Education Program Adult Treatment Panel III Guidelines. *J Am Coll Cardiol.* 2004;44:720–32.
9. Miller MR, Hankinson J, Brusasco V, et al. Standardisation of spirometry. ATS/ERS Task Force: standardisation of lung function testing. *Eur Respir J.* 2005;26:319–38.
10. National Cholesterol Education Program. *Third Report of the National Cholesterol Education Program (NCEP) Expert Panel on Detection, Evaluation, and Treatment of High Blood Cholesterol in Adults (Adult Treatment Panel III).* Washington, DC:2002. NIH Publication No. 02-5215.
11. National High Blood Pressure Education Program. *The Seventh Report of the Joint National Committee on Prevention, Detection, Evaluation, and Treatment of High Blood Pressure (JNC7).* Washington, DC:2003; 03-5233.
12. Pauwels RA, Buist AS, Calverly PM, et al. Global strategy for the diagnosis, management, and prevention of chronic obstructive pulmonary disease. NHLBI/WHO Global Initiative for Chronic Obstructive Lung Disease (GOLD) Workshop summary. *Am J Respir Crit Care Med* [Internet]. 2001 [cited 2007 June 15];163:1256–76. Available from: http//www.goldcopd.com (last major revision, November 2006).

13. Pellegrino R, Viegi G, Enright P, et al. Interpretive strategies for lung function tests. ATS/ERS Task Force: standardisation of lung function testing. *Eur Respir J.* 2005;26:948–68.
14. Pickering TG, Hall JE, Appel LJ, et al. Recommendations for blood pressure measurement in humans and experimental animals: Part 1: Blood pressure measurement in humans. *Hypertension.* 2005;45:142–61.
15. Smith Jr SC, Allen J, Blair SN, et al. AHA/ACC Guidelines. AHA/ACC guidelines for secondary prevention for patients with coronary and other atherosclerotic vascular disease: 2006 update. *Circulation.* 2006;113:2363–72.

4

Health-Related Physical Fitness Testing and Interpretation

As evidence rapidly continues to evolve regarding the numerous health benefits of physical activity and exercise, the focus on health-related physical fitness and physiologic fitness appears to have superseded that of skill-related physical fitness (13). The health-related components of physical fitness have a strong relationship with good health, are characterized by an ability to perform daily activities with vigor, and demonstrate the traits and capacities associated with low risk of premature development of the hypokinetic diseases (e.g., those associated with physical inactivity) (56). Both health-related and physiologic fitness measures are closely allied with disease prevention and health promotion and can be modified through regular physical activity and exercise. A fundamental goal of primary and secondary intervention programs is promotion of health; therefore, such programs should focus on enhancement of health-related and physiologic components of physical fitness.

PURPOSES OF HEALTH-RELATED FITNESS TESTING

Measurement of physical fitness is a common and appropriate practice in preventive and rehabilitative exercise programs. The purposes of health-related fitness testing in such programs include the following:

- Educating participants about their present health-related fitness status relative to health-related standards and age- and sex-matched norms
- Providing data that are helpful in development of exercise prescriptions to address all fitness components
- Collecting baseline and follow-up data that allow evaluation of progress by exercise program participants
- Motivating participants by establishing reasonable and attainable fitness goals
- Stratifying cardiovascular risk

BASIC PRINCIPLES AND GUIDELINES

The information obtained from health-related physical fitness testing, in combination with the individual's health and medical information, is used by the health and fitness professional to help an individual achieve specific fitness goals. An ideal health-related physical fitness test is reliable, valid, relatively inexpensive, and easy to administer. The test should yield results that are indicative of the current state of fitness, reflect change from physical activity or exercise intervention, and be directly comparable to normative data.

PRETEST INSTRUCTIONS

All pretest instructions should be provided and adhered to before arrival at the testing facility. Certain steps should be taken to ensure client safety and comfort before administering a health-related fitness test. A minimal recommendation is that individuals complete a questionnaire such as the Physical Activity Readiness Questionnaire (PAR-Q; see Fig. 2.1) or the ACSM/AHA form (see Fig. 2.2). A listing of preliminary instructions for all clients can be found in Chapter 3 under Participant Instructions, page 57. These instructions may be modified to meet specific needs and circumstances.

TEST ORDER

The following should be accomplished before the participant arrives at the test site:

- Assure all forms, score sheets, tables, graphs, and other testing documents are organized and available for the test's administration
- Calibrate all equipment a minimum of once each month to ensure accuracy (e.g., metronome, cycle ergometer, treadmill, sphygmomanometer, skinfold calipers)
- Organize equipment so that tests can follow in sequence without stressing the same muscle group repeatedly
- Provide informed consent form (see Fig. 3.1)
- Maintain room temperature of 68°F to 72°F (20°C–22°C) and humidity of <60%

When multiple tests are to be administered, the organization of the testing session can be very important, depending on what physical fitness components are to be evaluated. Resting measurements such as heart rate (HR), blood pressure (BP), height, weight, and body composition should be obtained first. Resting measurements should be followed (in order) by tests of cardiorespiratory (CR) endurance, muscular fitness, and flexibility when all fitness components are assessed in a single session. Testing CR endurance after assessing muscular fitness (which elevates HR) can produce inaccurate results about an individual's CR endurance status, particularly when tests using HR to predict aerobic fitness are used. Likewise, dehydration resulting from CR endurance tests might influence body composition values if measured by bioelectrical impedance analysis (BIA). Because certain medications, such as β-blockers, which lower HR, will affect some fitness test results, use of these medications should be noted.

TEST ENVIRONMENT

The test environment is important for test validity and reliability. Test anxiety, emotional problems, food in the stomach, bladder distention, room temperature, and ventilation should be controlled as much as possible. To minimize anxiety, the test procedures should be explained adequately, and the test environment should be quiet and private. The room should be equipped with a comfortable seat and/or examination table to be used for resting BP and HR and/or electro-cardiographic (ECG) recordings. The demeanor of personnel should be one of relaxed confidence to put the subject at ease. Testing procedures should not be rushed, and all procedures must be explained clearly before initiating the process. These seemingly minor tasks are accomplished easily and are important in achieving valid and reliable test results.

BODY COMPOSITION

It is well established that excess body fat, particularly when located centrally around the abdomen, is associated with hypertension, the metabolic syndrome, type 2 diabetes, stroke, coronary artery disease, and hyperlipidemia (49). Approx-imately two thirds of American adults are classified as overweight (body mass index [BMI] ≥25), and about 32% are classified as obese (BMI ≥30) (51). In the years 1960 to 1962, 1971 to 1974, 1976 to 1980, 1988 to 1994, 1999 to 2000, and 2003 to 2004, the prevalence of obesity in the United States was 13.4%, 14.5%, 15%, 23.3%, 30.9%, and 32.2%, respectively (19,51). The more than twofold increase in adult obesity between 1980 and 2004 coincides with an alarming trend in the prevalence of overweight children in the United States and other developed nations, who displayed an increase from ~4% in 1970 to 15% in 2000 to 17% in 2004 (51,52,68). This more than fourfold increase in the past three decades shows no signs of abatement (51,52). Moreover, in 2003 to 2004, significant differences in obesity prevalence remained by race/ethnicity. Approximately 30% of non-Hispanic white adults were obese as were 45% of non-Hispanic black adults and 36.8% of Mexican Americans (51). Consequently, efforts to address health dispar-ities related to obesity and its comorbidities should be emphasized.

Basic body composition can be expressed as the relative percentage of body mass that is fat and fat-free tissue using a two-compartment model. Body com-position can be estimated with both laboratory and field techniques that vary in terms of complexity, cost, and accuracy. Different assessment techniques are briefly reviewed in this section; however, the detail associated with obtaining measurements and calculating estimates of body fat for all of these techniques is beyond the scope of this text. More detailed descriptions of each technique are available in Chapter 12 of the *ACSM Resource Manual for Guidelines for Exercise Testing and Prescription*, 6th ed. and elsewhere (28,37,62). Before collecting data for body composition assessment, the technician must be trained, be routinely practiced in the techniques, and already have demonstrated reliability in his or her measurements, independent of the technique being used. Experience can be accrued under the direct supervision of a highly qualified mentor in a controlled testing environment.

ANTHROPOMETRIC METHODS

Measurements of height, weight, circumferences, and skinfolds are used to estimate body composition. Although skinfold measurements are more difficult than other anthropometric procedures, they provide a better estimate of body fatness than those based only on height, weight, and circumferences (43).

Body Mass Index

The BMI, or Quetelet index, is used to assess weight relative to height and is calculated by dividing body weight in kilograms by height in meters squared $(kg \cdot m^{-2})$. For most people, obesity-related health problems increase beyond a BMI of 25, and the *Expert Panel on the Identification, Evaluation, and Treatment of Overweight and Obesity in Adults* (54) lists a BMI of 25.0 to 29.9 $kg \cdot m^{-2}$ for overweight and a BMI of ≥ 30.0 $kg \cdot m^{-2}$ for obesity. Although BMI fails to distinguish between body fat, muscle mass, or bone, an increased risk of hypertension, total cholesterol/high-density lipoprotein (HDL) cholesterol ratio, coronary disease, and mortality are associated with a BMI >30 $kg \cdot m^{-2}$ (Table 4.1) (59). A BMI of <18.5 $kg \cdot m^{-2}$ also increases the risk of cardiovascular disease and is responsible for the lower portion of the J-shaped curve of BMI versus cardiovascular risk. The use of specific BMI values to predict percentage body fat and health risk can be found in Table 4.2 (22). Because of the relatively large standard error of estimating percent fat from BMI ($\pm 5\%$ fat) (43), other methods of body composition assessment should be used to predict body fatness during a fitness assessment.

Circumferences

The pattern of body fat distribution is recognized as an important predictor of the health risks of obesity (69). Android obesity, which is characterized by more

TABLE 4.1. CLASSIFICATION OF DISEASE RISK BASED ON BODY MASS INDEX (BMI) AND WAIST CIRCUMFERENCE

| | | DISEASE RISK[a] RELATIVE TO NORMAL WEIGHT AND WAIST CIRCUMFERENCE | |
| | | MEN, ≤102 cm | MEN, >102 cm |
	BMI $(kg \cdot m^{-2})$	WOMEN, ≤88 cm	WOMEN, >88 cm
Underweight	<18.5	—	—
Normal	18.5–24.9	—	—
Overweight	25.0–29.9	Increased	High
Obesity, class			
I	30.0–34.9	High	Very high
II	35.0–39.9	Very high	Very high
III	≥40	Extremely high	Extremely high

[a]Disease risk for type 2 diabetes, hypertension, and cardiovascular disease. Dashes (—) indicate that no additional risk at these levels of BMI was assigned. Increased waist circumference can also be a marker for increased risk even in persons of normal weight.

Modified from Expert Panel. Executive summary of the clinical guidelines on the identification, evaluation, and treatment of overweight and obesity in adults. *Arch Intern Med.* 1998;158:1855-67.

TABLE 4.2. PREDICTED BODY FAT PERCENTAGE BASED ON BODY MASS INDEX (BMI) FOR AFRICAN-AMERICAN AND WHITE ADULTS[a]

BMI (kg · m^{-2})	HEALTH RISK	20–39 Yr	40–59 Yr	60–79 Yr
Men				
<18.5	Elevated	<8%	<11%	<13%
18.6–24.9	Average	8%–19%	11%–21%	13%–24%
25.0–29.9	Elevated	20%–24%	22%–27%	25%–29%
>30	High	≥25%	≥28%	≥30%
Women				
<18.5	Elevated	<21%	<23%	<24%
18.6–24.9	Average	21%–32%	23%–33%	24%–35%
25.0–29.9	Elevated	33%–38%	34%–39%	36%–41%
>30	High	≥39%	≥40%	≥42%

[a]Note: Standard error of estimate is ±5% for predicting percent body fat from BMI (based on a four-compartment estimate of body fat percentage).

From Gallagher D, Heymsfield SB, Heo M, et al. Healthy percentage body fat ranges: an approach for developing guidelines based on body mass index. *Am J Clin Nutr.* 2000;72:694-701.

fat on the trunk (abdominal fat), provides an increased risk of hypertension, metabolic syndrome, type 2 diabetes, dyslipidemia, coronary artery disease, and premature death compared with individuals who demonstrate gynoid or gynecoid obesity (fat distributed in the hip and thigh) (20).

Girth measurements may be used to predict body composition, and equations are available for both sexes and a range of age groups (66,67). The accuracy may be within 2.5% to 4% of the actual body composition if the subject possesses similar characteristics of the original validation population and the girth measurements are precise. A cloth tape measure with a spring-loaded handle (e.g., Gulick tape measure) reduces skin compression and improves consistency of measurement. Duplicate measurements are recommended at each site and should be obtained in a rotational instead of a consecutive order. The average of the two measures is used provided each measure is within 5 mm. Box 4.1 contains a description of the common sites.

The waist-to-hip ratio (WHR) is the circumference of the waist divided by the circumference of the hips (Box 4.1, buttocks/hips measure) and has been used as a simple method for determining body fat distribution (8). Health risk increases with WHR, and standards for risk vary with age and sex. For example, health risk is *very high* for young men when WHR is more than 0.95 and for young women when WHR is more than 0.86. For people 60 to 69 years old, the WHR values are greater than 1.03 for men and greater than 0.90 for women for the same risk classification (20,28).

The waist circumference can be used alone as an indicator of health risk because abdominal obesity is the primary issue. The Expert Panel on the Identification, Evaluation and Treatment of Overweight and Obesity in Adults provided a classification of disease risk based on both BMI and waist circumference as shown in Table 4.1 (54). Furthermore, a newer risk stratification scheme for

BOX 4.1	Standardized Description of Circumference Sites and Procedures

Abdomen:
With the subject standing upright and relaxed, a horizontal measure is taken at the greatest anterior extension of the abdomen, usually at the level of the umbilicus.

Arm:
With the subject standing erect and arms hanging freely at the sides with hands facing the thigh, a horizontal measure is taken midway between the acromion and olecranon processes.

Buttocks/hips:
With the subject standing erect and feet together, a horizontal measure is taken at the maximal circumference of buttocks. This measure is used for the hip measure in a waist/hip measure.

Calf:
With the subject standing erect (feet apart ~20 cm), a horizontal measure is taken at the level of the maximum circumference between the knee and the ankle, perpendicular to the long axis.

Forearm:
With the subject standing, arms hanging downward but slightly away from the trunk and palms facing anteriorly, a measure perpendicular to the long axis at the maximal circumference.

Hips/thigh:
With the subject standing, legs slightly apart (~10 cm), a horizontal measure is taken at the maximal circumference of the hip/proximal thigh, just below the gluteal fold.

Midthigh
With the subject standing and one foot on a bench so the knee is flexed at 90 degrees, a measure is taken midway between the inguinal crease and the proximal border of the patella, perpendicular to the long axis.

Waist:
With the subject standing, arms at the sides, feet together, and abdomen relaxed, a horizontal measure is taken at the narrowest part of the torso (above the umbilicus and below the xiphoid process). The National Obesity Task Force (NOTF) suggests obtaining a horizontal measure directly above the iliac crest as a method to enhance standardization. Unfortunately, current formulae are not predicated on the NOTF suggested site.

PROCEDURES
- All measurements should be made with a flexible yet inelastic tape measure.
- The tape should be placed on the skin surface without compressing the subcutaneous adipose tissue. >

> **Box 4.1. continued**

- If a Gulick spring-loaded handle is used, the handle should be extended to the same marking with each trial.
- Take duplicate measures at each site, and retest if duplicate measurements are not within 5 mm.
- Rotate through measurement sites or allow time for skin to regain normal texture.

Modified from Callaway CW, Chumlea WC, Bouchard C. Circumferences. In: Lohman TG, Roche AF, Martorell R, editors. *Anthropometric Standardization Reference Manual.* Champaign (IL): Human Kinetics; 1988;39–54.

adults based on waist circumference has been proposed (Table 4.3) (7). This can be used alone or in conjunction with BMI to evaluate chronic disease risk (Table 4.1). All assessments should include a minimum of either waist circumference or BMI, but preferably both, for risk stratification.

Skinfold Measurements

Body composition determined from skinfold measurements correlates well ($r =$ 0.70–0.90) with body composition determined by hydrodensitometry (62). The principle behind this technique is that the amount of subcutaneous fat is proportional to the total amount of body fat. It is assumed that close to one third of the total fat is located subcutaneously. The exact proportion of subcutaneous-to-total fat varies with sex, age, and ethnicity (61). Therefore, regression equations used to convert sum of skinfolds to percent body fat must consider these variables for greatest accuracy. Box 4.2 presents a standardized description of skinfold sites and procedures. Refer to the *ACSM Resource Manual*, 6th ed. for additional descriptions of the skinfold sites. To improve the accuracy of the measurement, it is recommended that one train with a skilled technician, use video media that demonstrate proper technique, participate in workshops, and accrue experience in a supervised practical environment. The accuracy of predicting percent fat from skinfolds is approximately ±3.5% assuming that appropriate techniques and equations have been used (28).

Factors that may contribute to measurement error within skinfold assessment include poor technique and/or an inexperienced evaluator, an extremely obese or

TABLE 4.3. CRITERIA FOR WAIST CIRCUMFERENCE IN ADULTS

	WAIST CIRCUMFERENCE cm (IN)	
RISK CATEGORY	WOMEN	MEN
Very low	<70 cm (27.5 in)	<80 cm (31.5 in)
Low	70–89 (28.5–35.0)	80–99 (31.5–39.0)
High	90–109 (35.5–43.0)	100–120 (39.5–47.0)
Very high	>110 (43.5)	>120 (47.0)

From Bray GA. Don't throw the baby out with the bath water. *Am J Clin Nutr.* 2004;70(3):347–9.

BOX 4.2	Standardized Description of Skinfold Sites and Procedures

SKINFOLD SITE

Abdominal	Vertical fold; 2 cm to the right side of the umbilicus
Triceps	Vertical fold; on the posterior midline of the upper arm, halfway between the acromion and olecranon processes, with the arm held freely to the side of the body
Biceps	Vertical fold; on the anterior aspect of the arm over the belly of the biceps muscle, 1 cm above the level used to mark the triceps site
Chest/pectoral	Diagonal fold; one half the distance between the anterior axillary line and the nipple (men), or one third of the distance between the anterior axillary line and the nipple (women)
Medial calf	Vertical fold; at the maximum circumference of the calf on the midline of its medial border
Midaxillary	Vertical fold; on the midaxillary line at the level of the xiphoid process of the sternum (An alternate method is a horizontal fold taken at the level of the xiphoid/ sternal border in the midaxillary line.)
Subscapular	Diagonal fold (at a 45-degree angle); 1 to 2 cm below the inferior angle of the scapula
Suprailiac	Diagonal fold; in line with the natural angle of the iliac crest taken in the anterior axillary line immediately superior to the iliac crest
Thigh	Vertical fold; on the anterior midline of the thigh, midway between the proximal border of the patella and the inguinal crease (hip)

PROCEDURES

- All measurements should be made on the right side of the body with the subject standing upright.
- The caliper should be placed directly on the skin surface, 1 cm away from the thumb and finger, perpendicular to the skinfold, and halfway between the crest and the base of the fold.
- A pinch should be maintained while reading the caliper.
- Wait 1 to 2 seconds (not longer) before reading caliper.
- Take duplicate measures at each site, and retest if duplicate measurements are not within 1 to 2 mm.
- Rotate through measurement sites, or allow time for skin to regain normal texture and thickness.

extremely lean subject, and an improperly calibrated caliper (tension should be set at ~12 g·mm^{-2}) (27). Various regression equations have been developed to predict body density or percent body fat from skinfold measurements. For example, Box 4.3 lists generalized equations that allow calculation of body density without a loss in prediction accuracy for a wide range of individuals (27,33). However, if a population-specific equation is needed, Heyward and Stolarczyk provide a quick reference guide to match the client to the correct equation based on sex, age, ethnicity, fatness, and sport (28).

BOX 4.3   Generalized Skinfold Equations

MEN
- **Seven-Site Formula** (chest, midaxillary, triceps, subscapular, abdomen, suprailiac, thigh)
  Body density = 1.112 − 0.00043499 (sum of seven skinfolds)
  $\qquad$ + 0.00000055 (sum of seven skinfolds)^2
  $\qquad$ − 0.00028826 (age) *[SEE 0.008 or ~3.5% fat]*
- **Three-Site Formula** (chest, abdomen, thigh)
  Body density = 1.10938 − 0.0008267 (sum of three skinfolds)
  $\qquad$ + 0.0000016 (sum of three skinfolds)^2
  $\qquad$ − 0.0002574 (age) *[SEE 0.008 or ~3.4% fat]*
- **Three-Site Formula** (chest, triceps, subscapular)
  Body density = 1.1125025 − 0.0013125 (sum of three skinfolds)
  $\qquad$ + 0.0000055 (sum of three skinfolds)^2
  $\qquad$ − 0.000244 (age) *[SEE 0.008 or ~3.6% fat]*

WOMEN
- **Seven-Site Formula** (chest, midaxillary, triceps, subscapular, abdomen, suprailiac, thigh)
  Body density = 1.097 − 0.00046971 (sum of seven skinfolds)
  $\qquad$ + 0.00000056 (sum of seven skinfolds)^2
  $\qquad$ − 0.00012828 (age) *[SEE 0.008 or ~3.8% fat]*
- **Three-Site Formula** (triceps, suprailiac, thigh)
  Body density = 1.099421 − 0.0009929 (sum of three skinfolds)
  $\qquad$ + 0.0000023 (sum of three skinfolds)^2
  $\qquad$ − 0.0001392 (age) *[SEE 0.009 or ~3.9% fat]*
- **Three-Site Formula** (triceps, suprailiac, abdominal)
  Body density = 1.089733 − 0.0009245 (sum of three skinfolds)
  $\qquad$ + 0.0000025 (sum of three skinfolds)^2
  $\qquad$ − 0.0000979 (age) *[SEE 0.009 or ~3.9% fat]*

Adapted from Jackson AS, Pollock ML. Practical assessment of body composition. *Phys Sport Med.* 1985;13:76–90. Pollock ML, Schmidt DH, Jackson AS. Measurement of cardiorespiratory fitness and body composition in the clinical setting. *Comp Ther.* 1980;6:12–7.

DENSITOMETRY

Body composition can be estimated from a measurement of whole body density, using the ratio of body mass to body volume. In this technique, which has been used as a reference or criterion standard for assessing body composition, the body is divided into two components: the fat mass (FM) and the fat-free mass (FFM). The limiting factor in the measurement of body density is the accuracy of the body volume measurement because body mass is measured simply as body weight. Body volume can be measured by hydrodensitometry (underwater) weighing and by plethysmography.

Hydrodensitometry (Underwater) Weighing

This technique of measuring body composition is based on Archimedes' principle, which states that when a body is immersed in water, it is buoyed by a counterforce equal to the weight of the water displaced. This loss of weight in water allows calculation of body volume. Bone and muscle tissue are denser than water, whereas fat tissue is less dense. Therefore, a person with more FFM for the same total body mass weighs more in water and has a higher body density and lower percentage of body fat. Although hydrostatic weighing is a standard method for measuring body volume and hence, body composition, it requires special equipment, the accurate measurement of residual volume, and significant cooperation by the subject (23). For a more detailed explanation of the technique, see Chapter 17 of *ACSM's Resource Manual for Guidelines for Exercise Testing and Prescription*.

Plethysmography

Body volume also can be measured by air rather than water displacement. One commercial system uses a dual-chamber plethysmograph that measures body volume by changes in pressure in a closed chamber. This technology shows promise and generally reduces the anxiety associated with the technique of hydrodensitometry (16,23,43). For a more detailed explanation of the technique, see Chapter 17 of *ACSM's Resource Manual for Guidelines for Exercise Testing and Prescription*.

Conversion of Body Density to Body Composition

Percent body fat can be estimated once body density has been determined. Two of the most common prediction equations used to estimate percent body fat from body density are derived from the two-component model of body composition (9,65):

$$\% \text{ fat} = \frac{457}{\text{Body Density}} - 414.2$$

$$\% \text{ fat} = \frac{495}{\text{Body Density}} - 450$$

Each method assumes a slightly different density of both fat and FFM. Ongoing research using the three- and four-component models of body composition provides a variety of newer equations that should increase the accuracy of the estimate of percent fat when applied to different populations. These equations

TABLE 4.4. POPULATION-SPECIFIC FORMULAS FOR CONVERSION OF BODY DENSITY (Db) TO PERCENT BODY FAT

POPULATION	AGE	SEX	% BODY FAT[a]
Race			
American Indian	18–60	Female	(4.81/Db)–4.34
Black	18–32	Male	(4.37/Db)–3.93
	24–79	Female	(4.85/Db)–4.39
Hispanic	20–40	Female	(4.87/Db)–4.41
Japanese Native	18–48	Male	(4.97/Db)–4.52
		Female	(4.76/Db)–4.28
	61–78	Male	(4.87/Db)–4.41
		Female	(4.95/Db)–4.50
White	7–12	Male	(5.30/Db)–4.89
		Female	(5.35/Db)–4.95
	13–16	Male	(5.07/Db)–4.64
		Female	(5.10/Db)–4.66
	17–19	Male	(4.99/Db)–4.55
		Female	(5.05/Db)–4.62
	20–80	Male	(4.95/Db)–4.50
		Female	(5.01/Db)–4.57
Levels of body fatness			
Anorexia	15–30	Female	(5.26/Db)–4.83
Obese	17–62	Male	(5.00/Db)–4.56

[a]Percent body fat is obtained by multiplying the value calculated from the equation by 100.

Adapted from Heyward VH, Stolarczyk LM. *Applied Body Composition Assessment.* Champaign (IL): Human Kinetics; 1996. p. 12.

(Table 4.4) are likely to improve over time as additional studies are done on larger samples within each population group (28).

OTHER TECHNIQUES

Additional assessment techniques of dual energy x-ray absorptiometry (DEXA) and total body electrical conductivity (TOBEC) are reliable and accurate measures of body composition, but these techniques are not popular for general health fitness testing because of cost and the need for highly trained personnel (62). Techniques of BIA and near-infrared intercadence are used for general health fitness testing. Generally, the accuracy of BIA is similar to skinfolds, as long as a stringent protocol is followed and the equations programmed into the analyzer are valid and accurate for the populations being tested (26). Near-infrared intercadence requires additional research to substantiate the validity and accuracy for body composition assessment (46). Detailed explanations of these techniques are found in Chapter 12 of *ACSM's Resource Manual for Guidelines for Exercise Testing and Prescription.*

BODY COMPOSITION NORMS

There are no universally accepted norms for body composition; however, Tables 4.5 and 4.6, which are based on selected populations, provide percentile values for percent body fat in men and women, respectively. A consensus opinion for an

TABLE 4.5. BODY COMPOSITION (% BODY FAT) FOR MEN

%	20–29	30–39	40–49	50–59	60–69	70–79	
99	4.2	7.0	9.2	10.9	11.5	13.6	
95	6.3	9.9	12.8	14.4	15.5	15.2	VL[a]
90	7.9	11.9	14.9	16.7	17.6	17.8	
85	9.2	13.3	16.3	18.0	18.8	19.2	
80	10.5	14.5	17.4	19.1	19.7	20.4	E
75	11.5	15.5	18.4	19.9	20.6	21.1	
70	12.7	16.5	19.1	20.7	21.3	21.6	
65	13.9	17.4	19.9	21.3	22.0	22.5	
60	14.8	18.2	20.6	22.1	22.6	23.1	G
55	15.8	19.0	21.3	22.7	23.2	23.7	
50	16.6	19.7	21.9	23.2	23.7	24.1	
45	17.4	20.4	22.6	23.9	24.4	24.4	
40	18.6	21.3	23.4	24.6	25.2	24.8	F
35	19.6	22.1	24.1	25.3	26.0	25.4	
30	20.6	23.0	24.8	26.0	26.7	26.0	
25	21.9	23.9	25.7	26.8	27.5	26.7	
20	23.1	24.9	26.6	27.8	28.4	27.6	P
15	24.6	26.2	27.7	28.9	29.4	28.9	
10	26.3	27.8	29.2	30.3	30.9	30.4	
5	28.9	30.2	31.2	32.5	32.9	32.4	
1	33.3	34.3	35.0	36.4	36.8	35.5	VP
n =	1826	8373	10442	6079	1836	301	

Total n = 28,857

Norms are based on Cooper Clinic patients.

[a]Very Lean—No less than 3% body fat is recommended for males.

VL, very lean; E, excellent; G, good; F, fair; P, poor; VP, very poor.

Reprinted with permission from the Cooper Institute, Dallas, Texas. For more information: www.cooperinstitute.org.

exact percentage body-fat value associated with optimal health risk has yet to be defined; however, a range 10% to 22% and 20% to 32% for men and women, respectively, is considered satisfactory for health (42).

CARDIORESPIRATORY FITNESS

Cardiorespiratory fitness is related to the ability to perform large muscle, dynamic, moderate-to-high intensity exercise for prolonged periods. Performance of such exercise depends on the functional state of the respiratory, cardiovascular, and skeletal muscle systems. Cardiorespiratory fitness is considered health-related because (a) low levels of CR fitness have been associated with a markedly increased risk of premature death from all causes and specifically from cardiovascular disease, (b) increases in CR fitness are associated with a reduction in death from all causes, and (c) high levels of CR fitness are associated with

TABLE 4.6. BODY COMPOSITION (% BODY FAT) FOR WOMEN

%	20–29	30–39	40–49	50–59	60–69	70–79	
				AGE			
99	9.8	11.0	12.6	14.6	13.9	14.6	
95	13.6	14.0	15.6	17.2	17.7	16.6	VL[a]
90	14.8	15.6	17.2	19.4	19.8	20.3	
85	15.8	16.6	18.6	20.9	21.4	23.0	
80	16.5	17.4	19.8	22.5	23.2	24.0	E
75	17.3	18.2	20.8	23.8	24.8	25.0	
70	18.0	19.1	21.9	25.1	25.9	26.2	
65	18.7	20.0	22.8	26.0	27.0	27.7	
60	19.4	20.8	23.8	27.0	27.9	28.6	G
55	20.1	21.7	24.8	27.9	28.7	29.7	
50	21.0	22.6	25.6	28.8	29.8	30.4	
45	21.9	23.5	26.5	29.7	30.6	31.3	
40	22.7	24.6	27.6	30.4	31.3	31.8	F
35	23.6	25.6	28.5	31.4	32.5	32.7	
30	24.5	26.7	29.6	32.5	33.3	33.9	
25	25.9	27.7	30.7	33.4	34.3	35.3	
20	27.1	29.1	31.9	34.5	35.4	36.0	P
15	28.9	30.9	33.5	35.6	36.2	37.4	
10	31.4	33.0	35.4	36.7	37.3	38.2	
5	35.2	35.8	37.4	38.3	39.0	39.3	
1	38.9	39.4	39.8	40.4	40.8	40.5	VP
n =	1360	3597	3808	2366	849	136	

Total n = 12,116

Norms are based on Cooper Clinic patients.

[a]Very Lean—No less than 10–13% body fat is recommended for females.

VL, very lean; E, excellent; G, good; F, fair; P, poor; VP, very poor.

Reprinted with permission from the Cooper Institute, Dallas, Texas. For more information: www.cooperinstitute.org.

higher levels of habitual physical activity, which in turn are associated with many health benefits (5,6,63). The assessment of CR fitness is an important part of a primary or secondary prevention program.

THE CONCEPT OF MAXIMAL OXYGEN UPTAKE

Maximal oxygen uptake ($\dot{V}O_{2max}$) is accepted as the criterion measure of CR fitness. Maximal oxygen uptake is the product of the maximal cardiac output (L blood·min^{-1}) and arterial-venous oxygen difference (mL O_2 per L blood). Significant variation in $\dot{V}O_{2max}$ across populations and fitness levels results primarily from differences in maximal cardiac output; therefore, $\dot{V}O_{2max}$ is closely related to the functional capacity of the heart.

Open-circuit spirometry is used to measure $\dot{V}O_{2max}$. In this procedure, the subject breathes through a low-resistance valve with his/her nose occluded (or through a nonlatex foam mask) while pulmonary ventilation and expired fractions of oxygen (O_2) and carbon dioxide (CO_2) are measured. Modern automated systems provide ease of use and a detailed printout of test results that save time and effort (15). However, attention to detail relative to calibration is still essential to obtain accurate results. Administration of the test and interpretation of results should be reserved for professional personnel with a thorough understanding of exercise science. Because of the costs associated with the equipment, space, and personnel needed to carry out these tests, direct measurement of $\dot{V}O_{2max}$ generally is reserved for research or clinical settings.

When direct measurement of $\dot{V}O_{2max}$ is not feasible or desirable, a variety of submaximal and maximal exercise tests can be used to estimate $\dot{V}O_{2max}$. These tests have been validated by examining (a) the correlation between directly measured $\dot{V}O_{2max}$ and the $\dot{V}O_{2max}$ estimated from physiologic responses to submaximal exercise (e.g., HR at a specified power output); or (b) the correlation between directly measured $\dot{V}O_{2max}$ and test performance (e.g., time to run 1 or 1.5 miles [1.6 or 2.4 km] or time to volitional fatigue using a standard graded exercise test protocol).

MAXIMAL VERSUS SUBMAXIMAL EXERCISE TESTING

The decision to use a maximal or submaximal exercise test depends largely on the reasons for the test and the availability of appropriate equipment and personnel. $\dot{V}O_{2max}$ can be estimated using conventional exercise test protocols, by considering test duration at a given workload on an ergometer, and by using the prediction equations found in Chapter 7. The user would need to consider the population being tested and the standard error of the associated equation. Maximal tests have the disadvantage of requiring participants to exercise to the point of volitional fatigue and might require medical supervision (Chapter 2) and emergency equipment. However, maximal exercise testing offers increased sensitivity in the diagnosis of coronary artery disease in asymptomatic individuals and provides a better estimate of $\dot{V}O_{2max}$ (Chapter 5). Additionally, the use of open circuit spirometry during maximal exercise testing allows for the accurate assessment of anaerobic threshold and the measurement of $\dot{V}O_{2max}$.

Practitioners commonly rely on submaximal exercise tests to assess CR fitness because maximal exercise testing is not always feasible in the health and fitness setting. The basic aim of submaximal exercise testing is to determine the HR response to one or more submaximal work rates and uses the results to predict $\dot{V}O_{2max}$. Although the primary purpose of the test has traditionally been to predict $\dot{V}O_{2max}$ from the HR-workload relationship, it is important to obtain additional indices of the client's response to exercise. The practitioner should use the various submaximal measures of HR, BP, workload, rating of perceived exertion (RPE), and other subjective indices as valuable information regarding one's functional response to exercise. This information can be used to evaluate submaximal exercise responses over time in a controlled environment and to fine-tune an exercise prescription.

The most accurate estimate of $\dot{V}O_{2max}$ is achieved if all of the following assumptions are met. Subjects with diabetes may have a blunted HR response to exercise and may not have an age-normal maximal HR (32). Estimates of $\dot{V}O_{2max}$ from the HR response to submaximal exercise tests are based on these assumptions:

- A steady-state HR is obtained for each exercise work rate and is consistent each day.

- A linear relationship exists between HR and work rate.
- The maximal work load is indicative of the $\dot{V}O_{2max}$.
- The maximal HR for a given age is uniform.
- Mechanical efficiency (i.e., $\dot{V}O_2$ at a given work rate) is the same for everyone.
- The subject is not on medications that alter HR.

MODES OF TESTING

Commonly used modes for exercise testing include field tests, treadmill tests, cycle ergometry tests, and step tests. Medical supervision may be required for moderate or high-risk individuals for each of these modes. Refer to Figure 2.4 for exercise testing and supervision guidelines. There are advantages and disadvantages of each mode:

- *Field tests* consist of walking or running a certain distance in a given time (i.e., 12-minute and 1.5-mile [2.4-km] run tests, and the 1- and 6-minute walk test). The advantages of field tests are that they are easy to administer to large numbers of individuals at one time and little equipment (e.g., a stopwatch) is needed. The disadvantages are that they all potentially could be maximal tests, and by their nature, are unmonitored for BP and HR. An individual's level of motivation and pacing ability also can have a profound impact on test results. These all-out run tests may be inappropriate for sedentary individuals or individuals at increased risk for cardiovascular and musculoskeletal complications. However, $\dot{V}O_{2max}$ can be estimated from test results.
- *Motor driven treadmills* can be used for submaximal and maximal testing and often are used for diagnostic testing. They provide a common form of exercise (i.e., walking) and can accommodate the least fit to the fittest individuals across the continuum of walking to running speeds. Nevertheless, a practice session might be necessary in some cases to permit habituation and reduce anxiety. On the other hand, treadmills usually are expensive, not easily transportable, and make some measurements (e.g., BP) more difficult. Treadmills must be calibrated to ensure the accuracy of the test. In addition, holding on to the support rail should not be permitted to ensure accuracy of the metabolic work.
- *Mechanically braked cycle ergometers* are excellent test modalities for submaximal and maximal testing. They are relatively inexpensive, easily transportable, and allow BP and the ECG (if appropriate) to be measured easily. The main disadvantage is that cycling is a less familiar mode of exercise, often resulting in limiting localized muscle fatigue. Cycle ergometers provide a non–weight-bearing test modality in which work rates are easily adjusted in small work-rate increments, and subjects tend to be least anxious using this device. The cycle ergometer must be calibrated and the subject must maintain the proper pedal rate because most tests require that HR be measured at specific work rates. Electronic cycle ergometers can deliver the same work rate across a range of pedal rates, but calibration might require special equipment not available in most laboratories. Some electronic fitness cycles cannot be calibrated and should not be used for testing.

- *Step testing* is an inexpensive modality for predicting CR fitness by measuring the HR response to stepping at a fixed rate and/or a fixed step height or by measuring postexercise recovery HR. Step tests require little or no equipment; steps are easily transportable; stepping skill requires little practice; the test usually is of short duration; and stepping is advantageous for mass testing (45). Postexercise (recovery) HR decreases with improved CR fitness, and test results are easy to explain to participants (36). Special precautions might be needed for those who have balance problems or are extremely deconditioned. Some single-stage step tests require an energy cost of seven to nine metabolic equivalents (METs), which may exceed the maximal capacity of the participant (2). The workload must be appropriate to the fitness level of the client. In addition, inadequate compliance to the step cadence and excessive fatigue in the lead limb may diminish the value of a step test. Most tests are unmonitored because of the difficulty of measuring HR and BP during a step test.

Field Tests

Two of the most widely used running tests for assessing CR fitness are the Cooper 12-minute test and the 1.5-mile (2.4-km) test for time. The objective in the 12-minute test is to cover the greatest distance in the allotted time period; for the 1.5-mile (2.4-km) test, it is to run the distance in the shortest period of time. $\dot{V}O_{2max}$ can be estimated from the equations in Chapter 7.

The Rockport One-Mile Fitness Walking Test has gained wide popularity as an effective means for estimating CR fitness. In this test, an individual walks 1 mile (1.6 km) as fast as possible, preferably on a track or a level surface, and HR is obtained in the final minute. An alternative is to measure a 10-second HR immediately on completion of the 1-mile (1.6 km) walk, but this may overestimate the $\dot{V}O_{2max}$ compared with when HR is measured during the walk. $\dot{V}O_{2max}$ is estimated from a regression equation (found in Chapter 7) based on weight, age, sex, walk time, and HR (38). In addition to independently predicting morbidity and mortality (4), the 6-minute walk test has been used to evaluate CR fitness within some clinical patient populations (e.g., persons with chronic heart failure or pulmonary disease). Even though the test is considered submaximal, it may result in near maximal performance for those with low fitness levels or disease. Patients completing <300 meters during the 6-minute walk demonstrate a limited short-term survival (10). Several multivariate equations are available to predict peak $\dot{V}O_2$ from the 6-minute walk; however, the following equation requires minimal clinical information (10):

- Peak $\dot{V}O_2 = \dot{V}O_2$ mL$\cdot$kg$^{-1}\cdot$min^{-1} = [0.02 × distance (m)]
  $-$ [0.191 × age (yr)] $-$ [0.07 × weight (kg)]
  $+$ [0.09 × height (cm)] + [0.26 × RPP (× 10^{-3})] + 2.45

  Where m = distance in meters; y = year; kg = kilogram; cm = centimeter; RPP = rate pressure product (HR × systolic BP in mm Hg)
- $R^2 = 0.65$ SEE = 2.68

Submaximal Exercise Tests

Both single-stage and multistage submaximal exercise tests are available to estimate $\dot{V}O_{2max}$ from simple HR measurements. Accurate measurement of HR is critical for valid testing. Although HR obtained by palpation is used commonly, the accuracy of this method depends on the experience and technique of the evaluator. It is recommended that an ECG, HR monitor, or a stethoscope be used to determine HR. The use of a relatively inexpensive HR monitor can reduce a significant source of error in the test. The submaximal HR response is easily altered by several environmental (e.g., heat and/or humidity, Chapter 7), dietary (e.g., caffeine, time since last meal), and behavioral (e.g., anxiety, smoking, previous activity) factors. These variables must be controlled to have a valid estimate that can be used as a reference point in a person's fitness program. In addition, the test mode (e.g., cycle, treadmill, or step) should be consistent with the primary activity used by the participant to address specificity of training issues. Standardized procedures for submaximal testing are presented in Box 4.4. Although there are no specific submaximal protocols for treadmill testing, several stages from any of the treadmill protocols found in Chapter 5 can be used to assess submaximal exercise responses. Pre-exercise test instructions were presented in Chapter 3.

Cycle Ergometer Tests

The Astrand-Rhyming cycle ergometer test is a single-stage test lasting 6 minutes (3). For the population studied, these researchers observed that at 50% of $\dot{V}O_{2max}$ the average HR was 128 and 138 beats $\cdot$ min^{-1} for men and women, respectively. If a woman was working at a $\dot{V}O_2$ of 1.5 L $\cdot$ min^{-1} and her HR was 138 beats $\cdot$ min^{-1}, then her $\dot{V}O_{2max}$ was estimated to be 3.0 L $\cdot$ min^{-1}. The suggested work rate is based on sex and an individual's fitness status as follows:

men, unconditioned: 300 or 600 kg $\cdot$ m $\cdot$ min^{-1} (50 or 100 watts)
men, conditioned: 600 or 900 kg $\cdot$ m $\cdot$ min^{-1} (100 or 150 watts)
women, unconditioned: 300 or 450 kg $\cdot$ m $\cdot$ min^{-1} (50 or 75 watts)
women, conditioned: 450 or 600 kg $\cdot$ m $\cdot$ min^{-1} (75 or 100 watts)

The pedal rate is set at 50 rpm. The goal is to obtain HR values between 125 and 170 beats·min^{-1}, and HR is measured during the fifth and sixth minute of work. The average of the two heart rates is then used to estimate $\dot{V}O_{2max}$ from a nomogram (Fig. 4.1). This value must then be adjusted for age (because maximal HR decreases with age) by multiplying the $\dot{V}O_{2max}$ value by the following correction factors (2):

AGE	CORRECTION FACTOR
15	1.10
25	1.00
35	0.87
40	0.83
45	0.78
50	0.75
55	0.71
60	0.68
65	0.65

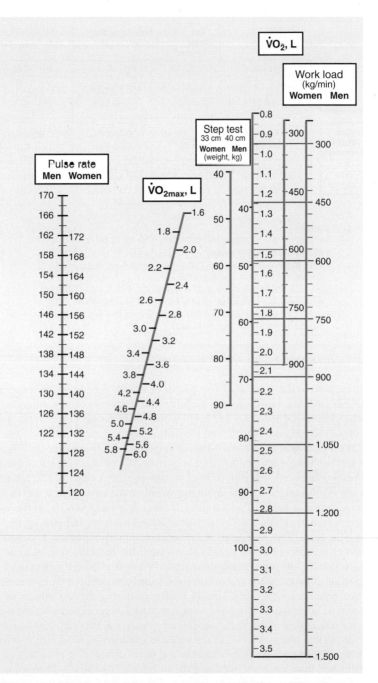

FIGURE 4.1. Modified Astrand-Ryhming nomogram. (Used with permission from Astrand PO, Ryhming I. A nomogram for calculation of aerobic capacity [physical fitness] from pulse rate during submaximal work. *J Appl Physiol.* 1954;7:218–21.)

	1st stage	150 kgm/min (0.5 kg)		
	HR: <80	**HR: 80–89**	**HR: 90–100**	**HR: >100**
2nd stage	750 kgm/min (2.5 kg)*	600 kgm/min (2.0 kg)	450 kgm/min (1.5 kg)	300 kgm/min (1.0 kg)
3rd stage	900 kgm/min (3.0 kg)	750 kgm/min (2.5 kg)	600 kgm/min (2.0 kg)	450 kgm/min (1.5 kg)
4th stage	1050 kgm/min (3.5 kg)	900 kgm/min (3.0 kg)	750 kgm/min (2.5 kg)	600 kgm/min (2.0 kg)

Directions:

1 Set the 1st work rate at 150 kgm/min (0.5 kg at 50 rpm)
2 If the HR in the third minute of the stage is:
    <80, set the 2nd stage at 750 kgm/min (2.5 kg at 50 rpm)
    80-89, set the 2nd stage at 600 kgm/min (2.0 kg at 50 rpm)
    90-100, set the 2nd stage at 450 kgm/min (1.5 kg at 50 rpm)
    >100, set the 2nd stage at 300 kgm/min (1.0 kg at 50 rpm)
3 Set the 3rd and 4th (if required) according to the work rates in the columns below the 2nd loads

FIGURE 4.2. YMCA cycle ergometry protocol. Resistance settings shown here are appropriate for an ergometer with a flywheel of 6 m·rev^{-1}.

In contrast to the single-stage test, Maritz et al. (44) measured HR at a series of submaximal work rates and extrapolated the response to the subject's age-predicted maximal HR. This has become one of the most popular assessment techniques to estimate $\dot{V}O_{2max}$, and the YMCA test is a good example (24). The YMCA protocol uses two to four 3-minute stages of continuous exercise (Fig. 4.2). The test is designed to raise the steady-state HR of the subject to between 110 beats·min^{-1} and 70% HRR (85% of the age-predicted maximal HR) for at least two consecutive stages. It is important to remember that two consecutive HR measurements must be obtained within this HR range to predict $\dot{V}O_{2max}$. In the YMCA protocol, each work rate is performed for at least 3 minutes, and HRs are recorded during the final 15 to 30 seconds of the second and third minutes. The work rate should be maintained for an additional minute if the two HRs vary by more than 5 beats·min^{-1}. The test administrator should recognize the error associated with age-predicted maximal HR and monitor the subject throughout the test to ensure the test remains submaximal. The HR measured during the last minute of each steady-state stage is plotted against work rate. The line generated from the plotted points is then extrapolated to the age-predicted maximal HR (e.g., 220 – age), and a perpendicular line is dropped to the x-axis to estimate the work rate that would have been achieved if the person had worked to maximum (Fig. 4.3). $\dot{V}O_{2max}$ can be estimated from the work rate using the formula in Chapter 7. These equations are valid to estimate oxygen consumption at submaximal steady-state workloads from 300 to 1,200 kg·m·min^{-1}; therefore, caution must be used if extrapolating to workloads outside of this range. The two lines noted as ±1 SD in Figure 4.3

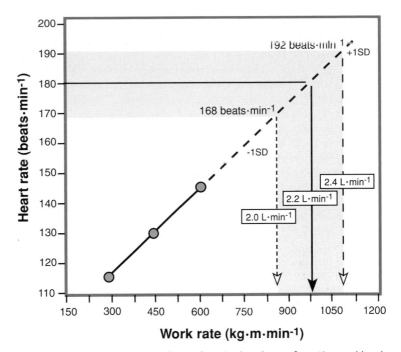

FIGURE 4.3. Heart rate responses to three submaximal work rates for a 40-year-old, sedentary woman weighing 64 kg. $\dot{V}O_{2max}$ was estimated by extrapolating the heart rate (HR) response to the age-predicted maximal HR of 180 beats·min^{-1} (based on 220 − age). The work rate that would have been achieved at that HR was determined by dropping a line from that HR value to the x-axis. $\dot{V}O_{2max}$ is estimated using the formula in Chapter 7 and expressed in L·min^{-1}, was 2.2 L·min^{-1}. The other two lines estimate what the $\dot{V}O_{2max}$ would have been if the subject's true maximal HR was ±1 SD from the 180 beats·min^{-1} value.

show what the estimated $\dot{V}O_{2max}$ would be if the subject's true maximal HR were 168 or 192 beats·min^{-1}, rather than 180 beats·min^{-1}. Part of the error involved in estimating $\dot{V}O_{2max}$ from submaximal HR responses occurs because the formula (220 – age) can provide only an estimate of maximal HR (standard deviation of formula = 12 to 15 beats·min^{-1}) (70). In addition, errors can be attributed to inaccurate pedaling cadence (workload) and imprecise steady-state heart rates.

Treadmill Tests

The primary exercise modality for submaximal exercise testing traditionally has been the cycle ergometer, although treadmills have been used in many settings. The same endpoint (70% HRR or 85% of age-predicted maximal HR) is used, and the stages of the test should be 3 minutes or longer to ensure a steady-state HR response at each stage. The HR values are extrapolated to age-predicted maximal HR, and $\dot{V}O_{2max}$ is estimated using the formula in Chapter 7 from the highest speed and/or grade that would have been achieved if the person had worked to maximum. Most common treadmill protocols (Chapter 5) can be used, but the duration of each stage should be at least 3 minutes.

Step Tests

Step tests have also been used to estimate $\dot{V}O_{2max}$. Astrand and Ryhming (3) used a single-step height of 33 cm (13 in) for women and 40 cm (15.7 in) for men at a rate of 22.5 steps·min^{-1}. These tests require oxygen uptakes of about 25.8 and 29.5 mL·kg^{-1}·min^{-1}, respectively. Heart rate is measured as described for the cycle test, and $\dot{V}O_{2max}$ is estimated from the nomogram (Fig. 4.1). In contrast, Maritz et al. (44) used a single-step height of 12 inches (30.5 cm) and four-step rates to systematically increase the work rate. A steady-state HR was measured for each step rate, and a line formed from these HR values was extrapolated to age-predicted maximal HR; the maximal work rate was determined as described for the YMCA cycle test. $\dot{V}O_{2max}$ can be estimated from the formula for stepping in Chapter 7. Such step tests should be modified to suit the population being tested. The Canadian Home Fitness Test has demonstrated that such testing can be performed on a large scale and at low cost (2,3,24,36,38,44,64).

Instead of estimating $\dot{V}O_{2max}$ from HR responses to several submaximal work rates, a wide variety of step tests have been developed to categorize cardiovascular fitness on the basis of a person's recovery HR following a standardized step test. The 3-Minute YMCA Step Test is a good example of such a test. This test uses a 12-inch (30.5 cm) bench, with a stepping rate of 24 steps·min^{-1} (estimated oxygen cost of 25.8 mL·kg^{-1}·min^{-1}). After exercise is completed, the subject immediately sits down and HR is counted for 1 minute. Counting must start within 5 seconds at the end of exercise. Heart rate values are used to obtain a qualitative rating of fitness from published normative tables (24).

CARDIORESPIRATORY TEST SEQUENCE AND MEASURES

A minimum of HR, BP, and RPE should be measured during exercise tests. After the initial screening process, selected baseline measurements should be obtained before the start of the exercise test. Taking a resting ECG before exercise testing assumes that trained personnel are available to interpret the ECG and provide medical guidance. An ECG is not necessary when diagnostic testing is not being done and when apparently healthy individuals are being tested with submaximal tests. The sequence of measures is listed in Box 4.4.

Heart rate can be determined using several techniques, including radial or carotid pulse palpation, auscultation with a stethoscope, or the use of HR monitors. The pulse palpation technique involves "feeling" the pulse by placing the first and second fingers over an artery (usually the radial artery located near the thumb side of the wrist or the carotid artery located in the neck near the larynx). The pulse is typically counted for 15 seconds, and then multiplied by four, to determine the per-minute HR. Although the carotid pulse might be easier to obtain, one should not press too hard with the palpating fingers because this could produce a marked bradycardia in the presence of a hypersensitive carotid sinus reflex. For the auscultation method, the bell of the stethoscope should be placed to the left of the sternum just above the level of the nipple. This method is most accurate when the heart sounds are clearly audible and the subject's torso is relatively stable. Heart rate telemetry monitors (heart rate watches) with chest electrodes have proved to be accurate and reliable, provided there is no outside

BOX 4.4	General Procedures for Submaximal Testing of Cardiorespiratory Fitness

1. Obtain resting heart rate and BP immediately before exercise in the exercise posture.
2. The client should be familiarized with the ergometer. If using a cycle ergometer, properly position the client on the ergometer (i.e., upright posture, five-degree bend in the knee at maximal leg extension, hands in proper position on handlebars).
3. The exercise test should begin with a two- to three-minute warm-up to acquaint the client with the cycle ergometer and prepare him or her for the exercise intensity in the first stage of the test.
4. A specific protocol should consist of 2- or 3-minute stages with appropriate increments in work rate.
5. Heart rate should be monitored at least two times during each stage, near the end of the second and third minutes of each stage. If heart rate >110 beats $\cdot$ min^{-1}, steady-state heart rate (i.e., two heart rates within 5 beats $\cdot$ min^{-1}) should be reached before the workload is increased.
6. Blood pressure should be monitored in the last minute of each stage and repeated (verified) in the event of a hypotensive or hypertensive response.
7. Perceived exertion and additional rating scales should be monitored near the end of the last minute of each stage using either the 6–20 or 0–10 scale (Table 4.8).
8. Client appearance and symptoms should be monitored and recorded regularly.
9. The test should be terminated when the subject reaches 70% heart rate reserve (85% of age-predicted maximal heart rate), fails to conform to the exercise test protocol, experiences adverse signs or symptoms, requests to stop, or experiences an emergency situation.
10. An appropriate cool-down/recovery period should be initiated consisting of either:
    a. Continued exercise at a work rate equivalent to that of the first stage of the exercise test protocol or lower; or
    b. A passive cool-down if the subject experiences signs of discomfort or an emergency situation occurs
11. All physiologic observations (e.g., heart rate, BP, signs and symptoms) should be continued for at least 5 minutes of recovery unless abnormal responses occur, which would warrant a longer posttest surveillance period. Continue low-level exercise until heart rate and BP stabilize, but not necessarily until they reach pre-exercise levels.

electrical interference (e.g., emissions from the display consoles of computerized exercise equipment) (39). Many electronic cycles and treadmills have embedded this HR technology into the equipment.

Blood pressure should be measured at heart level with the subject's arm relaxed and not grasping a handrail (treadmill) or handlebar (cycle ergometer). To help ensure accurate readings, the use of an appropriate-sized BP cuff is important. The rubber bladder of the BP cuff should encircle at least 80% of the subject's upper arm. If the subject's arm is large, a normal-size adult cuff will be too small, thus resulting in an erroneous elevated reading (the converse is also true). Blood pressure measurements should be taken with a mercury sphygmomanometer adjusted to eye level or a recently calibrated aneroid manometer. Systolic and diastolic BP measurements can be used as indicators for stopping an exercise test (see next section). To obtain accurate BP measures during exercise, follow the guidelines in Chapter 3 (Box 3.4) for resting BP; however, obtain BP in the exercise position. In addition, if the fourth Korotkoff sound can not be discerned, the fifth Korotkoff sound should be obtained. During exercise, it is advisable to obtain the first, fourth, and fifth Korotkoff sounds.

RPE can be a valuable indicator for monitoring an individual's exercise tolerance. Although perceived exertion ratings correlate with exercise HRs and work rates, large interindividual variability in RPE with both healthy as well as cardiac patients mandates caution in the universal application of the scales (71). Borg's RPE scale was developed to allow the exerciser to subjectively rate his or her feelings during exercise, taking into account personal fitness level, environmental conditions, and general fatigue levels (50). Ratings can be influenced by psychological factors, mood states, environmental conditions, exercise modes, and age, which reduce its utility (60). Currently, two RPE scales are widely used: the original or category scale, which rates exercise intensity on a scale of 6 to 20, and the category-ratio scale of 0 to 10. Both RPE scales are shown in Table 4.7. Either scale is appropriate as a subjective tool.

During exercise testing, the RPE can be used as an indication of impending fatigue. Most apparently healthy subjects reach their subjective limit of fatigue at an RPE of 18 to 19 (very, very hard) on the category Borg scale or 9 to 10 (very, very strong) on the category-ratio scale; therefore, RPE can be used to monitor progress toward maximal exertion during exercise testing (48).

TEST TERMINATION CRITERIA

Graded exercise testing, whether maximal or submaximal, is a safe procedure when subject screening and testing guidelines (Chapter 2) are adhered to. Occasionally, for safety reasons, the test may have to be terminated before the subject reaches a measured $\dot{V}O_{2max}$, volitional fatigue, or a predetermined endpoint (i.e., 50% to 70% HRR or 70% to 85% age-predicted maximal HR). Because of the individual variation in maximal HR, the upper limit of 85% of an estimated maximal HR may result in a maximal effort for some individuals. General indications— those that do not rely on physician involvement or ECG monitoring—for stopping an exercise test are outlined in Box 4.5. More specific termination criteria for clinical or diagnostic testing are provided in Chapter 5.

TABLE 4.7. CATEGORY AND CATEGORY-RATIO SCALES FOR RATINGS OF PERCEIVED EXERTION

CATEGORY SCALE	CATEGORY-RATIO SCALE	
6 No exertion at all	0 Nothing at all	
7 Extremely light	0.3	
8	0.5 Extremely weak	Just noticeable
9 Very light	0.7	
10	1 Very weak	
11 Light	1.5	
12	2 Weak	Light
13 Somewhat hard	2.5	
14	3 Moderate	
15 Hard (heavy)	4	
16	5 Strong	Heavy
17 Very hard	6	
18	7 Very strong	
19 Extremely hard	8	
20 Maximal exertion	9	
	10 Extremely strong	"Maximal"
	11	
	ⸯ	
	● Absolute maximum	Highest possible

Copyright Gunnar Borg. Reproduced with permission. For correct use of the Borg scales, it is necessary to follow the administration and instructions given in Borg G. *Borg's Perceived Exertion and Pain Scales*. Champaign (IL): Human Kinetics; 1998.

BOX 4.5	**General Indications for Stopping an Exercise Test in Low-Risk Adults**[a]

- Onset of angina or anginalike symptoms
- Drop in systolic BP of >10 mm Hg from baseline BP despite an increase in workload
- Excessive rise in BP: systolic pressure >250 mm Hg or diastolic pressure >115 mm Hg
- Shortness of breath, wheezing, leg cramps, or claudication
- Signs of poor perfusion: light-headedness, confusion, ataxia, pallor, cyanosis, nausea, or cold and clammy skin
- Failure of heart rate to increase with increased exercise intensity
- Noticeable change in heart rhythm
- Subject requests to stop
- Physical or verbal manifestations of severe fatigue
- Failure of the testing equipment

[a]Assumes that testing is nondiagnostic and is being performed without direct physician involvement or ECG monitoring. For clinical testing, Box 5–2 provides more definitive and specific termination criteria.

INTERPRETATION OF RESULTS

Table 4.8 provides normative values for $\dot{V}O_{2max}$ ($mL \cdot kg^{-1} \cdot min^{-1}$), with specific reference to age and sex. Research suggests that a $\dot{V}O_{2max}$ below the twentieth percentile for age and sex, which is often indicative of a sedentary lifestyle, is associated with an increased risk of death from all causes (5). In a comparison of the fitness status of any one individual to published norms, the accuracy of the classification is dependent on the similarities between the populations and methodology (estimated versus measured $\dot{V}O_{2max}$; maximal versus submaximal, etc.). Although submaximal exercise testing is not as precise as maximal exercise testing, it provides a reasonably accurate reflection of an individual's fitness at a lower cost and reduced risk, and requires less time and effort on the part of the subject.

Some of the assumptions inherent in a submaximal test are more easily met (e.g., steady-state HR can be verified), whereas others (e.g., estimated maximal HR) introduce unknown errors into the prediction of $\dot{V}O_{2max}$. When an individual

TABLE 4.8. PERCENTILE VALUES FOR MAXIMAL AEROBIC POWER

				MALES					
	AGE 20–29				AGE 30–39				
%	Balke Treadmill (time)	Max $\dot{V}O_2$ (mL/kg/ min)	12 min Run (miles)	1.5 Mile Run (time)	Balke Treadmill (time)	Max $\dot{V}O_2$ (mL/kg/ min)	12 min Run (miles)	1.5 Mile Run (time)	
99	32:00	61.2	2.02	8:22	30:00	58.3	1.94	8:49	
95	28:31	56.2	1.88	9:10	27:11	54.3	1.82	9:31	S
90	27:00	54.0	1.81	9:34	26:00	52.5	1.77	9:52	
85	26:00	52.5	1.77	9:52	24:45	50.7	1.72	10:14	
80	25:00	51.1	1.73	10:08	23:30	47.5	1.67	10:38	E
75	23:40	49.2	1.68	10:34	22:30	47.5	1.63	10:59	
70	23:00	48.2	1.65	10:49	22:00	46.8	1.61	11:09	
65	22:00	46.8	1.61	11:09	21:00	45.3	1.57	11:34	
60	21:15	45.7	1.58	11:27	20:20	44.4	1.55	11:49	G
55	21:00	45.3	1.57	11:34	20:00	43.9	1.53	11:58	
50	20:00	43.9	1.53	11:58	19:00	42.4	1.49	12:25	
45	19:26	43.1	1.51	12:11	18:15	41.4	1.46	12:44	
40	18:50	42.2	1.49	12:29	18:00	41.0	1.45	12:53	F
35	18:00	41.0	1.45	12:53	17:00	39.5	1.41	13:25	
30	17:30	40.3	1.43	13:08	16:15	38.5	1.38	13:48	
25	17:00	39.5	1.41	13:25	15:40	37.6	1.36	14:10	
20	16:00	38.1	1.37	13:58	15:00	36.7	1.33	14:33	P
15	15:00	36.7	1.33	14:33	14:00	35.2	1.29	15:14	
10	14:00	35.2	1.29	15:14	13:00	33.8	1.25	15:56	
5	12:00	32.3	1.21	16:46	11:10	31.1	1.18	17:30	
1	8:00	26.6	1.05	20:55	8:00	26.6	1.05	20:55	VP
		n = 2,606				n = 13,158			

Total n = 15,764

S, Superior; E, excellent; G, good; F, fair; P, poor; VP, very poor.

TABLE 4.8. PERCENTILE VALUES FOR MAXIMAL AEROBIC POWER (*Continued*)

MALES

	AGE 40–49				AGE 50–59				
%	Balke Treadmill (time)	Max $\dot{V}O_2$ (mL/kg/min)	12 min Run (miles)	1.5 Mile Run (time)	Balke Treadmill (time)	Max $\dot{V}O_2$ (mL/kg/min)	12 min Run (miles)	1.5 Mile Run (time)	
99	29:06	57.0	1.90	9:02	27:15	54.3	1.82	9:31	
95	26:16	52.9	1.79	9:47	24:00	49.7	1.69	10:27	S
90	25:00	51.1	1.73	10:09	22:00	46.8	1.61	11:09	
85	23:14	48.5	1.66	10:44	20:31	44.6	1.55	11:45	
80	22:00	46.8	1.61	11:09	19:35	43.3	1.52	12:08	E
75	21:02	45.4	1.58	11:32	18:32	41.8	1.47	12:37	
70	20:15	44.2	1.54	11:52	18:00	41.0	1.45	12:53	
65	20:00	43.9	1.53	11:58	17:00	39.5	1.41	13:25	
60	19:00	42.4	1.49	12:25	16:10	38.3	1.38	13:53	G
55	18:02	41.0	1.45	12:53	16:00	38.1	1.37	13:58	
50	17:34	40.4	1.44	13:05	15:02	36.7	1.33	14:33	
45	17:00	39.5	1.41	13:25	14:56	36.6	1.33	14:35	
40	16:12	38.4	1.38	13:50	14:00	35.2	1.29	15:14	F
35	15:38	37.6	1.36	14:10	13:05	33.9	1.26	15:53	
30	15:00	36.7	1.33	14:33	12:38	33.2	1.24	16:16	
25	14:20	35.7	1.31	15:00	12:00	32.3	1.21	16:46	
20	13:35	34.6	1.28	15:32	11:10	31.1	1.18	17:30	P
15	12:45	33.4	1.24	16:09	10:15	29.8	1.14	18:22	
10	11:40	31.8	1.20	17:04	9:15	28.4	1.10	19:24	
5	10:00	29.4	1.13	18:39	7:30	25.8	1.03	21:40	
1	7:00	25.1	1.01	22:22	4:20	21.3	0.90	27:08	VP
	n = 16,534				n = 9,102				

Total n = 25,636

S, Superior; E, excellent; G, good; F, fair; P, poor; VP, very poor.

Reprinted with permission from the Cooper Institute, Dallas, TX. For more information: www.cooperinstitute.org.

is given repeated submaximal exercise tests over a period of weeks or months and the HR response to a fixed work rate decreases over time, it is likely that the individual's CR fitness has improved, independent of the accuracy of the $\dot{V}O_{2max}$ prediction. Despite differences in test accuracy and methodology, virtually all evaluations can establish a baseline and be used to track relative progress.

MUSCULAR STRENGTH AND MUSCULAR ENDURANCE

Muscular strength and endurance are health-related fitness components that may improve or maintain the following:

- Bone mass, which is related to osteoporosis
- Glucose tolerance, which is related to type 2 diabetes
- Musculotendinous integrity, which is related to a lower risk of injury, including low-back pain

TABLE 4.8. PERCENTILE VALUES FOR MAXIMAL AEROBIC POWER (*Continued*)

	MALES								
	AGE 60–69				AGE 70–79				
%	Balke Treadmill (time)	Max $\dot{V}O_2$ (mL/kg/min)	12 min Run (miles)	1.5 Mile Run (time)	Balke Treadmill (time)	Max $\dot{V}O_2$ (mL/kg/min)	12 min Run (miles)	1.5 Mile Run (time)	
99	25:02	51.1	1.74	10:09	24:00	49.7	1.69	10:27	
95	21:33	46.1	1.60	11:20	19:00	42.4	1.49	12:25	S
90	19:30	43.2	1.51	12:10	17:00	39.5	1.41	13:25	
85	18:00	41.0	1.45	12:53	16:00	38.1	1.37	13:57	
80	17:00	39.5	1.41	13:25	14:34	36.0	1.32	14:52	E
75	16:00	38.1	1.37	13:58	13:25	34.4	1.27	15:38	
70	15:00	36.7	1.33	14:33	12:27	33.0	1.23	16:22	
65	14:30	35.9	1.31	14:55	12:00	32.3	1.21	16:46	
60	13:51	35.0	1.29	15:20	11:00	30.9	1.17	17:37	G
55	13:04	33.9	1.26	15:53	10:30	30.2	1.15	18:05	
50	12:30	33.1	1.23	16:19	10:00	29.4	1.13	18:39	
45	12:00	32.3	1.21	16:46	9:20	28.5	1.11	19:19	
40	11:21	31.4	1.19	17:19	9:00	28.0	1.09	19:43	F
35	10:49	30.6	1.17	17:49	8:21	27.1	1.07	20:28	
30	10:00	29.4	1.13	18:39	7:38	26.0	1.04	21:28	
25	9:29	28.7	1.11	19:10	7:00	25.1	1.01	22:22	
20	8:37	27.4	1.08	20:13	6:00	23.7	0.97	23:55	P
15	7:33	25.9	1.03	21:34	5:00	22.2	0.93	25:49	
10	6:20	24.1	0.99	23:27	4:00	20.8	0.89	27:55	
5	4:55	22.1	0.93	25:58	3:00	19.3	0.85	30:34	
1	2:29	18.6	0.83	31:59	2:00	17.9	0.81	33:30	VP
	n = 2,682				n = 467				

Total n = 3,149

S, Superior; E, excellent; G, good; F, fair; P, poor; VP, very poor.

Reprinted with permission from the Cooper Institute, Dallas, TX. For more information: www.cooperinstitute.org.

- The ability to carry out the activities of daily living, which is related to self-esteem
- The FFM and resting metabolic rate, which are related to weight management

The ACSM has melded the terms *muscular strength* and *muscular endurance* into a category termed *muscular fitness* and included it as an integral portion of total health-related fitness in a position stand on the quantity and quality of exercise to achieve and maintain fitness (1). Muscular strength refers to *the ability of the muscle to exert force* (56). Muscular endurance is *the muscle's ability to continue to perform for successive exertions or many repetitions* (56). Traditionally, tests allowing few (<3) repetitions of a task before reaching momentary muscular fatigue have been considered strength measures, whereas those in which numerous repetitions (>12) are performed before momentary muscular fatigue were considered measures of muscular endurance. However, the performance of a maximal repetition range (i.e., 4, 6, 8) also can be used to assess strength.

TABLE 4.8. PERCENTILE VALUES FOR MAXIMAL AEROBIC POWER (Continued)

	FEMALES								
	AGE 20–29				AGE 30–39				
%	Balke Treadmill (time)	Max $\dot{V}O_2$ (mL/kg/min)	12 min Run (miles)	1.5 Mile Run (time)	Balke Treadmill (time)	Max $\dot{V}O_2$ (mL/kg/min)	12 min Run (miles)	1.5 Mile Run (time)	
99	27:43	55.0	1.84	9:23	26:00	52.5	1.77	9:52	
95	24:24	50.2	1.71	10:20	22:06	46.9	1.62	11:08	S
90	22:30	47.5	1.63	10:59	20:34	44.7	1.56	11:43	
85	21:00	45.3	1.57	11:34	19:03	42.5	1.50	12:23	
80	20:04	44.0	1.54	11:56	18:00	41.0	1.45	12:53	E
75	19:42	43.4	1.52	12:07	17:30	40.3	1.43	13:08	
70	18:06	41.1	1.46	12:51	16:30	38.8	1.39	13:41	
65	17:45	40.6	1.44	13:01	16:00	38.1	1.37	13.58	
60	17:00	39.5	1.41	13:25	15:02	36.7	1.33	14:33	G
55	16:00	38.1	1.37	13:58	15:00	36.7	1.33	14:33	
50	15:30	37.4	1.35	14:15	14:00	35.2	1.29	15:14	
45	15:00	36.7	1.33	14:33	13:30	34.5	1.27	15:35	
40	14:11	35.5	1.30	15:05	13:00	33.8	1.25	15:56	F
35	13:36	34.6	1.27	15:32	12:03	32.4	1.21	16:43	
30	13:00	33.8	1.25	15:56	12:00	32.3	1.21	16:46	
25	12:04	32.4	1.22	16:43	11:00	30.9	1.17	17:38	
20	11:30	31.6	1.19	17:11	10:20	29.9	1.15	18:18	P
15	10:42	30.5	1.16	17:53	9:39	28.9	1.12	19:01	
10	10:00	29.4	1.13	18:39	8:36	27.4	1.08	20:13	
5	7:54	26.4	1.05	21:05	7:16	25.5	1.02	21:57	
1	5:14	22.6	0.94	25:17	5:20	22.7	0.94	25:10	VP
	n = 1,350				n = 4,394				

Total n = 5,744

S, Superior; E, excellent; G, good; F, fair; P, poor; VP, very poor.

Reprinted with permission from the Cooper Institute, Dallas, TX. For more information: www.cooperinstitute.org.

RATIONALE

Performing fitness tests to assess muscular strength and muscular endurance before commencing exercise training or as part of a fitness screening evaluation can provide valuable information on a client's baseline fitness level. For example, muscular fitness test results can be compared with established standards and can be helpful in identifying weaknesses in certain muscle groups or muscle imbalances that could be targeted in exercise training programs. The information obtained during baseline muscular fitness assessments can also serve as a basis for designing individualized exercise training programs. An equally useful application of fitness testing is to show a client's progressive improvements over time as a result of the training program and thus provide feedback that is often beneficial in promoting long-term exercise adherence.

TABLE 4.8. PERCENTILE VALUES FOR MAXIMAL
AEROBIC POWER (*Continued*)

	FEMALES								
	AGE 40–49				**AGE 50–59**				
%	**Balke Treadmill (time)**	**Max $\dot{V}O_2$ (mL/kg/ min)**	**12 min Run (miles)**	**1.5 Mile Run (time)**	**Balke Treadmill (time)**	**Max $\dot{V}O_2$ (mL/kg/ min)**	**12 min Run (miles)**	**1.5 Mile Run (time)**	
99	25:00	51.1	1.74	10:09	21:00	45.3	1.57	11:34	
95	20:56	45.2	1.57	11:35	17:16	39.9	1.42	13:16	S
90	19:00	42.4	1.49	12:25	16:00	38.1	1.37	13:58	
85	17:20	40.0	1.43	13:14	15:00	36.7	1.33	14:33	
80	16:34	38.9	1.40	13:38	14:00	35.2	1.29	15:14	E
75	16:00	38.1	1.37	13:58	13:15	34.1	1.26	15:47	
70	15:00	36.7	1.33	14:33	12:23	32.9	1.23	16:26	
65	14:14	35.6	1.30	15:03	12:00	32.3	1.21	16:46	
60	13:56	35.1	1.29	15:17	11:23	31.4	1.19	17:19	G
55	13:02	33.8	1.25	15:56	11:00	30.9	1.17	17:38	
50	12:39	33.3	1.24	16:13	10:30	30.2	1.15	18:05	
45	12:00	32.3	1.21	16:46	10:00	29.4	1.13	18:39	
40	11:30	31.6	1.19	17:11	9:30	28.7	1.11	19:10	F
35	11:00	30.9	1.17	17:38	9:00	28.0	1.09	19:43	
30	10:10	29.7	1.14	18:26	8:30	27.3	1.07	20:17	
25	10:00	29.4	1.13	18:39	8:00	26.6	1.05	20:55	
20	9:00	28.0	1.09	19:43	7:15	25.5	1.02	21:57	P
15	8:07	26.7	1.06	20:49	6:40	24.6	1.00	22:53	
10	7:21	25.6	1.03	21:52	6:00	23.7	0.97	23:55	
5	6:17	24.1	0.98	23:27	4:48	21.9	0.92	26:15	
1	4:00	20.8	0.89	27:55	3:00	19.3	0.85	30:34	VP
	n = 4,834				n = 3,103				

Total n = 7,937

S, Superior; E, excellent; G, good; F, fair; P, poor; VP, very poor.

Reprinted with permission from the Cooper Institute, Dallas, TX. For more information: www.cooperinstitute.org.

PRINCIPLES

Muscle function tests are very specific to the muscle group tested, the type of contraction, the velocity of muscle movement, the type of equipment, and the joint range of motion. Results of any one test are specific to the procedures used, and no single test exists for evaluating total body muscular endurance or muscular strength. Unfortunately, few muscle endurance or strength tests control for repetition duration (speed of movement) or range of motion, thus results are difficult to interpret. Individuals should participate in familiarization/practice sessions with the equipment and adhere to a specific protocol (including a predetermined repetition duration and range of motion) to obtain a reliable score that can be used to track true physiologic adaptations over time. Moreover, proper warm-up consisting of 5 to 10 minutes of brief cardiovascular exercise, light stretching, and several light repetitions of the

TABLE 4.8. PERCENTILE VALUES FOR MAXIMAL
AEROBIC POWER (Continued)

	FEMALES							
	AGE 60–69				AGE 70–79			
%	Balke Treadmill (time)	Max $\dot{V}O_2$ (mL/kg/min)	12 min Run (miles)	1.5 Mile Run (time)	Balke Treadmill (time)	Max $\dot{V}O_2$ (mL/kg/min)	12 min Run (miles)	1.5 Mile Run (time)	
99	19:00	42.4	1.49	12:25	19:00	42.4	1.49	12:25	
95	15:09	36.9	1.34	14:28	15:00	36.7	1.33	14:33	S
90	13:33	34.6	1.27	15:32	12:50	33.5	1.25	16:06	
85	12:28	33.0	1.23	16:22	11:46	32.0	1.20	16:57	
80	12:00	32.3	1.21	16:46	10:30	30.2	1.15	18:05	E
75	11:04	31.0	1.18	17:34	10:00	29.4	1.13	18:39	
70	10:30	30.2	1.15	18:05	9:15	28.4	1.10	19:24	
65	10:00	29.4	1.13	18:39	8:43	27.6	1.08	20:02	
60	9:44	29.1	1.12	18:52	8:00	26.6	1.05	20:54	G
55	9:11	28.3	1.10	19:29	7:37	26.0	1.04	21:45	
50	8:40	27.5	1.08	20:08	7:00	25.1	1.01	22:22	
45	8:15	26.9	1.06	20:38	6:39	24.6	1.00	22:54	
40	8:00	26.6	1.05	20:55	6:05	23.8	0.98	23:47	F
35	7:14	25.4	1.02	22:03	5:28	22.9	0.95	24:54	
30	6:52	24.9	1.01	22:34	5:00	22.2	0.93	25:49	
25	6:21	24.2	0.99	23:20	4:45	21.9	0.92	26:15	
20	6:00	23.7	0.97	23:55	4:16	21.2	0.90	27:17	P
15	5:25	22.8	0.95	25:02	4:00	20.8	0.89	27:55	
10	4:40	21.7	0.92	26:32	3:00	19.3	0.85	30:34	
5	3:30	20.1	0.87	29:06	2:00	17.9	0.81	33:32	
1	2:10	18.1	0.82	33:05	1:00	16.4	0.77	37:26	VP
	n = 1,088				n = 209				

Total n = 1,297

S, superior; E, excellent; G, good; F, fair; P, poor; VP, very poor.

Reprinted with permission from the Cooper Institute, Dallas, Texas. For more information:www.cooperinstitute.org

specific testing exercise should precede muscular fitness testing. This increases muscle temperature and localized blood flow as well as promotes appropriate cardiovascular responses to exercise. A summary of standardized conditions include:

- Strict posture
- Consistent repetition duration (movement speed)
- Full range of motion
- Use of spotters (when necessary)
- Equipment familiarization
- Proper warm-up

A change in one's muscular fitness over time can be based on the absolute value of the external load or resistance (e.g., newtons, kilograms [kg], or pounds

[lb]), but when comparisons are made between individuals, the values should be expressed as relative values (per kilogram of body weight [kg/kg]). In both cases, caution must be used in the interpretation of the scores because the norms may not include a representative sample of the individual being measured, a standardized protocol may be absent, or the exact test being used (free weight versus machine weight) may differ.

MUSCULAR STRENGTH

Although muscular strength refers to the external force (properly expressed in newtons, although kilograms and pounds are commonly used as well) that can be generated by a specific muscle or muscle group, it is commonly expressed in terms of resistance lifted. Strength can be assessed either statically (no overt muscular movement or limb movement) or dynamically (movement of an external load or body part, in which the muscle changes length). Static or isometric strength can be measured conveniently using a variety of devices, including cable tensiometers and handgrip dynamometers. Unfortunately, measures of static strength are specific to both the muscle group and joint angle involved in testing; therefore, their utility in describing overall muscular strength is limited. Peak force development in such tests is commonly referred to as the maximum voluntary contraction (MVC).

Traditionally, the one-repetition maximum (1-RM), the greatest resistance that can be moved through the full range of motion in a controlled manner with good posture, has been the standard for dynamic strength assessment. However, a multiple RM can be used, such as 4- or 8-RM, as a measure of muscular strength, which may allow the participant to integrate evaluation into their training program. For example, if one were training with 6- to 8-RM, the performance of a 6-RM to momentary muscular fatigue would provide an index of strength changes over time, independent of the true 1-RM. Estimating a 1-RM from such tests is problematic and generally not necessary. The number of lifts one can perform at a fixed percent of a 1-RM for different muscle groups (e.g., leg press versus bench press) varies tremendously, thus rendering an estimate of 1-RM impractical (29,31). However, the true 1-RM is still a popular measure (41). Valid measures of general upper-body strength include the 1-RM values for bench press or military press. Corresponding indices of lower-body strength include 1-RM values for leg press or leg extension. Norms, based on resistance lifted divided by body mass for the bench press and leg press are provided in Tables 4.9 and 4.10, respectively. The following represents the basic steps in 1-RM (or any multiple RM) testing following familiarization/practice sessions (41):

1. The subject should warm up by completing several submaximal repetitions.
2. Determine the 1-RM (or any multiple RM) within four trials with rest periods of 3 to 5 minutes between trials.
3. Select an initial weight that is within the subject's perceived capacity (~50%–70% of capacity).
4. Resistance is progressively increased by 2.5 to 20 kg until the subject cannot complete the selected repetition(s); all repetitions should be performed at the same speed of movement and range of motion to instill consistency between trials.
5. The final weight lifted successfully is recorded as the absolute 1-RM or multiple RM.

TABLE 4.9. UPPER BODY STRENGTH[a]

MALES

Bench Press Weight Ratio $= \dfrac{\text{weight pushed in lbs}}{\text{body weight in lbs}}$

%	<20	20–29	30–39	40–49	50–59	60+	
99	>1.76	>1.63	>1.35	>1.20	>1.05	>.94	
95	1.76	1.63	1.35	1.20	1.05	.94	S
90	1.46	1.48	1.24	1.10	.97	.89	
85	1.38	1.37	1.17	1.04	.93	.84	
80	1.34	1.32	1.12	1.00	.90	.82	E
75	1.29	1.26	1.08	.96	.87	.79	
70	1.24	1.22	1.04	.93	.84	.77	
65	1.23	1.18	1.01	.90	.81	.74	
60	1.19	1.14	.98	.88	.79	.72	G
55	1.16	1.10	.96	.86	.77	.70	
50	1.13	1.06	.93	.84	.75	.68	
45	1.10	1.03	.90	.82	.73	.67	
40	1.06	.99	.88	.80	.71	.66	F
35	1.01	.96	.86	.78	.70	.65	
30	.96	.93	.83	.76	.68	.63	
25	.93	.90	.81	.74	.66	.60	
20	.89	.88	.78	.72	.63	.57	P
15	.86	.84	.75	.69	.60	.56	
10	.81	.80	.71	.65	.57	.53	
5	.76	.72	.65	.59	.53	.49	
1	<.76	<.72	<.65	<.59	<.53	<.49	VP
n	60	425	1,909	2,090	1,279	343	

Total n = 6,106

FEMALES

AGE

%	<20	20–29	30–39	40–49	50–59	60+	
99	>.88	>1.01	>.82	>.77	>.68	>.72	
95	.88	1.01	.82	.77	.68	.72	S
90	.83	.90	.76	.71	.61	.64	
85	.81	.83	.72	.66	.57	.59	
80	.77	.80	.70	.62	.55	.54	E
75	.76	.77	.65	.60	.53	.53	
70	.74	.74	.63	.57	.52	.51	
65	.70	.72	.62	.55	.50	.48	
60	.65	.70	.60	.54	.48	.47	G
55	.64	.68	.58	.53	.47	.46	
50	.63	.65	.57	.52	.46	.45	
45	.60	.63	.55	.51	.45	.44	
40	.58	.59	.53	.50	.44	.43	F

(Continued)

TABLE 4.9. UPPER BODY STRENGTH[a] (Continued)

FEMALES AGE

35	.57	.58	.52	.48	.43	.41	
30	.56	.56	.51	.47	.42	.40	
25	.55	.53	.49	.45	.41	.39	
20	.53	.51	.47	.43	.39	.38	P
15	.52	.50	.45	.42	.38	.36	
10	.50	.48	.42	.38	.37	.33	
5	.41	.44	.39	.35	.31	.26	
1	<.41	<.44	<.39	<.35	<.31	<.26	VP
n	20	191	379	333	189	42	

Total n = 1,154

S, superior; E, excellent; G, good; F, fair; P, poor; VP, very poor.

[a]One repetition maximum bench press, with bench press weight ratio = weight pushed in pounds/body weight in pounds.

Reprinted with permission from The Cooper Institute, Dallas, Texas. For more information: www.cooperinstitute.org.

TABLE 4.10. LEG STRENGTH[a]

PERCENTILE	AGE				
	20–29	30–39	40–49	50–59	60+
Men					
90	2.27	2.07	1.92	1.80	1.73
80	2.13	1.93	1.82	1.71	1.62
70	2.05	1.85	1.74	1.64	1.56
60	1.97	1.77	1.68	1.58	1.49
50	1.91	1.71	1.62	1.52	1.43
40	1.83	1.65	1.57	1.46	1.38
30	1.74	1.59	1.51	1.39	1.30
20	1.63	1.52	1.44	1.32	1.25
10	1.51	1.43	1.35	1.22	1.16
Women					
90	1.82	1.61	1.48	1.37	1.32
80	1.68	1.47	1.37	1.25	1.18
70	1.58	1.39	1.29	1.17	1.13
60	1.50	1.33	1.23	1.10	1.04
50	1.44	1.27	1.18	1.05	0.99
40	1.37	1.21	1.13	0.99	0.93
30	1.27	1.15	1.08	0.95	0.88
20	1.22	1.09	1.02	0.88	0.85
10	1.14	1.00	0.94	0.78	0.72

[a]One repetition maximum leg press with leg press weight ratio = weight pushed/body weight.

Adapted from Institute for Aerobics Research, Dallas, 1994. Study population for the data set was predominantly white and college educated. A Universal DVR machine was used to measure the 1-RM. The following may be used as descriptors for the percentile rankings: well above average (90), above average (70), average (50), below average (30), and well below average (10).

Isokinetic testing involves the assessment of maximal muscle tension through-out a range of joint motion set at a constant angular velocity (e.g., 60 angles/sec). Equipment that allows control of the speed of joint rotation (degrees/sec) as well as the ability to test movement around various joints (e.g., knee, hip, shoulder, elbow) is available from commercial sources. Such devices measure peak rotational force or torque, but an important drawback is that this equipment is extremely expensive compared with other strength-testing modalities (25).

MUSCULAR ENDURANCE

Muscular endurance is the ability of a muscle group to execute repeated contractions over a period of time sufficient to cause muscular fatigue, or to maintain a specific percentage of the MVC for a prolonged period of time. If the total number of repetitions at a given amount of resistance is measured, the result is termed *absolute muscular endurance*. If the number of repetitions performed at a percentage of the 1-RM (e.g., 70%) is used both pre- and posttesting, the result is termed *relative muscular endurance*. Simple field tests such as a curl-up (crunch) test (12,25) or the maximum number of push-ups that can be performed without rest (12) may be used to evaluate the endurance of the abdominal muscle groups and upper-body muscles, respectively. Although scientific data to support a cause-effect relationship between abdominal strength and low back pain are lacking, poor abdominal strength or endurance is commonly thought to contribute to muscular low back pain (17,18). Procedures for conducting the push-up and curl-up (crunch) muscular endurance tests are given in Box 4.6, and fitness categories are provided in Tables 4.11 and 4.12, respectively.

Resistance-training equipment also can be adapted to measure muscular endurance by selecting an appropriate submaximal level of resistance and measuring the number of repetitions or the duration of static contraction before fatigue. For example, the YMCA bench-press test involves performing standardized

---

BOX 4.6 | **Push-up and Curl-up (Crunch) Test Procedures for Measurement of Muscular Endurance**

PUSH-UP

1. The push-up test is administered with male subjects starting in the standard "down" position (hands pointing forward and under the shoulder, back straight, head up, using the toes as the pivotal point) and female subjects in the modified "knee push-up" position (legs together, lower leg in contact with mat with ankles plantar-flexed, back straight, hands shoulder width apart, head up, using the knees as the pivotal point).
2. The subject must raise the body by straightening the elbows and return to the "down" position, until the chin touches the mat. The stomach should not touch the mat.
3. For both men and women, the subject's back must be straight at all times and the subject must push up to a straight arm position. ➤

> Box 4.6. continued

4. The maximal number of push-ups performed consecutively without rest is counted as the score.
5. The test is stopped when the client strains forcibly or is unable to maintain the appropriate technique within two repetitions.

CURL-UP (CRUNCH)

1. The individual assumes a supine position on a mat with the knees at 90 degrees. The arms are at the side, palms facing down with the middle fingers touching a piece of masking tape. A second piece of masking tape is placed 10 cm apart.[a] Shoes remain on during the test.
2. A metronome is set to 50 beats $\cdot$ min^{-1} and the individual does slow, controlled curl-ups to lift the shoulder blades off the mat (trunk makes a 30-degree angle with the mat) in time with the metronome at a rate of 25 per minute. The test is done for 1 minute. The low back should be flattened before curling up.
3. Individual performs as many curl-ups as possible without pausing, to a maximum of 25.[b]

[a]Alternatives include (a) having the hands held across the chest, with the head activating a counter when the trunk reaches a 30-degree position (17) and placing the hands on the thighs and curling up until the hands reach the knee caps (18). Elevation of the trunk to 30 degrees is the important aspect of the movement.

[b]An alternative includes doing as many curl-ups as possible in 1 minute.

From Canadian Society for Exercise Physiology. *Canadian Physical Activity, Fitness & Lifestyle Approach: CSEP-Health & Fitness Program's Appraisal & Counseling Strategy.* 3rd ed. Ottawa (ON): Canadian Society for Exercise Physiology; 2003, with permission.

TABLE 4.11. FITNESS CATEGORIES BY AGE GROUPS AND SEX FOR PUSH-UPS

| CATEGORY | AGE | | | | | | | | | |
| | 20–29 | | 30–39 | | 40–49 | | 50–59 | | 60–69 | |
SEX	M	F	M	F	M	F	M	F	M	F
Excellent	36	30	30	27	25	24	21	21	18	17
Very good	35	29	29	26	24	23	20	20	17	16
	29	21	22	20	17	15	13	11	11	12
Good	28	20	21	19	16	14	12	10	10	11
	22	15	17	13	13	11	10	7	8	5
Fair	21	14	16	12	12	10	9	6	7	4
	17	10	12	8	10	5	7	2	5	2
Needs improvement	16	9	11	7	9	4	6	1	4	1

M, male; F, female.

Source: Canadian Physical Activity, Fitness & Lifestyle Approach: CSEP-Health & Fitness Program's Appraisal & Counseling Strategy, 3rd ed, ©2003. Used with permission from the Canadian Society for Exercise Physiology.

TABLE 4.12. FITNESS CATEGORIES BY AGE GROUPS AND SEX FOR PARTIAL CURL-UP

CATEGORY	AGE									
	20–29		30–39		40–49		50–59		60–69	
SEX	M	F	M	F	M	F	M	F	M	F
Excellent	25	25	25	25	25	25	25	25	25	25
Very good	24	24	24	24	24	24	24	24	24	24
	21	18	18	19	18	19	17	19	16	17
Good	20	17	17	18	17	18	16	18	15	16
	16	14	15	10	13	11	11	10	11	8
Fair	15	13	14	9	12	10	10	9	10	7
	11	5	11	6	6	4	8	6	6	3
Needs improvement	10	4	10	5	5	3	7	5	5	2

M, male; F, female.

Source: Canadian Physical Activity, Fitness & Lifestyle Approach: CSEP-Health & Fitness Program's Appraisal & Counseling Strategy, 3rd ed, ©2003. Used with permission from the Canadian Society for Exercise Physiology.

repetitions at a rate of 30 lifts or reps·min^{-1}. Men are tested using an 80-pound (36.3-kg) barbell and women using a 35-pound (15.9-kg) barbell. Subjects are scored by the number of successful repetitions completed (24). The YMCA test is an excellent example of a test that attempts to control for repetition duration and posture alignment, thus possessing high reliability. Normative data for the YMCA bench press test are presented in Table 4.13.

TABLE 4.13. YMCA BENCH PRESS TEST: TOTAL LIFTS

CATEGORY	AGE											
	18–25		26–35		36–45		46–55		56–65		>65	
SEX	M	F	M	F	M	F	M	F	M	F	M	F
Excellent	64	66	61	62	55	57	47	50	41	42	36	30
	44	42	41	40	36	33	28	29	24	24	20	18
Good	41	38	37	34	32	30	25	24	21	21	16	16
	34	30	30	29	26	26	21	20	17	17	12	12
Above average	33	28	29	28	25	24	20	18	14	14	10	10
	29	25	26	24	22	21	16	14	12	12	9	8
Average	28	22	24	22	21	20	14	13	11	10	8	7
	24	20	21	18	18	16	12	10	9	8	7	5
Below average	22	18	20	17	17	14	11	9	8	6	6	4
	20	16	17	14	14	12	9	7	5	5	4	3
Poor	17	13	16	13	12	10	8	6	4	4	3	2
	13	9	12	9	9	6	5	2	2	2	2	0
Very poor	<10	6	9	6	6	4	2	1	1	1	1	0

M, male. F, female.

Reprinted with permission from Golding LA, editor. *YMCA Fitness Testing and Assessment Manual*, 4th ed. Champaign (IL): Human Kinetics; 2000.

SPECIAL CONSIDERATIONS

Older Adults

The number of older adults in the United States is expected to increase exponentially over the next several decades. As people are living longer, it is becoming increasingly more important to find ways to extend active, healthy lifestyles and reduce physical frailty in later years. Assessing muscular strength, muscular endurance, and other aspects of health-related physical fitness in older adults can aid in detecting physical weaknesses and yield important information used to design exercise programs that improve strength before serious functional limitations occur. The Senior Fitness Test (SFT) was developed in response to a need for improved assessment tools for older persons (58). The test was designed to assess the key physiologic parameters (e.g., strength, endurance, agility, and balance) needed to perform common everyday physical activities that are often difficult in later years. One aspect of the SFT is the 30-second chair-stand test. This test, and others of the SFT, meets scientific standards for reliability and validity, is simple and easy to administer in the "field" setting, and has accompanying performance norms for older men and women ages 60 to 94 years based on a study of more than 7,000 older Americans (58). This test has been shown to correlate well with other muscular fitness tests, such as the 1-RM. Two specific tests included in the SFT, the 30-second chair stand and the single arm curl, can be used by the health/fitness professional to safely and effectively assess muscular strength and muscular endurance in most older adults.

Coronary-Prone Clients

Moderate-intensity resistance training performed 2 to 3 days per week has been shown to be effective for improving muscular fitness, preventing and managing a variety of chronic medical conditions, modifying coronary risk factors, and enhancing psychosocial well-being for persons with and without cardiovascular disease. Consequently, authoritative professional health organizations, including the American Heart Association and ACSM, support the inclusion of resistance training as an adjunct to endurance-type exercise in their current recommendations and guidelines on exercise for individuals with cardiovascular disease (55).

The absence of anginal symptoms, ischemic ST-segment changes on the ECG, abnormal hemodynamics, and complex ventricular dysrhythmias suggests that both moderate-to-high intensity (e.g., 40%–80% 1-RM) resistance testing and training can be performed safely by cardiac patients deemed low risk (e.g., persons without resting or exercise-induced evidence of myocardial ischemia, severe left ventricular dysfunction, or complex ventricular dysrhythmias, and with normal or near-normal CR fitness; see Box 2.3). Moreover, despite concerns that resistance exercise elicits abnormal cardiovascular "pressor responses" in patients with coronary artery disease and/or controlled hypertension, studies have found that strength testing and resistance training in these patients elicit HR and BP responses that appear to fall within clinically acceptable limits. Specific data on the safety of muscular fitness testing in moderate-to-high–risk cardiac patients, especially those with poor left ventricular function, are limited and require additional investigation (55).

Contemporary exercise guidelines suggest that contraindications to muscular strength and muscular endurance testing should include unstable angina, uncontrolled hypertension (systolic BP $\geq$160 mm Hg and/or diastolic BP $\geq$100 mm Hg), uncontrolled dysrhythmias, a recent history of heart failure that has not been evaluated and effectively treated, severe stenotic or regurgitant valvular disease, and hypertrophic cardiomyopathy. Because patients with myocardial ischemia or poor left ventricular function may develop wall-motion abnormalities or serious ventricular arrhythmias during resistance-related exertion, moderate to good left ventricular function and CR fitness (>5 or 6 METs) without anginal symptoms or ischemic ST segment changes have been suggested as additional prerequisites for participation in traditional resistance-training programs and, thus, for testing of muscular strength and muscular endurance (21,55). As with graded exercise testing, the risk of a serious cardiac event during muscular strength and muscular endurance testing can be minimized by proper preparticipation screening and close supervision by health/fitness instructors.

Children and Adolescents

Along with CR fitness, flexibility, and body composition, muscular fitness is recognized as an important component of health-related fitness in children and adolescents. The benefits of enhancing muscular strength and muscular endurance in youth include developing proper posture, reducing the risk of injury, improving body composition, and enhancing motor performance skills such as sprinting and jumping. Assessing muscular strength and muscular endurance with the push-up and abdominal curl-up is common practice in most physical education programs, YMCA/YWCA recreation programs, and youth sport centers. Standardized testing procedures have been developed for youth, and normative data for children and teenagers are available in most physical education text books.

When properly administered, different muscular fitness measures can be used to assess a child's strengths and weaknesses, develop a personalized fitness program, track progress, and motivate participants. Conversely, unsupervised or poorly administered muscular fitness assessments may not only discourage youth from participating in fitness activities, but may also result in injury. Qualified fitness professionals should demonstrate the proper performance of each skill, provide an opportunity for each child to practice a few repetitions of each skill, and offer guidance and instruction when necessary. In addition, it is important and usually required to obtain informed consent from the parent or legal guardian before initiating muscular fitness testing. The informed consent includes information on potential benefits and risks, the right to withdraw at any time, and issues regarding confidentiality.

When assessing muscular fitness in youth, it is important to avoid the "pass-fail" mentality that may discourage some boys and girls from participating. Instead, consider referring to the assessment as a "challenge" in which all participants can feel good about their performance and get excited about monitoring their progress. Fitness professionals should also understand that children are not simply "miniature" adults. Because children are physically and psychologically less mature than adults, the assessment of any physical fitness measure requires special considerations. Fitness professionals should develop a friendly rapport with each child, and the exercise area should be nonthreatening. Because most children have limited experience performing maximum exertion, fitness professionals should reassure children that they can safely perform exercise at a high level of exertion. Moreover, positive encouragement serves as a useful motivational tool to help ensure a valid test outcome.

FLEXIBILITY

Flexibility is the ability to move a joint through its complete range of motion. It is important in athletic performance (e.g., ballet, gymnastics) and in the ability to carry out the activities of daily living. Consequently, maintaining flexibility of all joints facilitates movement; in contrast, when an activity moves the structures of a joint beyond a joint's shortened range of motion, tissue damage can occur.

Flexibility depends on several specific variables, including distensibility of the joint capsule, adequate warm-up, and muscle viscosity. Additionally, compliance ("tightness") of various other tissues, such as ligaments and tendons, affects the range of motion. Just as muscular strength is specific to the muscles involved, flexibility is joint specific; therefore, no single flexibility test can be used to evaluate total body flexibility. Laboratory tests usually quantify flexibility in terms of range of motion, expressed in degrees. Common devices for this purpose include various goniometers, electrogoniometers, the Leighton flexometer, inclinometers, and tape measures. Comprehensive instructions are available for the evaluation of flexibility of most anatomic joints (14,53). Visual estimates of range of motion can be useful in fitness screening but are inaccurate relative to directly measured range of motion. These estimates can include neck and trunk flexibility, hip flexibility, lower-extremity flexibility, shoulder flexibility, and postural assessment. A more precise measurement of joint range of motion can be assessed at most anatomic joints following strict procedures (14,53) and the proper use of a goniometer. Accurate measurements require in-depth knowledge of bone, muscle, and joint anatomy, as well as experience in administering the evaluation. Table 4.14 provides normative range of motion values for select anatomic joints. Additional information can be found in the ACSM Resource Manual.

The sit-and-reach test has been used commonly to assess low-back and hip-joint flexibility; however, its relationship to predict the incidence of low-back pain is limited (35). The sit-and-reach test is suggested to be a better measure of hamstring flexibility than low-back flexibility (34). However, the relative importance of hamstring flexibility to activities of daily living and sports performance requires the inclusion of the sit-and-reach test for health-related fitness testing until a criterion measure evaluation of low-back flexibility is available. Although limb- and torso-length disparity may affect the sit-and-reach scoring, modified testing that establishes an individual zero point for each participant has not enhanced the predictive index for low-back flexibility or low-back pain (11,30,47).

Poor lower-back and hip flexibility may, in conjunction with poor abdominal strength/endurance or other causative factors, contribute to development of muscular low-back pain; however, this hypothesis remains to be substantiated (57). Methods for administering the sit-and-reach test are presented in Box 4.7. Normative data for two sit-and-reach tests are presented in Tables 4.15 and 4.16.

TABLE 4.14. RANGE OF MOTION OF SELECT SINGLE JOINT MOVEMENTS (DEGREES)

SHOULDER GIRDLE

Flexion	90–120	Extension	20–60
Abduction	80–100		
Horizontal abduction	30–45	Horizontal adduction	90–135
Medial rotation	70–90	Lateral rotation	70–90

ELBOW

Flexion	135–160		
Supination	75–90	Pronation	75–90

TRUNK

Flexion	120–150	Extension	20–45
Lateral flexion	10–35	Rotation	20–40

HIP

Flexion	90–135	Extension	10–30
Abduction	30–50	Adduction	10–30
Medial rotation	30–45	Lateral rotation	45–60

KNEE

Flexion	130–140	Extension	5–10

ANKLE

Dorsiflexion	15–20	Plantarflexion	30–50
Inversion	10–30	Eversion	10–20

Adapted from Norkin C, Levangie P. *Joint Structure and Function: A Comprehensive Approach*. 2nd ed. Philadelphia (PA): Davis FA; 1992.

BOX 4.7 Trunk Flexion (Sit-and-Reach) Test Procedures

Pretest: Participant should perform a short warm-up before this test and include some stretches (e.g., modified hurdler's stretch). It is also recommended that the participant refrain from fast, jerky movements, which may increase the possibility of an injury. The participant's shoes should be removed.

1. For the Canadian Trunk Forward Flexion test, the client sits without shoes and the soles of the feet flat against the flexometer (sit-and-reach box) at the 26-cm mark. Inner edges of the soles are placed within 2 cm of the measuring scale. For the YMCA sit-and-reach test, a yardstick is placed on the floor and tape is placed across it at a right angle to the 15-inch mark. The participant sits with the yardstick between the legs, with legs extended at right angles to the taped line on the floor. Heels of the feet should touch the edge of the taped line and be about 10 to 12 inches apart. (Note the zero point at the foot/box interface and use the appropriate norms.) >

> Box 4.7. continued

2. The participant should slowly reach forward with both hands as far as possible, holding this position ~2 seconds. Be sure that the participant keeps the hands parallel and does not lead with one hand. Fingertips can be overlapped and should be in contact with the measuring portion or yardstick of the sit-and-reach box.
3. The score is the most distant point (in centimeters or inches) reached with the fingertips. The best of two trials should be recorded. To assist with the best attempt, the participant should exhale and drop the head between the arms when reaching. Testers should ensure that the knees of the participant stay extended; however, the participant's knees should not be pressed down. The participant should breathe normally during the test and should not hold his or her breath at any time. Norms for the Canadian test are presented in Table 4.15. Note that these norms use a sit-and-reach box in which the zero point is set at the 26-cm mark. If you are using a box in which the zero point is set at 23 cm (e.g., Fitnessgram), subtract 3 cm from each value in this table. The norms for the YMCA test are presented in Table 4.16.

From Golding LA, editor. *YMCA Fitness Testing and Assessment Manual.* 4th ed. Champaign (IL): Human Kinetics; 2000; Canadian Society for Exercise Physiology. *Canadian Physical Activity, Fitness & Lifestyle Approach: CSEP-Health & Fitness Program's Appraisal & Counseling Strategy.* 3rd ed. Ottawa (ON): Canadian Society for Exercise Physiology; 2003.

TABLE 4.15. FITNESS CATEGORIES BY AGE GROUPS FOR TRUNK FORWARD FLEXION USING A SIT-AND-REACH BOX (cm)[a]

| CATEGORY | AGE | | | | | | | | | |
| | 20–29 | | 30–39 | | 40–49 | | 50–59 | | 60–69 | |
SEX	M	F	M	F	M	F	M	F	M	F
Excellent	40	41	38	41	35	38	35	39	33	35
Very good	39	40	37	40	34	37	34	38	32	34
	34	37	33	36	29	34	28	33	25	31
Good	33	36	32	35	28	33	27	32	24	30
	30	33	28	32	24	30	24	30	20	27
Fair	29	32	27	31	23	29	23	29	19	26
	25	28	23	27	18	25	16	25	15	23
Needs improvement	24	27	22	26	17	24	15	24	14	22

M, male; F, female.

[a]Note: These norms are based on a sit-and-reach box in which the zero point is set at 26 cm. When using a box in which the zero point is set at 23 cm, subtract 3 cm from each value in this table.

Source: *Canadian Physical Activity, Fitness & Lifestyle Approach: CSEP-Health & Fitness Program's Appraisal & Counseling Strategy,* 3rd ed, © 2003. Used with permission from the Canadian Society for Exercise Physiology.

TABLE 4.16. PERCENTILES BY AGE GROUPS AND SEX FOR YMCA SIT-AND-REACH TEST (INCHES)

	AGE										
PERCENTILE	18–25		26–35		36–45		46–55		56–65		>65	
SEX	M	F	M	F	M	F	M	F	M	F	M	F
90	22	24	21	23	21	22	19	21	17	20	17	20
80	20	22	19	21	19	21	17	20	15	19	15	18
70	19	21	17	20	17	19	15	18	13	17	13	17
60	18	20	17	20	16	18	14	17	13	16	12	17
50	17	19	15	19	15	17	13	16	11	15	10	15
40	15	18	14	17	13	16	11	14	9	14	9	14
30	14	17	13	16	13	15	10	14	9	13	8	13
20	13	16	11	15	11	14	9	12	7	11	7	11
10	11	14	9	13	7	12	6	10	5	9	4	9

M, male; F, female.

The following may be used as descriptors for the percentile rankings: well above average (90), above average (70), average (50), below average (30), and well below average (10).

Reprinted with permission from Golding LA, editor. *YMCA Fitness Testing and Assessment Manual.* 4th ed. Champaign (IL): Human Kinetics; 2000;200–211.

A COMPREHENSIVE HEALTH FITNESS EVALUATION

A typical fitness assessment includes the following:

- Prescreening/risk stratification
- Resting HR, BP, height, weight, BMI, ECG (if appropriate)
- Body composition
  - Waist circumference
  - Skinfold assessment
- Cardiorespiratory fitness
  - Submaximal YMCA cycle ergometer test or treadmill test
- Muscular strength
  - 1-, 4-, 6-, or 8-RM upper body (bench press) and lower body (leg press)
- Muscular endurance
  - Curl-up test
  - Push-up test
- Flexibility
  - Sit-and-reach test or goniometric measures of isolated anatomic joints

Additional evaluations may be administered; however, the aforementioned components of a fitness evaluation represent a comprehensive assessment that can be performed within 1 hour. The data accrued from the evaluation should be interpreted by a competent professional and conveyed to the client. This information is central to the development of a client's short- and long-term goals, as well as forming the basis for the initial exercise prescription and subsequent evaluations to monitor progress.

REFERENCES

1. American College of Sports Medicine. Position Stand: The recommended quantity and quality of exercise for developing and maintaining cardiorespiratory and muscular fitness, and flexibility in healthy adults. *Med Sci Sports Exerc.* 1998;30:975–91.
2. Astrand PO. Aerobic work capacity in men and women with special reference to age. *Acta Physiol Scand.* 1960;49(suppl):45–60.
3. Astrand PO, Ryhming I. A nomogram for calculation of aerobic capacity (physical fitness) from pulse rate during submaximal work. *J Appl Physiol.* 1954;7:218–21.
4. Bittner V, Weiner DH, Yusuf S, et al. Prediction of mortality and morbidity with a 6-minute walk test in patients with left ventricular dysfunction. *JAMA.* 1993;270:1702–7.
5. Blair SN, Kohl HW, Barlow CE, et al. Changes in physical fitness and all-cause mortality: a prospective study of healthy and unhealthy men. *JAMA.* 1995;273:1093–8.
6. Blair SN, Kohl HW, Paffenbarger Jr RS, et al. Physical fitness and all-cause mortality: a prospective study of healthy men and women. *JAMA.* 1989;262:2395–2401.
7. Bray GA. Don't throw the baby out with the bath water. *Am J Clin Nutr.* 2004;79:347–9.
8. Bray GA, Gray DS. Obesity. Part I. Pathogenesis. *West J Med.* 1988;149:429–41.
9. Brozek J, Grade F, Anderson J. Densitometric analysis of body composition: revision of some quantitative assumptions. *Ann N Y Acad Sci.* 1963;110:113–40.
10. Cahalin LP, Mathier MA, Semigran MJ, et al. The six minute walk test predicts peak oxygen uptake and survival in patients with advanced heart failure. *Chest.* 1996;110:325–32.
11. Cailliet R. *Low Back Pain Syndrome.* Philadelphia (PA): FA Davis; 1988. p. 175–9.
12. Canadian Society for Exercise Physiology. *The Canadian Physical Activity, Fitness & Lifestyle Approach: CSEP-Health & Fitness Program's Health-Related Appraisal & Counseling Strategy.* 3rd ed. Canadian Society for Exercise Physiology, 2003;Ontario, Canada.
13. Caspersen CJ, Powell KE, Christenson GM. Physical activity, exercise, and physical fitness: definitions and distinctions for health-related research. *Public Health Rep.* 1985;100:126–31.
14. Clarkson H. *Musculoskeletal Assessment, Joint Range of Motion and Manual Muscle Strength.* Baltimore: Lippincott Williams & Wilkins; 1999.
15. Davis JA, editor. Direct determination of aerobic power. In: Maud PJ, Foster C, editors. *Physiological Assessment of Human Fitness.* Champaign (IL): Human Kinetics; 1995. p. 9–17.
16. Dempster P, Aitkens S. A new air displacement method for the determination of human body composition. *Med Sci Sports Exerc.* 1995;27:1692–7.
17. Diener MH, Golding LA, Diener D. Validity and reliability of a one-minute half sit-up test of abdominal muscle strength and endurance. *Sports Med Training Rehab.* 1995;6:5–119.
18. Faulkner RA, Sprigings EJ, McQuarrie A, et al. A partial curl-up protocol for adults based on an analysis of two procedures. *Can J Sport Sci.* 1989;14:135–41.
19. Flegal KM, Carroll MD, Ogden CL, et al. Prevalence and trends in obesity among US adults, 1999–2000. *JAMA.* 2002;288:1723–7.
20. Folsom AR, Kaye SA, Sellers TA, et al. Body fat distribution and 5-year risk of death in older women. *JAMA.* 1993;269:483–7.
21. Franklin BA, Gordon NF. *Contemporary Diagnosis and Management in Cardiovascular Exercise.* Newton (PA): Handbooks in Health Care; 2005.
22. Gallagher D, Heymsfield SB, Heo M, et al. Healthy percentage body fat ranges: an approach for developing guidelines based on body mass index. *Am J Clin Nutr.* 2000;72:694–701.
23. Going BS. Densitometry. In: Roche AF, Heymsfield SB, Lohman TG, editors. *Human Body Composition.* Champaign (IL): Human Kinetics; 1996. p. 3–23.
24. Golding LA, editor. *YMCA Fitness Testing and Assessment Manual.* Champaign (IL): Human Kinetics; 1989.
25. Graves JE, Pollock ML, Bryant CX. Assessment of muscular strength and endurance. In: Roitman JL, editor. *ACSM's Resource Manual for Guidelines for Exercise Testing and Prescription.* 4th ed. Baltimore (MD): Lippincott Williams & Wilkins; 2001. p. 376–80.
26. Hendel HW, Gotfredsen A, Hojgaard L, et al. Change in fat-free mass assessed by bioelectrical impedance, total body potassium and dual energy x-ray absorptiometry during prolonged weight loss. *Scand J Clin Lab Invest.* 1996;56:671–9.
27. Heyward VH. Practical body composition assessment for children, adults, and older adults. *Int J Sport Nutr.* 1998;8:285–307.
28. Heyward VH, Stolarczyk LM, editors. *Applied Body Composition Assessment.* Champaign (IL): Human Kinetics; 1996. 12 p.

29. Hoeger WW, Barette SL, Hale DR. Relationship between repetition and selected percentages of one repetition maximum. *J Appl Sport Sci Res.* 1987;1:11–3.
30. Hoeger WW, Hopkins DR. A comparison of the sit and reach and the modified sit and reach in the measurement of flexibility in women. *Res Q Exerc Sport.* 1992;63:191–5.
31. Hoeger WW, Hopkins DR, Barette SL. Relationship between repetitions and selected percentages of one repetition maximum: a comparison between untrained and trained males and females. *J Appl Sport Sci Res.* 1990;4:47–54.
32. Hornsby WG, Albright AL. Diabetes. In: Durstine JL, Moore GE, editors. *ACSM's Exercise Management for Persons with Chronic Diseases and Disabilities.* 2nd ed. Champaign (IL): Human Kinetics; 2003. p. 137.
33. Jackson AS, Pollock ML. Practical assessment of body composition. *Phys Sport Med.* 1985;13(3):76–90.
34. Jackson AW, Baker AA. The relationship of the sit and reach test to criterion measures of hamstring and back flexibility in young females. *Res Q Exerc Sport.* 1986;57(3):183–6.
35. Jackson AW, Morrow Jr JR, Brill PA, et al. Relations of sit-up and sit-and-reach tests to low back pain in adults. *J Orthop Sports Phys Ther.* 1998;27:22–6.
36. Jette M, Campbell J, Mongeon J, et al. The Canadian Home Fitness Test as a predictor for aerobic capacity. *Can Med Assoc J.* 1976;114:680–2.
37. Kaminsky LA, editor. *ACSM's Resource Manual for Guidelines for Exercise Testing and Prescription.* Baltimore (MD): Lippincott Williams & Wilkins; 2005.
38. Kline GM, Porcari JP, Hintermeister R, et al. Estimation of VO_{2max} from a one-mile track walk, gender, age, and body weight. *Med Sci Sports Exerc.* 1987;19:253–59.
39. Leger L, Thivierge M. Heart rate monitors: validity, stability and functionality. *Phys Sport Med.* 1988;16:143–51.
40. Liemohn WP, Sharpe GL, Wasserman JF. Lumbosacral movement in the sit-and-reach and in Cailliet's protective-hamstring stretch. *Spine.* 1994;19:2127–30.
41. Logan P, Fornasiero D, Abernathy P. Protocols for the assessment of isoinertial strength. In: Fore CJ, editor. *Physiological tests for elite athletes.* Champaign (IL): Human Kinetics; 2000. p. 200–21.
42. Lohman TG. Body composition methodology in sports medicine. *Phys Sportsmed.* 1982;10:47–58.
43. Lohman TG, Houtkooper L, Going SB. Body fat measurement goes high-tech. *ACSM's Health Fitness J.* 1997;1(1):30–5.
44. Maritz JS, Morrison JF, Peter J. A practical method of estimating an individual's maximal oxygen uptake. *Ergonomics.* 1961;4:97–122.
45. McConnell TR. Cardiorespiratory assessment of apparently healthy populations. In: Roitman JL, editor. *ACSM Resource Manual for Guidelines for Exercise Testing and Prescription.* 4th ed. Baltimore (MD): Williams & Wilkins; 2001. p. 361–75.
46. Mclean KP, Skinner JS. Validity of Futrex-5000 for body composition determination. *Med Sci Sports Exerc.* 1992;24:253–8.
47. Minkler S, Patterson P. The validity of the modified sit-and-reach test in college-age students. *Res Q Exerc Sport.* 1994;65:189–92.
48. Morgan W, Borg GA. Perception of effort in the prescription of physical activity. In: Nelson T, editor. *Mental Health and Emotional Aspects of Sports.* Chicago (IL): American Medical Association; 1976. p. 126–9.
49. National Institutes of Health. Health implications of obesity. *Ann Intern Med.* 1985;163:1073–7.
50. Noble BJ, Borg GA, Jacobs I, et al. A category-ratio perceived exertion scale: relationship to blood and muscle lactates and heart rate. *Med Sci Sports Exerc.* 1983;15:523–8.
51. Ogden CL, Carroll MD, Curtin LR, et al. Prevalence of overweight and obesity in the United States, 1999–2004. *JAMA.* 2006;295:1549–55.
52. Ogden CL, Flegal KM, Carroll MD, et al. Prevalence and trends in overweight among US children and adolescents, 1999–2000. *JAMA.* 2002;288:1728–32.
53. Palmer ML, Epler ME, editors. *Fundamentals of Musculoskeletal Assessment Techniques.* 2nd ed. Philadelphia (PA): Lippincott-Raven; 1998.
54. Panel E. Executive summary of the clinical guidelines on the identification, evaluation, and treatment of overweight and obesity in adults. *Arch Intern Med.* 1998;158:1855–67.
55. Pollock ML, Franklin BA, Balady GK, et al. Resistance exercise in individuals with and without cardiovascular disease: benefits, rationale, safety, and prescription: an advisory from the American Heart Association. *Circulation.* 2000;101:828–33.
56. President's Council on Physical Fitness. Definitions: health, fitness, and physical activity. [Internet]. 2000. Available from http://www.fitness.gov/digest_Mar2000.htm

57. Protas EJ. Flexibility and range of motion. In: Roitman JL, editor. *ACSM's Resource Manual for Guidelines for Exercise Testing and Prescription.* Baltimore (MD): Lippincott Williams & Wilkins; 2001. p. 381–390.

58. Rikli R, Jones CJ. *Senior Fitness Test Manual.* Champaign (IL): Human Kinetics; 2001.

59. Rimm EB, Stampfer MJ, Giovannucci E, et al. Body size and fat distribution as predictors of coronary heart disease among middle-aged and older US men. *Am J Epidemiol.* 1995;141:1117–27.

60. Robertson RJ, Noble BJ. Perception of physical exertion: methods, mediators, and applications. *Exerc Sport Sci Rev.* 1997;25:407–52.

61. Roche AF. Anthropometry and ultrasound. In: Roche AF, Heymsfield SB, Lohman TG, editors. *Human Body Composition.* Champaign (IL): Human Kinetics; 1996. p. 167–89.

62. Roche AF, Heymsfield SB, Lohman TG, editors. *Human Body Composition.* Champaign (IL): Human Kinetics; 1996.

63. Sesso HD, Paffenbarger Jr RS, Lee IM. Physical activity and coronary heart disease in men: The Harvard Alumni Health Study. *Circulation.* 2000;102:975–80.

64. Shephard RJ, Thomas S, Weller I. The Canadian Home Fitness Test. 1991 update. *Sports Med.* 1991;11:358–66.

65. Siri WE. Body composition from fluid spaces and density. *Univ Calif Donner Lab Med Phys Rep;* March 1956.

66. Tran ZV, Weltman A. Generalized equation for predicting body density of women from girth measurements. *Med Sci Sports Exerc.* 1989;21:101–4.

67. Tran ZV, Weltman A. Predicting body composition of men from girth measurements. *Hum Biol.* 1988;60:167–75.

68. Troiano RP, Flegal KM. Overweight children and adolescents: description, epidemiology, and demographics. *Pediatrics.* 1988;101:497–504.

69. Van Itallie TB. Topography of body fat: relationship to risk of cardiovascular and other diseases. In: Lohman TG, Roche AF, Martorell R, editors. *Anthropometric Standardization Reference Manual.* Champaign (IL): Human Kinetics; 1988;143–149.

70. Wallace J. Principles of cardiorespiratory endurance programming. In: *ACSM's Resource Manual for Guidelines for Exercise Testing and Prescription.* 5th ed. Philadelphia (PA): Lippincott Williams & Wilkins; 2006. 342 p.

71. Whaley MH, Prubaker PH, Kaminsky LA, et al. Validity of rating of perceived exertion during graded exercise testing in apparently healthy adults and cardiac patients. *J Cardiopulm Rehabil.* 1997;17:261–7.

Clinical Exercise Testing

Standard graded exercise tests (GXTs) are used in clinical applications to assess a patient's ability to tolerate increasing intensities of exercise while electrocardiographic (ECG), hemodynamic, and symptomatic responses are monitored for manifestations of myocardial ischemia, electrical instability, or other exertion-related signs or symptoms. Gas exchange and ventilatory responses also are commonly assessed during the exercise test, particularly in patients with chronic heart failure, in those whom preoperative risk is indeterminate, among post-myocardial infarction (post-MI) patients who wish to return to occupational or leisure-time pursuits requiring vigorous physical activity, or in patients with known or suspected pulmonary limitations.

INDICATIONS AND APPLICATIONS

The exercise test may be used for diagnostic, prognostic, and therapeutic applications, especially in regard to exercise prescription (Chapters 7 and 8).

DIAGNOSTIC EXERCISE TESTING

Diagnostic exercise testing has the greatest utility in patients with an intermediate probability of angiographically significant atherosclerotic cardiovascular disease (CVD) as determined by age, sex, and symptoms (Table 5.1). Asymptomatic individuals generally represent those with a low likelihood (i.e., <10%) of significant CVD. Diagnostic exercise testing in asymptomatic individuals generally is not indicated, but may be useful when multiple risk factors are present (27), indicating at least a moderate risk of experiencing a serious cardiovascular event within 5 years (54). Among asymptomatic men, ST-segment depression, failure to reach 85% of the predicted maximal heart rate, and exercise capacity during peak or symptom-limited treadmill testing have been shown to provide additional prognostic information in age- and Framingham-risk score-adjusted models, particularly among those in the highest risk group (10-year predicted coronary risk ≥20%) (7). It also may be indicated in selected individuals who are about to start a vigorous exercise program (Chapter 2) or those involved in occupations in which acute cardiovascular events may affect public safety. In general, patients with a high probability of disease (e.g., typical angina, prior coronary revascularization, or myocardial infarction [MI]) are tested to assess residual

TABLE 5.1. PRETEST LIKELIHOOD OF ATHEROSCLEROTIC CARDIOVASCULAR DISEASE (CVD)[a]

AGE	SEX	TYPICAL/ DEFINITE ANGINA PECTORIS	ATYPICAL/ PROBABLE ANGINA PECTORIS	NONANGINAL CHEST PAIN	ASYMPTOMATIC
30–39	Men	Intermediate	Intermediate	Low	Very low
	Women	Intermediate	Very low	Very low	Very low
40–49	Men	High	Intermediate	Intermediate	Low
	Women	Intermediate	Low	Very low	Very low
50–59	Men	High	Intermediate	Intermediate	Low
	Women	Intermediate	Intermediate	Low	Very low
60–69	Men	High	Intermediate	Intermediate	Low
	Women	High	Intermediate	Intermediate	Low

[a]No data exist for patients who are <30 or >69 years, but it can be assumed that prevalence of CVD increases with age. In a few cases, patients with ages at the extremes of the decades listed may have probabilities slightly outside the high or low range. High indicates >90%; intermediate, 10%–90%; low, <10%; and very low, <5%.

Reprinted with permission from Gibbons RJ, Balady GJ, Bricker JT, et al. Pretest Likelihood of Atherosclerotic Cardiovascular Disease (CVD). ACC/AHA 2002 Guideline Update for Exercise Testing; a report of the American College of Cardiology/ American Heart Association Task Force on Practice Guidelines; Committee on Exercise Testing, 2002. *Circulation.* 2002;106(14):1883–92.

myocardial ischemia, threatening ventricular arrhythmias, and prognosis rather than for diagnostic purposes. Exercise electrocardiography for diagnostic purposes is less accurate in women largely because of a greater number of false-positive responses. Although differences in test accuracy between men and women may approximate 10% on average, the standard exercise test is considered the initial diagnostic evaluation of choice, regardless of sex (27). A truly positive exercise test requires a hemodynamically significant coronary lesion (e.g., >75% stenosis) (3), yet nearly 90% of acute MIs occur at the site of previously nonobstructive atherosclerotic plaques (21).

The use of maximal or sign/symptom-limited exercise testing has expanded greatly to help guide decisions regarding medical management and surgical therapy in a broad spectrum of patients. For example, immediate exercise testing of selected low-risk patients presenting to the emergency department with chest pain is now increasingly employed to "rule out myocardial infarction" (37) and help make decisions regarding which patients require additional diagnostic studies before hospital discharge (4). Generally, patients who may be safely discharged include those who are no longer symptomatic, and those with unremarkable resting and exercise ECGs and normal serial cardiac enzymes (e.g., no appreciable rise in the level of troponin).

EXERCISE TESTING FOR DISEASE SEVERITY AND PROGNOSIS

Exercise testing is useful for the evaluation of disease severity among persons with known or suspected CVD. Data derived from the exercise test are most useful when considered in context with other clinical data. Information related to demographics, risk factors, symptoms, functional capacity, exercise hemodynamics, and ECG findings at rest and during exercise must be considered together to reliably predict long-term mortality after exercise testing (29). The magnitude of ischemia caused by a coronary lesion generally is proportional to the degree of ST-segment depression, the number of ECG leads involved, and the duration of ST-segment depression in recovery. It is inversely proportional to the ST slope, the double product at which the ST-segment depression occurs, and the maximal heart rate, systolic blood pressure, and metabolic equivalent (MET) level achieved. Several numeric indices of prognosis have been proposed and are discussed in Chapter 6 (6,38).

EXERCISE TESTING AFTER MYOCARDIAL INFARCTION

Exercise testing after MI can be performed before or soon after hospital discharge for prognostic assessment, activity prescription, and evaluation of further medical therapy or interventions, including coronary revascularization. Submaximal tests may be used before hospital discharge at 4 to 6 days after acute MI. Low-level exercise testing provides sufficient data to make recommendations about the patient's ability to safely perform activities of daily living and serves as a guide for early ambulatory exercise therapy. Symptom-limited tests are usually performed at more than 14 days after MI (27). As contemporary therapies have led to dramatic reductions in mortality after MI, the use of exercise testing in the evaluation of prognosis has changed. Patients who have not undergone coronary revascularization and are unable to undergo exercise testing appear to have the worst prognosis. Other indicators of adverse prognosis in the post-MI patient include ischemic ST-segment depression at a low level of exercise (particularly if accompanied by reduced left ventricular systolic function); functional capacity of <5 METs; and a hypotensive blood pressure response to exercise.

FUNCTIONAL EXERCISE TESTING

Exercise testing is useful to determine functional capacity. This information can be valuable for activity counseling, exercise prescription, return to work evaluations, disability assessment, and to help estimate prognosis. Functional capacity can be evaluated based on percentile ranking (based on apparently healthy men and women) as presented in Table 4-8. Exercise capacity also may be reported as the percentage of expected METs for age using a nomogram (Fig. 5.1), with 100% being normal (separate nomograms are provided for referred men with suspected CVD and in healthy men) (41). Normal standards for exercise capacity based on directly measured maximal oxygen consumption $\dot{V}O_{2max}$ are also available for women and by age (2). When using a particular regression equation for estimating percentage of normal exercise capacity achieved, factors such as population specificity, exercise mode, and whether exercise capacity was measured directly or estimated should be considered.

Previous studies in persons without known CVD have identified a low level of aerobic fitness as an independent risk factor for all-cause and cardiovascular mortality (10,11). In 1994, investigators extended these analyses to 527 men with

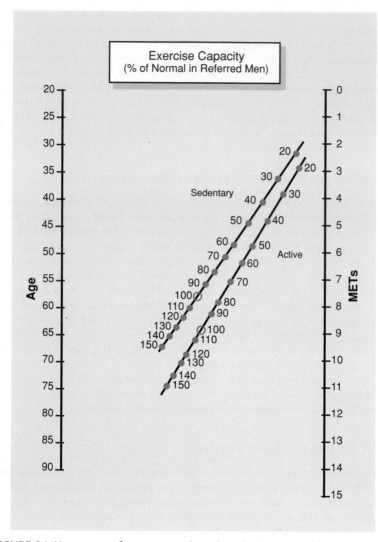

FIGURE 5.1. Nomograms of percent normal exercise capacity in men with suspected coronary artery disease who were referred for clinical exercise testing and in healthy men. (Reprinted from Morris CK, Myers J, Froelicher VF, et al. Nomogram based on metabolic equivalents and age for assessing aerobic exercise capacity in men. *J Am Coll Cardiol.* 1993;22:175–82, with permission.) (continued)

cardiovascular disease who were referred to an outpatient cardiac rehabilitation program (52). Oxygen uptake at peak exercise on a cycle ergometer was directly measured 13 weeks after acute MI ($N = 312$) or coronary artery bypass surgery ($N = 215$). All tests were terminated at a comparable endpoint—that is, volitional fatigue. During an average follow-up of 6.1 years, 33 and 20 patients died of

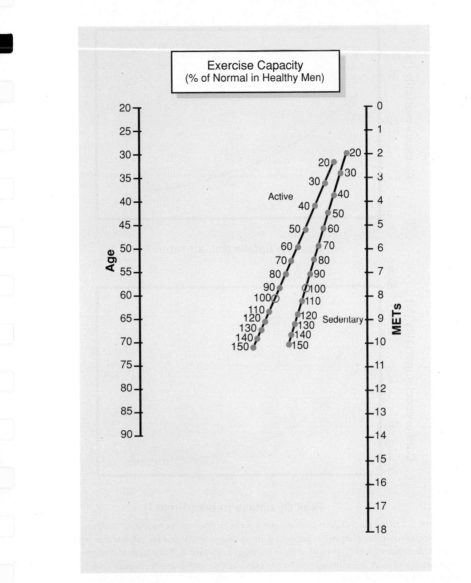

FIGURE 5.1. *Continued.*

cardiovascular and noncardiovascular cases, respectively. Figure 5.2 shows the inverse relationship between peak oxygen uptake ($\dot{V}O_{2peak}$) and subsequent mortality. Those with the highest cardiovascular and all-cause mortality averaged ≤4.4 METs. In contrast, there were no deaths among patients who averaged ≤9.2 METs.

Another study (44) reported on 3,679 men with coronary disease who were referred for treadmill exercise testing for clinical reasons. Those with an exercise capacity of ≤4.9 METs had a relative risk of death of 4.1 compared with those

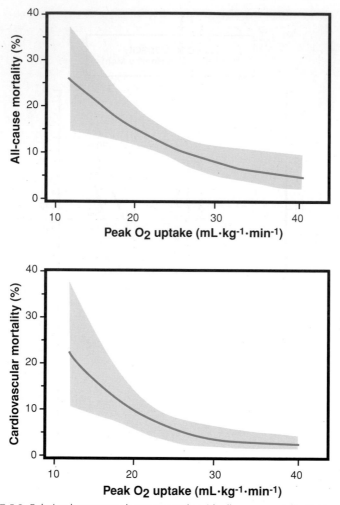

FIGURE 5.2. Relation between peak oxygen uptake with all-cause mortality (*top*) and cardiovascular mortality (*bottom*) in patients with coronary artery disease (*shaded area represents 95% confidence limits*). (Modified from Vanhees L, Fagard R, Thijs L, et al. Prognostic significance of peak exercise capacity in patients with coronary artery disease. *J Am Coll Cardiol*. 1994;23:358–63.)

with a fitness level ≤10.7 METs over the average follow-up of 6.2 years. For every 1-MET increase in exercise capacity, there was a 12% improvement in survival. Similarly, findings from the National Exercise and Heart Disease Project among post-MI patients demonstrated that every 1-MET increase after the training period conferred an approximate 10% reduction in mortality from any cause, regardless of the study group assignment, over a 19-year follow-up (18).

More recently, researchers extended these data to men (33) and women (32) with known CVD who were referred for exercise-based cardiac rehabilitation. Directly measured ($\dot{V}O_{2peak}$) during a progressive cycle ergometer test to exhaustion at program entry proved to be a powerful predictor of cardiovascular and all cause mortality. The cutoff points above which there was a marked survival benefit were 13 mL·kg·min^{-1} (3.7 METs) in women and 15 mL·kg·min^{-1} (4.3 METs) in men. For each 1 mL·kg·min^{-1} increase in aerobic capacity, there was a 9% and 10% reduction in cardiac mortality in men and women, respectively. Other investigators have now reported that exercise capacity, expressed as METs, is a better predictor of 2- and 5-year mortality than left ventricular ejection fraction in patients with ST-elevation MI treated with percutaneous coronary intervention (20). Collectively, these data highlight the value of exercise capacity in risk stratifying patients with and without known CVD (23), and suggest that those with a reduced exercise tolerance should be encouraged to engage in a structured exercise program or other lifestyle physical activity to increase their cardiorespiratory fitness (24).

EXERCISE TEST MODALITIES

The treadmill and cycle ergometer are the most commonly used modalities for clinical exercise testing. Treadmill testing provides a more common form of physiologic stress (e.g., walking) in which subjects are more likely to attain a slightly higher oxygen consumption ($\dot{V}O_2$) and peak heart rate than during cycle ergometer testing (28,43). The treadmill should have handrails for balance and stability, but tight gripping of the handrails can reduce the accuracy of estimated exercise capacity and the quality of the ECG recording, and should be discouraged. However, it may be necessary for some individuals to hold the handrails lightly for balance. An emergency stop button should be readily available to supervising staff.

Cycle ergometers are less expensive, require less space, and make less noise than treadmills. Incremental work rates on an electronically braked cycle ergometer are more sensitive than mechanically braked ergometers because the work rate can be maintained over a wide range of pedal rates. Because there is less movement of the patient's arms and thorax during cycling, it is easier to obtain better-quality ECG recordings and blood pressure measurements. However, stationary cycling is an unfamiliar method of exercise for many and is highly dependent on patient motivation. Thus, the test may end prematurely (i.e., because of localized leg fatigue) before a cardiopulmonary endpoint has been achieved. Lower values for $\dot{V}O_{2max}$ during cycle ergometer testing (versus treadmill testing) can range from 5% to 25%, depending on the participant's habitual activity, physical conditioning, and leg strength (28,43,47).

Arm ergometry is an alternative method of exercise testing for patients who cannot perform leg exercise. Because a smaller muscle mass is used during arm ergometry, $\dot{V}O_{2max}$ during arm exercise is generally 20% to 30% lower than that obtained during treadmill testing (22). Although this test has diagnostic utility

(8), it has been largely replaced by the nonexercise pharmacologic stress techniques that are described later in this chapter. Arm ergometer tests can be used for activity counseling and exercise prescription for certain disabled populations (e.g., spinal cord injury) and individuals who perform primarily dynamic upper-body work during occupational or leisure-time activities.

EXERCISE PROTOCOLS

The protocol employed during an exercise test should consider the purpose of the evaluation, the specific outcomes desired, and the characteristics of the individual being tested (e.g., age, symptomatology). Some of the most common exercise protocols and the predicted $\dot{V}O_2$ for each stage are illustrated in Figure 5.3. The Bruce treadmill test remains one of the most commonly used protocols; however, it employs relatively large increments (i.e., 2–3 METs per stage) every 3 minutes. Consequently, changes in physiologic responses tend to be less uniform, and exercise capacity may be markedly overestimated when it is predicted from exercise time or workload. Moreover, precise delineation of the ischemic ECG or anginal threshold is difficult. Protocols with larger increments (e.g., Bruce, Ellestad) are better suited for screening younger and/or physically active individuals, whereas protocols with smaller increments, such as Naughton or Balke-Ware (i.e., 1 MET per stage or lower), are preferable for older or deconditioned individuals and patients with chronic diseases.

The ramp protocol is an alternative approach to incremental exercise testing that has gained popularity in recent years, in which the work rate increases in a constant and continuous manner (31,42,43). Although ramp testing using a cycle ergometer has been available for many years, many of the major treadmill manufacturers recently developed controllers that ramp speed and grade. Both individualized (42) and standardized ramp tests, such as the BSU/Bruce ramp (31), have been used. The former test individualizes the rate of increase in intensity based on the subject, and the latter matches work rates to equivalent time periods on the commonly used Bruce protocol but increases in ramp fashion. Advantages of the ramp approach include the following (43):

- Avoidance of large and unequal increments in workload
- Uniform increase in hemodynamic and physiologic responses
- More accurate estimates of exercise capacity and ventilatory threshold
- Individualizes the test protocol (individualized ramp rate)
- Targeted test duration (applies only to individualized ramp protocols)

Whichever exercise protocol is chosen, it should be individualized so that the treadmill speed and increments in grade are based on the subject's perceived functional capacity. Ideally, increments in work rate should be chosen so that the total test time ranges between 8 and 12 minutes (2,14,27), assuming the endpoint is volitional fatigue. For example, increments of 10 to 15 watts ($1\ W = 6.12\ kg \cdot m \cdot min^{-1}$) per minute can be used on the cycle ergometer for elderly persons, deconditioned individuals, and patients with cardiovascular or pulmonary disease. Increases in treadmill grade of 1% to 3% per minute, with constant belt speeds of 1.5 to 2.5 mph (2.4–4.0 kph), can be used for such populations.

Although no longer widely used, submaximal testing can be an appropriate choice for predischarge, post-MI evaluations and for patients who may be at high risk for serious arrhythmias, abnormal blood pressure responses, or other adverse signs or symptoms. Submaximal tests can be useful for making activity recommendations, adjusting the medical regimen, and identifying the need for further diagnostic studies or interventions. These tests are generally terminated at a predetermined level, such as a heart rate of 120 beats $\cdot$ min^{-1}, perceived exertion of 13 (somewhat hard; 6–20 category scale), or a MET level of 5, but this may vary based on the patient and clinical judgment. When performed in this manner, submaximal tests may be useful in risk stratifying post-MI patients.

UPPER-BODY EXERCISE TESTING

An arm cycle ergometer can be purchased as such or modified from an existing stationary cycle ergometer by replacing the pedals with handles and mounting the unit on a table at shoulder height. Similar to leg cycle ergometers, these can be braked either mechanically or electrically. Work rates are adjusted by altering the cranking rates and/or resistance against the flywheel. Work rate increments of 10 W every 2 to 3 minutes, at a cranking rate of 50 to 60 revolutions per minute (rpm), have been applied to a broad spectrum of patients (9). Arm ergometry is best performed in the seated position with the fulcrum of the handle adjusted to shoulder height. ECG leads should be placed to minimize muscle artifact from upper-body movement. Blood pressure can be measured in an inactive arm while the subject continues cranking with the other or having the subject crank with both arms and pause briefly between stages (i.e., immediately after cessation of exercise). However, systolic blood pressures taken by the standard cuff method immediately after arm crank ergometry are likely to underestimate "true" physiologic responses (30). Systolic blood pressure during arm crank ergometry can be approximated using a Doppler stethoscope to measure the difference in ankle pressure (at the dorsalis pedis artery) at rest and during exercise.

TESTING FOR RETURN TO WORK

The decision to return to work after a cardiac event is a complex one, with about 15% to 20% of patients failing to resume work (50). National and cultural customs, local economic conditions, numerous nonmedical variables, employer stereotypes, and worker attitudes may govern failure to return to work. To counteract these deterrents, job modifications should be explored and implemented to facilitate the resumption of gainful employment.

Work assessment and counseling are useful in optimizing return-to-work decisions. Early discussion of work-related issues with patients, preferably before hospital discharge, may help establish reasonable return-to-work expectations. Discussion with the patient could include a job history analysis to (a) ascertain job aerobic requirements and potential cardiac demands, (b) establish tentative

FUNCTIONAL CLASS	CLINICAL STATUS	O₂ COST ml/kg/min	METS	BICYCLE ERGOMETER	BRUCE		RAMP	
					3 MIN STAGES MPH / %AGR			
		73.5	21					
		70	20	FOR 70 KG BODY WEIGHT Kpm/min (WATTS)	5.5	20		
		66.5	19					
		63	18					
		59.5	17		5.0	18		
		56.0	16					
NORMAL AND I	HEALTHY, DEPENDENT ON AGE, ACTIVITY	52.5	15				PER 30 SEC MPH / %GR	
		49.0	14	1500 (246)	4.2	16		
							3.0	25.0
		45.5	13				3.0	24.0
				1350 (221)			3.0	23.0
		42.0	12				3.0	22.0
							3.0	21.0
		38.5	11	1200 (197)			3.0	20.0
							3.0	19.0
	SEDENTARY HEALTHY	35.0	10	1050 (172)	3.4	14	3.0	18.0
							3.0	17.0
		31.5	9				3.0	16.0
				900 (148)			3.0	15.0
		28.0	8				3.0	14.0
				750 (123)			3.0	13.0
							3.0	12.0
		24.5	7		2.5	12	3.0	11.0
				600 (98)			3.0	10.0
		21.0	6				3.0	9.0
II							3.0	8.0
	LIMITED	17.5	5	450 (74)			3.0	7.0
							3.0	6.0
					1.7	10	3.0	5.0
	SYMPTOMATIC	14.0	4	300 (49)			3.0	4.0
III							3.0	3.0
		10.5	3				3.0	2.0
				150 (24)			3.0	1.0
		7.0	2				3.0	0
							2.5	0
							2.0	0
							1.5	0
IV		3.5	1				1.0	0
							0.5	0

FIGURE 5.3. Common exercise protocols and associated metabolic costs of each stage.

TREADMILL PROTOCOLS

METS	BRUCE RAMP (PER MIN) MPH / %GR	DALKE WARE	USAFSAM	"SLOW" USAFSAM	MODIFIED BALKE	ACIP	MOD. NAUGHTON (CHF)
21	5.8 / 20						
20	5.6 / 19	%GRADE AT 3.3 MPH 1 MIN STAGES					
19							
18	5.3 / 18						
17	5.0 / 18						
16	4.8 / 17		MPH / %GR			MPH / %GR	
15		26, 25, 24	3.3 25			3.4 24.0	
14	4.5 / 16	23			MPH / %GR	3.1 24.0	MPH / %GR
13	4.2 / 16	22, 21	3.3 20		3.0 25	3.0 21.0	3.0 25
12	4.1 / 15	20, 19, 18			3.0 22.5		3.0 22.5
12					3.0 20		3.0 20
11	3.8 / 14	17, 16	3.3 15		3.0 17.5	3.0 17.5	3.0 17.5
10	3.4 / 14	15		MPH / %GR	3.0 15		3.0 15
9	3.1 / 13	14, 13		2 25		3.0 14.0	3.0 12.5
8	2.8 / 12	12, 11	3.3 10	2 20	3.0 12.5		
7	2.5 / 12	10, 9			3.0 10	3.0 10.5	3.0 10
6	2.3 / 11	8, 7		2 15	3.0 7.5	3.0 7.0	3.0 7.5
5	2.1 / 10	6, 5	3.3 5	2 10	3.0 5	3.0 3.0	2.0 10.5
4	1.7 / 10	4, 3		2 5	3.0 2.5	2.5 2.0	2.0 7.0
3	1.3 / 5	2, 1	3.3 0		3.0 0	2.0 0.0	2.0 3.5
2			2.0 0	2 0	2.0 0		1.5 0
1	1.0 / 0						1.0 0

time lines for work evaluation and return to work, (c) individualize rehabilitation according to job demands, and (d) determine special work-related needs or job contacts (50). The appropriate time to return to work varies with type of cardiac event or intervention, associated complications, and prognosis.

The value of a symptom-limited treadmill or cycle ergometer GXT in evaluating and counseling patients on return-to-work status is well established (50). First, the patient's responses can help assess prognosis. Second, measured or estimated MET capacity can be compared with the estimated aerobic requirements of the patient's job to assess expected relative energy demands (1). For most patients, physical demands are considered appropriate if the 8-hour energy expenditure requirement averages ≤50% peak METs and peak job demands (e.g., 5–45 minutes) are within guidelines prescribed for a home exercise program (e.g., 80% peak METs or lower). Most contemporary job tasks require only very-light-to-light aerobic requirements (50).

A GXT can provide valuable data on return-to-work status for the majority of cardiac patients. However, some patients may benefit from further functional testing if job demands differ substantially from those evaluated with the GXT, especially patients with borderline physical work capacity in relationship to the anticipated job demands, those with concomitant left ventricular dysfunction, and/or those concerned about resuming a physically demanding job. Job tasks that may evoke disproportionate myocardial demands compared with a GXT include those requiring static muscular contraction, work combined with temperature stress, and intermittent heavy work (50).

Tests simulating the task(s) in question can be administered when insufficient information is available to determine a patient's ability to resume work within a reasonable degree of safety. For patients at risk for serious arrhythmias or silent or symptomatic myocardial ischemia on the job, ambulatory ECG monitoring may be considered. Specialized work simulators (e.g., Baltimore Therapeutic and Valpar work simulators) also are available (53), although simple, inexpensive tests can be set up to evaluate types of work not evaluated with a GXT (50). A weight-carrying test can be used to evaluate tolerance for light to heavy static work combined with light dynamic work and is typically performed to assess appropriateness for returning to occupational activities.

MEASUREMENTS DURING EXERCISE TESTING

Common variables assessed during clinical exercise testing include heart rate and blood pressure, ECG changes, subjective ratings, and signs and symptoms. Expired gases and ventilatory responses also are commonly evaluated during the exercise test, particularly in certain groups, such as patients with heart failure and/or pulmonary disease.

HEART RATE AND BLOOD PRESSURE

Heart rate and blood pressure responses should be measured before, during, and after the GXT. Table 5.2 indicates the recommended frequency and sequence of these measures. A standardized procedure should be adopted for each laboratory so that baseline measures can be assessed more accurately when repeat testing is performed.

TABLE 5.2. RECOMMENDED MONITORING INTERVALS ASSOCIATED WITH EXERCISE TESTING

VARIABLE	BEFORE EXERCISE TEST	DURING EXERCISE TEST	AFTER EXERCISE TEST
ECG	Monitored continuously; recorded supine position and posture of exercise	Monitored continuously; recorded during the last 15 s of each stage (interval protocol) or the last 15 s of each 2-min period (ramp protocols)	Monitored continuously; recorded immediately postexercise, during the last 15 s of first min of recovery, and then every 2 min thereafter
HR[b]	Monitored continuously; recorded supine position and posture of exercise	Monitored continuously; recorded during the last 5 s of each min	Monitored continuously; recorded during the last 5 s of each min
BP[a,b]	Measured and recorded in supine position and posture of exercise	Measured and recorded during the last 45 s of each stage (interval protocol) or the last 45 s of each 2-min period (ramp protocols)	Measured and recorded immediately postexercise and then every 2 min thereafter
Signs and symptoms	Monitored continuously; recorded as observed	Monitored continuously; recorded as observed	Monitored continuously; recorded as observed
RPE	Explain scale	Recorded during the last 5 s of each min	Obtain peak exercise value then not measured in recovery
Gas exchange	Baseline reading to assure proper operational status	Measured continuously	Generally not needed in recovery

ECG, electrocardiogram; HR, heart rate; BP, blood pressure; RPE, ratings of perceived exertion.

[a]An unchanged or decreasing systolic blood pressure with increasing workloads should be retaken (i.e., verified immediately).

[b]In addition, BP and HR should be assessed and recorded whenever adverse symptoms or abnormal ECG changes occur.

Adapted and used by permission from Brubaker PH, Kaminsky LA, Whaley MH. *Coronary Artery Disease*. Champaign (IL): Human Kinetics; 2002. p. 182.

BOX 5.1	Potential Sources of Error in Blood Pressure Assessment

- Inaccurate sphygmomanometer
- Improper cuff size
- Auditory acuity of technician
- Rate of inflation or deflation of cuff pressure
- Experience of technician
- Reaction time of technician
- Faulty equipment
- Improper stethoscope placement or pressure
- Background noise
- Allowing patient to hold treadmill handrails or flex elbow
- Certain physiologic abnormalities (e.g., damaged brachial artery, subclavian steal syndrome, arteriovenous fistula)

Although numerous devices have been developed to automate blood pressure measurements during exercise, these are generally prone to artifact. Thus, manual measurements (standard cuff method) remain the preferred technique. Boxes 3.4 and 5.1 suggest methods for blood pressure assessment at rest and potential sources of error during exercise, respectively. If systolic blood pressure appears to be decreasing with increasing exercise intensity, it should be retaken immediately (19). If a drop in systolic blood pressure of 10 mm Hg or more occurs with an increase in work rate, or if it decreases below the value obtained in the same position before testing, the test should be stopped, particularly if accompanied by adverse signs or symptoms (see Box 5.2 for test termination criteria). Anxious patients who demonstrate a drop in systolic blood pressure during the onset of exercise, without corresponding signs and symptoms, do not warrant test termination.

ELECTROCARDIOGRAPHIC MONITORING

A high-quality ECG is of paramount importance in an exercise test. Proper skin preparation lowers the resistance at the skin–electrode interface and thereby improves the signal-to-noise ratio. The general areas for electrode placement should be shaved, if necessary, and cleansed with an alcohol-saturated gauze pad. The superficial layer of skin then should be removed using light abrasion with fine-grain emery paper or gauze and electrodes placed according to standardized anatomic landmarks (Appendix C). Twelve leads are available; however, three leads—representing the inferior, anterior, and lateral cardiac distribution—are routinely monitored throughout the test, with 12-lead ECGs recorded at the end of each stage and at maximal exercise. Because electrodes placed on wrists and ankles obstruct exercise and cause artifact, the limb electrodes commonly are affixed to the torso at the base of the limbs for exercise testing (39). Because torso leads may give a slightly different ECG configuration when compared with the standard 12-lead resting ECG, use of torso leads should be noted on the ECG

BOX 5.2   Indications for Terminating Exercise Testing

ABSOLUTE INDICATIONS
- Drop in systolic blood pressure of >10 mm Hg from baseline[a] blood pressure despite an increase in workload when accompanied by other evidence of ischemia
- Moderately severe angina (defined as 3 on standard scale)
- Increasing nervous system symptoms (e.g., ataxia, dizziness, or near syncope)
- Signs of poor perfusion (cyanosis or pallor)
- Technical difficulties monitoring the ECG or systolic blood pressure
- Subject's desire to stop
- Sustained ventricular tachycardia
- ST elevation (+1.0 mm) in leads without diagnostic Q-waves (other than V_1 or aVR)

RELATIVE INDICATIONS
- Drop in systolic blood pressure of >10 mm Hg from baseline[a] blood pressure despite an increase in workload in the absence of other evidence of ischemia
- ST or QRS changes such as excessive ST depression (>2 mm horizontal or downsloping ST-segment depression) or marked axis shift
- Arrhythmias other than sustained ventricular tachycardia, including multifocal PVCs, triplets of PVCs, supraventricular tachycardia, heart block, or bradyarrhythmias
- Fatigue, shortness of breath, wheezing, leg cramps, or claudication
- Development of bundle-branch block or intraventricular conduction delay that cannot be distinguished from ventricular tachycardia
- Increasing chest pain
- Hypertensive response (systolic blood pressure of >250 mm Hg and/or a diastolic blood pressure of >115 mm Hg).

ECG, electrocardiogram; PVC, premature ventricular contraction.

[a]Baseline refers to a measurement obtained immediately before the test and in the same posture as the test is being performed.

Reprinted with permission from Gibbons RJ, Balady GJ, Bricker JT, et al. Pretest likelihood of atherosclerotic cardiovascular disease (CVD). ACC/AHA 2002 Guideline Update for Exercise Testing; a report of the American College of Cardiology/American Heart Association Task Force on Practice Guidelines; Committee on Exercise Testing, 2002. *Circulation.* 2002; 106(14):1883–92.

(39). Substantial breast tissue or abdominal adiposity may warrant modification of standard electrode placement to minimize movement artifact.

Signal-processing techniques have made it possible to average ECG waveforms and attenuate or eliminate electrical interference or muscle artifact, but caution is urged because signal averaging can actually distort the signal (40). Moreover, most manufacturers do not specify how such procedures modify the

ECG. Therefore, it is important to consider the real-time ECG data first, using filtered data to aid in the interpretation.

SUBJECTIVE RATINGS AND SYMPTOMS

The measurement of perceptual responses during exercise testing can provide useful clinical information. Somatic ratings of perceived exertion (RPE) and/or specific symptoms (e.g., degree of chest pain, burning, discomfort, dyspnea, lightheadedness, leg discomfort/pain) should be assessed routinely during clinical exercise tests. Patients are asked to provide subjective estimates during the last 15 seconds of each exercise stage (or every 2 minutes during ramp protocols) either verbally or manually. For example, the individual can provide a number verbally or point to a number if a mouthpiece or face mask precludes oral communication. The exercise technician should restate the number to confirm the correct rating. Either the 6–20 category scale or the 0–10 category-ratio scale (Chapter 4) may be used to assess RPE during exercise testing (12). Before the start of the exercise test, the patient should be given clear and concise instructions for use of the selected scale. Generic instructions for explaining either scale are provided in Chapter 4.

Use of alternative rating scales that are specific to subjective symptoms are recommended if subjects become symptomatic during exercise testing. Frequently used scales for assessing the patients' level of angina, claudication, and/or dyspnea can be found in Figure 5.4.

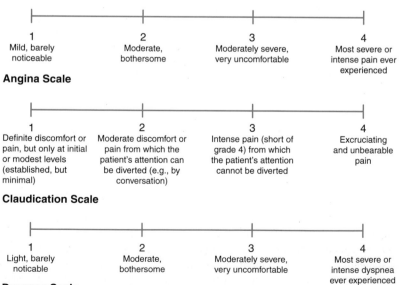

FIGURE 5.4. Frequently used scales for assessing the patient's level of angina (A), claudication (B), and dyspnea (C).

In general, ratings of ≥ 3 on the angina scale or a degree of chest discomfort that would cause the patient to stop normal daily activities are reasons to terminate the exercise test. However, higher levels of dyspnea or claudication may be acceptable during the exercise test (45).

GAS EXCHANGE AND VENTILATORY RESPONSES

Because of the inaccuracies associated with estimating oxygen consumption from work rate (i.e., treadmill speed and grade), many laboratories directly measure expired gases. The direct measurement of $\dot{V}O_2$ has been shown to be more reliable and reproducible than estimated values from treadmill or cycle ergometer work rates. Peak $\dot{V}O_2$ is the most accurate measurement of functional capacity and is a useful index of overall cardiopulmonary health (2). In addition, the measurement of $\dot{V}O_2$, carbon dioxide ($\dot{V}CO_2$) and the subsequent calculation of the respiratory exchange ratio (RER) can be used to determine total energy expenditure and substrate utilization during physical activity. The measurement of minute ventilation also should be made whenever gas exchange responses are obtained. Measurement of gas exchange and ventilation is not necessary for all clinical exercise testing, but the additional information can provide useful physiologic data. Because heart and lung diseases frequently manifest as ventilatory or gas exchange abnormalities during exercise, an integrated analysis of these measures can be useful for differential diagnosis (2). Furthermore, collection of gas exchange and ventilatory responses are increasingly being used in clinical trials to objectively assess the response to specific interventions. Situations in which gas exchange and ventilation measurements are appropriate include the following (27):

- When a precise cardiopulmonary response to a specific therapeutic intervention is required
- When the etiology of exercise limitation or dyspnea is uncertain
- When evaluation of exercise capacity in patients with heart failure is used to assist in the estimation of prognosis and assess the need for cardiac transplantation
- When a precise cardiopulmonary response is needed within a research context
- When assisting in the development of an appropriate exercise prescription for cardiac and/or pulmonary rehabilitation

BLOOD GASES

Pulmonary disease should be considered in patients who demonstrate dyspnea on exertion. As such, it is also important to measure gas partial pressures in these patients because oxygen desaturation may occur during exertion. Although measurement of partial pressure of oxygen in arterial blood (P_aO_2) and partial pressure of carbon dioxide in arterial blood (P_aCO_2) has been the standard in the past, the availability of oximetry has replaced the need to routinely draw arterial blood in most patients. In patients with pulmonary disease, measurements of oxygen saturation (S_aO_2) from oximetry at rest correlate reasonably well with S_aO_2 measured from arterial blood (95% confidence limits are $\pm 3\%$ to 5% saturation) (48). Carboxyhemoglobin (COHb) levels $>4\%$ and black skin may adversely affect the

BOX 5.3	Cognitive Skills Required to Competently Supervise Exercise Tests

- Knowledge of appropriate indications for exercise testing
- Knowledge of alternative physiologic cardiovascular tests
- Knowledge of appropriate contraindications, risks, and risk assessment of testing
- Knowledge to promptly recognize and treat complications of exercise testing
- Competence in cardiopulmonary resuscitation and successful completion of an American Heart Association–sponsored course in advance cardiovascular life support and renewal on a regular basis
- Knowledge of various exercise protocols and indications for each
- Knowledge of basic cardiovascular and exercise physiology, including hemodynamic response to exercise
- Knowledge of cardiac arrhythmia and the ability to recognize and treat serious arrhythmias
- Knowledge of cardiovascular drugs and how they can affect exercise performance, hemodynamics, and the electrocardiogram
- Knowledge of the effects of age and disease on hemodynamic and the electrocardiographic response to exercise
- Knowledge of principles and details of exercise testing, including proper lead placement and skin preparation
- Knowledge of endpoints of exercise testing and indications to terminate exercise testing

Adapted from Rodgers GP, Ayanian JZ, Balady GJ, et al. American College of Cardiology/American Heart Association clinical competence statement on stress testing. *Circulation.* 2000;102:1726-38.

accuracy of pulse oximeters (46,55), and most oximeters are inaccurate at an S_aO_2 of 85% or less. Arterial blood gases may be obtained if clinically warranted.

INDICATIONS FOR EXERCISE TEST TERMINATION

The absolute and relative indications for termination of an exercise test are listed in Box 5.2. Absolute indications are unambiguous, whereas relative indications may, in some instances, be superseded by clinical judgment.

POSTEXERCISE PERIOD

If maximal sensitivity is to be achieved with an exercise test, patients should assume a supine position during the postexercise period (36). Nevertheless, it is advantageous to record about 10 seconds of ECG data while the patient is in the upright position immediately after exercise for maximum clarity. In patients who are severely dyspneic, the supine posture may exacerbate the condition, and sitting may be a more appropriate posture. Having the patient perform a cool-down walk after the test may decrease the risk of hypotension but can attenuate the magnitude of ST-segment depression. When the test is being performed for nondiagnostic purposes, an active cooldown usually is preferable; for example, slow walking (1.0–1.5 mph or 2.4–4.0 kph) or continued cycling against minimal resistance. Monitoring should continue for at least five minutes after exercise or until ECG changes return to baseline and significant signs and symptoms resolve. Hemodynamic variables (heart rate and blood pressure) also should return to near-baseline levels before discontinuation of monitoring. ST-segment changes that occur only during the postexercise period are currently recognized to be an important diagnostic part of the test (49). In addition, the heart rate recovery from exercise has been shown to be an important prognostic marker (Chapter 6) (17,51).

IMAGING MODALITIES

Cardiac imaging modalities are indicated when ECG changes from standard exercise testing are nondiagnostic, it is important to quantify the extent and distribution of myocardial ischemia, or a positive or negative exercise ECG needs to be confirmed. Detailed recommendations for such testing are outlined in Tables 5.3 through 5.6.

EXERCISE ECHOCARDIOGRAPHY

Imaging modalities such as echocardiography can be combined with exercise ECG to increase the sensitivity and specificity of graded exercise testing, as well as to determine the extent of myocardium at risk as a result of ischemia. Echocardiographic images are obtained in four different views at rest and are compared with those obtained during cycle ergometry or immediately after treadmill exercise. Images must be obtained within 1 to 2 minutes after exercise because abnormal wall motion begins to normalize after this point.

Rest and stress images are compared side-by-side in a cine-loop display that is gated during systole from the QRS complex. Myocardial contractility normally increases with exercise, whereas ischemia causes hypokinetic, dyskinetic, or akinetic wall motion to develop or worsen in the affected segments. Advantages of exercise echocardiography over nuclear testing include a lower cost, the absence of exposure to low-level ionizing radiation, and a shorter amount of time for testing. Limitations include dependence on the operator for obtaining adequate, timely images. In addition, ~5% of patients have inadequate echocardiographic windows secondary to body habitus or lung interference, although sonicated contrast agents can be helpful to enhance endocardial definition in these conditions. Exercise echocardiography has a weighted mean sensitivity of 86%, specificity of 81%, and overall accuracy of 85% for the detection of CVD (16). Recommendations for the use of exercise echocardiography are outlined in Table 5.3.

EXERCISE NUCLEAR IMAGING

Exercise tests with nuclear imaging are performed with ECG monitoring. There are several different imaging protocols using only technetium (Tc)-99m

TABLE 5.3. INDICATIONS FOR EXERCISE ECHOCARDIOGRAPHY

CONDITION	ACC/AHA RECOMMENDATION
Diagnostic testing in patients with intermediate pretest probability of CVD and baseline ECG abnormalities including >1-mm ST depression or pre-excitation	Class I—level of evidence B (26)
Assessment of patients with stable angina who have had prior coronary revascularization	Class I—level of evidence B (26)
In-hospital or early-postdischarge assessment of patients after MI whenever baseline ST abnormalities are expected to compromise ECG interpretation	Class I—level of evidence B (5,16)
Assessment of functional significance of coronary lesions in planning percutaneous coronary intervention	Class I—level of evidence B (16,26)
Assessment for restenosis after revascularization in patients with atypical recurrent symptoms	Class I (16)
Assessment for restenosis after revascularization in patients with typical recurrent symptoms	Class IIa (16)
Detection of myocardial ischemia in women with an intermediate pretest likelihood of CVD	Class IIa (16)
In-hospital or early-postdischarge assessment of patients after MI in the absence of baseline ST abnormalities that are expected to compromise ECG interpretation	Class IIa (16)
Diagnostic testing in patients with high or low pretest probability of CVD and baseline ECG abnormalities including >1-mm ST depression or pre-excitation	Class IIb (16)
Diagnostic testing in patients with intermediate pretest probability of CVD who have <1-mm ST depression on resting ECG on digoxin or with LVH	Class IIb—level of evidence B (26)
Diagnostic testing in patients with normal resting ECG who are not taking digoxin	Class IIb—level of evidence B (26)
Diagnostic testing in patients with LBBB	Class IIb—level of evidence C (26)
Diagnostic testing in asymptomatic patients with severe coronary calcification on EBCT and have baseline ECG abnormalities including >1-mm ST depression or pre-excitation	Class IIb—level of evidence C (26)
Prognostic testing in asymptomatic patients with an intermediate or high risk Duke score on exercise–ECG testing	Class IIb—level of evidence C (26)
Diagnostic testing in patients with severe comorbidity that is likely to limit life expectancy or prevent coronary revascularization	Class III—level of evidence C (26)
Diagnostic testing in asymptomatic patients with LBBB	Class III—level of evidence C (26)
Diagnostic testing as the initial test in asymptomatic patients with normal resting ECG who are not taking digoxin	Class III—level of evidence C (26)

(continued)

TABLE 5.3. INDICATIONS FOR EXERCISE ECHOCARDIOGRAPHY
(*Continued*)

CONDITION	ACC/AHA RECOMMENDATION
Prognostic testing in asymptomatic patients with a low risk Duke score on exercise ECG testing	Class III—level of evidence C (26)

ACC, American College of Cardiology; AHA, American Heart Association; CVD, atherosclerotic cardiovascular disease; ECG, electrocardiogram; MI, myocardial infarction; LVH, left ventricular hypertrophy; LBBB, left bundle branch block; EBCT, electron beam computed tomography.

Classification of recommendations and level of evidence are expressed in the ACC/AHA format as follows: **Class I:** Conditions for which there is evidence and/or general agreement that the procedure or treatment is beneficial, useful, and effective. **Class II:** Conditions for which there is conflicting evidence and/or a divergence of opinion about the usefulness/efficacy of a procedure or treatment. **Class IIa:** Weight of evidence/opinion is in favor of usefulness/efficacy. **Class IIb:** Usefulness/efficacy is less well established by evidence/opinion. **Class III:** Conditions for which there is evidence and/or general agreement that the procedure/treatment is not useful/effective and in some cases may be harmful. In addition, the weight of evidence in support of the recommendation is listed as follows: **Level of Evidence A:** Data derived from multiple randomized clinical trials. **Level of Evidence B:** Data derived from a single randomized trial or nonrandomized studies. **Level of Evidence C:** Only consensus opinion of experts, case studies, or standard of care (34).

TABLE 5.4. INDICATIONS FOR EXERCISE NUCLEAR TESTING

CONDITION	ACC/AHA RECOMMENDATION
Diagnostic testing in patients with intermediate pretest probability of CVD and baseline ECG abnormalities including >1-mm ST depression or pre-excitation	Class I—level of evidence B (26,34)
Assessment of patients with stable angina who have had prior coronary revascularization	Class I—level of evidence B (26)
In-hospital or early-postdischarge assessment of patients after MI whenever baseline ST abnormalities are expected to compromise ECG interpretation	Class I—level of evidence B (5,26)
Assessment of myocardial viability for planning coronary revascularization	Class I—level of evidence B (34)
Assessment of functional significance of coronary lesions in planning percutaneous coronary intervention	Class I—level of evidence B (26,34)
Prognostic testing in asymptomatic patients with an intermediate Duke score on exercise ECG testing	Class I—level of evidence B (34)
Diagnostic or prognostic assessment of patients with abnormal resting ECG before undergoing noncardiac surgery	Class I—level of evidence B (34)
Assessment of patients with any intermediate risk predictor (mild angina, prior MI, diabetes, heart failure, or renal failure) AND abnormal baseline ECG with exercise capacity >4 METs before undergoing high-risk noncardiac surgery	Class I—level of evidence C (34)

(*continued*)

TABLE 5.4. INDICATIONS FOR EXERCISE NUCLEAR TESTING (*Continued*)

CONDITION	ACC/AHA RECOMMENDATION
Diagnostic testing as the initial test in patients who are considered high risk (defined as having diabetes or >20% 10-year risk of coronary event)	Class IIa—level of evidence B (34)
Detection of ischemia at 3–5 years after coronary revascularization in selected high-risk patients	Class IIa—level of evidence B (34)
Diagnostic testing in patients with intermediate pretest probability of CVD who have <1-mm ST depression on resting ECG on digoxin or with LVH	Class IIb—level of evidence B (26)
Diagnostic testing in patients with normal resting ECG who are not taking digoxin	Class IIb—level of evidence B (26)
Diagnostic testing in asymptomatic patients with severe coronary calcification on EBCT and have baseline ECG abnormalities including >1-mm ST depression or pre-excitation	Class IIb—level of evidence C (26,34)
Repeat testing to assess the adequacy of medical therapy in patients on cardioactive medications after initial abnormal perfusion imaging	Class IIb—level of evidence C (34)
Diagnostic testing in asymptomatic patients who have a high-risk occupation	Class IIb—level of evidence C (34)
Diagnostic testing in patients with severe comorbidity that is likely to limit life expectancy or prevent coronary revascularization	Class III—level of evidence C (26)
Diagnostic testing in patients with LBBB	Class III—level of evidence C (26)
Diagnostic testing as the initial test in asymptomatic patients with normal resting ECG who are not taking digoxin	Class III—level of evidence C (26)
Prognostic testing in asymptomatic patients with a low-risk Duke score on exercise ECG testing	Class III—level of evidence C (26)
Initial diagnostic or prognostic assessment of CVD in patients who require emergent noncardiac surgery	Class III—level of evidence C (34)

ACC, American College of Cardiology; AHA, American Heart Association; CVD, atherosclerotic cardiovascular disease; ECG, electrocardiogram; MI, myocardial infarction; LVH, left ventricular hypertrophy; EBCT, electron beam computed tomography; LBBB, left bundle branch block.

For ACC/AHA Recommendation definitions, see footnote to Table 5.3.

or thallous (thallium) chloride-201. A common protocol with technetium is to perform rest images 10 minutes after intravenous administration of technetium followed by exercise (or pharmacologic stress) 1 to 3 hours later. Stress images are obtained 10 minutes after injecting technetium, which is given ~1 minute before completion of peak exercise. Comparison of the rest and stress images permit differentiation of fixed versus transient perfusion abnormalities.

Technetium-99m permits higher dosing with less radiation exposure than thallium and results in improved images that are sharper and have less artifact and attenuation. Consequently, technetium is the preferred imaging agent when performing tomographic images of the heart using single-photon emission computed tomography (SPECT). SPECT images are obtained with a gamma

TABLE 5.5. INDICATIONS FOR DOBUTAMINE ECHOCARDIOGRAPHY

CONDITION	ACC/AHA RECOMMENDATION
Diagnostic testing in patients with intermediate pretest probability of CVD and baseline ECG abnormalities including >1-mm ST depression or pre-excitation	Class I—level of evidence B (26)
Diagnostic testing to evaluate the extent, severity, and location of ischemia in patients with stable angina and without LBBB or ventricularly paced rhythm who are unable to exercise	Class I—level of evidence B (26)
Assessment of patients with stable angina who have had prior coronary revascularization	Class I—level of evidence B (26)
In-hospital or early-postdischarge assessment of patients after MI whenever baseline ST abnormalities are expected to compromise ECG interpretation	Class I—level of evidence B (5,16)
Assessment of myocardial viability for planning coronary revascularization	Class I (16)
Assessment of functional significance of coronary lesions in planning percutaneous coronary intervention in patients unable to exercise	Class I—level of evidence B (16,26)
Assessment for restenosis after revascularization in patients with atypical recurrent symptoms	Class I (16)
Assessment for restenosis after revascularization in patients with typical recurrent symptoms	Class IIa (16)
Detection of coronary arteriopathy in patients who have undergone cardiac transplantation	Class IIa (16)
Detection of myocardial ischemia in women with an intermediate pretest likelihood of CVD	Class IIa (16)
In-hospital or early-postdischarge assessment of patients after MI in the absence of baseline ST abnormalities that are expected to compromise ECG interpretation	Class IIa (16)
Initial diagnostic testing in patients with normal resting ECG who are not taking digoxin and are able to exercise	Class IIb—level of evidence B (26)
Diagnostic testing in patients with LBBB whether or not they are able to exercise	Class IIb—level of evidence C (26)
Diagnostic testing in asymptomatic patients with severe coronary calcification on EBCT and who are unable to exercise	Class IIb—level of evidence C (26)
Diagnostic testing in patients with severe comorbidity that is likely to limit life expectancy or prevent coronary revascularization	Class III—level of evidence C (26)
Diagnostic testing in asymptomatic patients with LBBB	Class III—level of evidence C (26)
Diagnostic testing as the initial test in asymptomatic patients with normal resting ECG who are not taking digoxin	Class III—level of evidence C (16,26)
Prognostic testing in asymptomatic patients with a low-risk Duke score on exercise ECG testing	Class III—level of evidence C (26)

ACC, American College of Cardiology; AHA, American Heart Association; CVD, atherosclerotic cardiovascular disease; ECG, electrocardiogram; LBBB, left bundle branch block; MI, myocardial infarction; EBCT, electron beam computed tomography.

For ACC/AHA Recommendation definitions, see footnote to Table 5.3.

TABLE 5.6. INDICATIONS FOR PHARMACOLOGIC NUCLEAR STRESS TESTING

CONDITION	ACC/AHA RECOMMENDATION
Diagnostic testing in patients with intermediate pretest probability of CVD who are unable to exercise	Class I—level of evidence B (26,34)
Diagnostic testing to evaluate the extent, severity, and location of ischemia in patients with stable angina and without LBBB or ventricularly paced rhythm who are unable to exercise	Class I—level of evidence B (26)
Diagnostic testing in patients with an intermediate likelihood of CVD or intermediate-risk stratification with LBBB or electronically paced rhythm whether or not they are able to exercise	Class I—level of evidence B (34)
Assessment of patients with stable angina who have had prior coronary revascularization and are unable to exercise	Class I—level of evidence B (26)
In-hospital or early-postdischarge assessment of patients after MI in patients unable to exercise	Class I—level of evidence B (5)
Assessment of myocardial viability for planning coronary revascularization	Class I—level of evidence B (34)
Assessment of functional significance of coronary lesions in planning percutaneous coronary intervention in patients unable to exercise	Class I—level of evidence B (26,34)
Diagnostic or prognostic assessment in patients with abnormal resting ECG before undergoing noncardiac surgery who are unable to exercise	Class I—level of evidence B (34)
Assessment of patients with any intermediate or mild clinical risk predictor (mild angina, prior MI, diabetes, heart failure, or renal failure; age >75 years, abnormal ECG, rhythm other than sinus, history of cerebrovascular accident, uncontrolled hypertension) before undergoing high-risk noncardiac surgery in patients unable to exercise	Class I—level of evidence C (34)
Assessment of myocardial viability 4–10 days after MI for planning coronary revascularization	Class IIa—level of evidence C (5)
Detection of ischemia at 3–5 years after coronary revascularization in selected high-risk patients who are unable to exercise	Class IIa—level of evidence B (34)
Diagnostic testing in patients with low or high pretest probability of CVD and have either LBBB or electronically paced rhythm whether or not they are able to exercise	Class IIb (26)
Diagnostic testing in patients with normal resting ECG who are not taking digoxin	Class IIb—level of evidence B (26)
Diagnostic testing in asymptomatic patients with severe coronary calcification on EBCT and have LBBB or an electronically paced rhythm and are unable to exercise	Class IIb—level of evidence B (26,34)

(continued)

TABLE 5.6. INDICATIONS FOR PHARMACOLOGIC NUCLEAR STRESS TESTING (*Continued*)

CONDITION	ACC/AHA RECOMMENDATION
Repeat testing to assess the adequacy of medical therapy in patients on cardioactive medications after initial abnormal perfusion imaging in patients unable to exercise	Class IIb—level of evidence C (34)
Diagnostic testing in asymptomatic patients who have a high-risk occupation and are unable to exercise	Class IIb—level of evidence C (34)
Diagnostic testing in patients with severe comorbidity that is likely to limit life expectancy or prevent coronary revascularization	Class III—level of evidence C (26)
Diagnostic testing as the initial test in asymptomatic patients with normal resting ECG who are not taking digoxin	Class III—level of evidence C (26)
Prognostic testing in asymptomatic patients with a low-risk Duke score on exercise ECG testing	Class III—level of evidence C (26)

ACC, American College of Cardiology; AHA, American Heart Association; CVD, atherosclerotic cardiovascular disease; LBBB, left bundle branch block; MI, myocardial infarction; ECG, electrocardiogram; EBCT, electron beam computed tomography.

For ACC/AHA Recommendation definitions, see footnote to Table 5.3.

camera, which rotates 180 degrees around the patient, stopping at preset angles to record the image. Cardiac images then are displayed in slices from three different axes to allow visualization of the heart in three dimensions. Thus, multiple myocardial segments can be viewed individually, without the overlap of segments that occurs with planar imaging. Planar imaging is rarely performed and is generally reserved for those patients who exceed the weight limit of the SPECT imaging table. Perfusion defects that are present during exercise but not seen at rest suggest myocardial ischemia. Perfusion defects that are present during exercise and persist at rest suggest previous MI or scar. The extent and distribution of ischemic myocardium can be identified in this manner. Exercise nuclear SPECT imaging has a sensitivity of 87% and specificity of 73% for detecting CVD with ≥50% coronary stenosis (34). Recommendations for the use of exercise nuclear testing are outlined in Table 5.4.

The limitations of nuclear imaging include the exposure to low-level ionizing radiation. Furthermore, additional equipment and personnel are required for image acquisition and interpretation, including a nuclear technician to administer the radioactive isotope and acquire the images, and a physician trained in nuclear medicine to reconstruct and interpret the images.

PHARMACOLOGIC STRESS TESTING

Patients unable to undergo exercise stress testing for reasons such as deconditioning, peripheral vascular disease, orthopedic disabilities, neurologic disease, and concomitant illness may be evaluated by pharmacologic stress testing. The two most commonly used pharmacologic tests are dobutamine stress echocardiography and dipyridamole or adenosine stress nuclear scintigraphy. Some protocols include light exercise in combination with pharmacologic infusion.

Dobutamine elicits wall motion abnormalities by increasing heart rate and therefore myocardial oxygen demand. It is infused intravenously, and the dose is increased gradually until the maximal dose or an endpoint is achieved. Endpoints may include new or worsening wall-motion abnormalities, an adequate heart rate response, serious arrhythmias, angina, significant ST depression, intolerable side effects, and a significant increase or decrease in blood pressure. Atropine may be given if an adequate heart rate is not achieved or other endpoints have not been reached at peak dobutamine dose. Heart rate, blood pressure, ECG, and echocardiographic images are obtained throughout the infusion. Echocardiographic images are obtained similar to exercise echocardiography. A new or worsening wall motion abnormality constitutes a positive test for ischemia. Dobutamine stress echocardiography has a weighted mean sensitivity of 82%, specificity of 84%, and overall accuracy of 86% for the detection of CVD (16). Recommendations for the use of dobutamine stress testing are outlined in Table 5.5.

Vasodilators, such as dipyridamole and adenosine, commonly are used to assess coronary perfusion in conjunction with a nuclear imaging agent. Dipyridamole and adenosine cause maximal coronary vasodilation in normal epicardial arteries, but not in stenotic segments. As a result, a coronary steal phenomenon occurs, with a relatively increased flow to normal arteries and a relatively decreased flow to stenotic arteries. Nuclear perfusion imaging under resting conditions is then compared with imaging obtained after coronary vasodilation. Interpretation is similar to that for exercise nuclear testing. Severe side effects are uncommon, but both dipyridamole and adenosine may induce marked bronchospasm, particularly in patients with asthma or reactive airway disease. Thus, administration of these agents is contraindicated in such patients (34). The bronchospasm can be treated with theophylline, although this is rarely needed with adenosine because the latter's half-life is very short. Caffeine and other methylxanthines can block the vasodilator effects of dipyridamole and adenosine, and thus reduce the sensitivity of the test. Therefore, it is recommended that these agents be avoided for at least 24 hours before the stress test. The diagnostic accuracy of pharmacologic nuclear stress testing is similar to that of exercise nuclear stress testing as reported above (34). Recommendations for the use of pharmacologic nuclear stress testing are outlined in Table 5.6.

COMPUTED TOMOGRAPHY IN THE ASSESSMENT OF CORONARY ARTERY DISEASE

Advances in cardiac computed tomography (CT) offer additional methods for the clinical assessment of CVD. Although there are several types of cardiac CT, electron beam computed tomography (EBCT) has been available since 1987, and hence there are much scientific data regarding its application. EBCT is a highly sensitive method for the detection of coronary artery calcified plaque (15). However, it is important to understand that the presence of calcified plaque does not itself indicate the presence of a flow-obstructing coronary lesion; conversely, the absence of coronary calcium does not itself indicate the absence of atherosclerotic plaque. A coronary calcium score of zero makes the presence of atherosclerotic plaque, including vulnerable plaque, highly unlikely. It is associated with a low annual risk (0.1%) of a cardiovascular event in the next 2 to 5 years, whereas a high calcium score (>100) is associated with a high annual risk (>2%). Calcium scores correlate poorly with stenosis severity, although a score >400 is frequently associated with perfusion ischemia from obstructive CVD. Measurement of coronary artery calcium appears to improve risk prediction in individuals with an intermediate Framingham risk score (those with 10%–20% 10-year likelihood of a cardiovascular event). Thus, in clinically selected intermediate-risk patients, it may be reasonable to use EBCT to further refine risk prediction in an effort to establish more aggressive target values for lipid-lowering therapies (American College of Cardiology [ACC]/American Heart Association [AHA] Class IIb—level of evidence B) (5). However, the AHA recommends that the decision to pursue further diagnostic testing cannot be made from coronary calcium scores alone, but should be based on clinical history and other standard clinical criteria. Coronary artery calcium measurement may be reasonable in other clinical situations (AHA/ACC Class IIb—level of evidence B): the assessment of symptomatic patients in the setting of equivocal stress testing results, those with chest pain and equivocal or normal ECG and negative cardiac enzyme studies, and those with cardiomyopathy of uncertain cause. Because of concerns regarding the safety of repeated radiation exposure, serial imaging to assess for coronary calcium progression is not indicated at this time (AHA/ACC Class III—level of evidence C) (5).

Coronary CT angiography is an emerging noninvasive technique that can evaluate the coronary artery lumen and wall, and can be used to detect the presence of obstructive stenoses. Data to date demonstrate a high negative predictive value of this technique, and thus a normal coronary CT angiogram is highly reliable in excluding the presence of hemodynamically relevant coronary artery stenoses. Therefore, the AHA concludes that CT coronary angiography may be reasonable to use in ruling out coronary stenoses among symptomatic patients with a low to intermediate likelihood of CVD and may help avoid the need for invasive coronary angiography (ACC/AHA Class IIb—level of evidence B). Because of the associated high radiation doses, CT coronary angiography is not recommended to detect occult CVD in asymptomatic persons (ACC/AHA Class III—level of evidence C) (5).

SUPERVISION OF EXERCISE TESTING

Although exercise testing generally is considered a safe procedure, both acute MI and cardiac arrest have been reported and can be expected to occur at a combined rate of up to 1 per 2,500 tests (27). Accordingly, individuals who supervise exercise tests must have the cognitive and technical skills necessary to be competent to do so. The ACC, AHA, and American College of Physicians, with broad involvement from other professional organizations involved with exercise testing (including the American College of Sports Medicine), have outlined those cognitive skills needed to competently supervise exercise tests (49). These are presented in Box 5.3. In most cases, clinical exercise tests can be supervised by properly trained exercise physiologists, physical therapists, nurses, physician assistants, or medical technicians who are working under the direct supervision of a physician; that is, the physician must be in the immediate vicinity and available for emergencies (49). Several studies have demonstrated that the incidence of cardiovascular complications during exercise testing is no higher with experienced paramedical personnel than with direct physician supervision (25,35). In situations in which the patient is deemed to be at increased risk for an adverse event during exercise testing, the physician should be physically present in the exercise testing room to personally supervise the test. Such cases include, but are not limited to, patients undergoing symptom-limited testing following recent acute events (i.e., acute coronary syndrome or MI within 7–10 days), severe left ventricular dysfunction, severe valvular stenosis (e.g., aortic stenosis), or known complex arrhythmias (49).

REFERENCES

1. Ainsworth BE, Haskell WL, Whitt MC, et al. Compendium of physical activities: an update of activity codes and MET intensities. *Med Sci Sports Exerc.* 2000;32:S498–S516.
2. Ambrose JA, Tannenbaum MA, Alexopoulos D, et al. Angiographic progression of coronary artery disease and the development of myocardial infarction. *J Am Coll Cardiol.* 1988;12:56–62.
3. American Thoracic Society and American College of Chest Physicians. American Thoracic Society/American College of Chest Physicians Statement on Cardiopulmonary Exercise Testing. *Am J Respir Crit Care Med.* 2003;167:211–77.
4. Amsterdam EA, Kirk JD, Diercks DB, et al. Immediate exercise testing to evaluate low-risk patients presenting to the emergency department with chest pain. *J Am Coll Cardiol.* 2002;40:251–6.
5. Antman EM, Anbe DT, Armstrong PW, et al. ACC/AHA guidelines for the management of patients with ST-elevation myocardial infarction: a report of the American College of Cardiology/American Heart Association Task Force on Practice Guidelines (Committee to Revise the 1999 Guidelines for the Management of Patients with Acute Myocardial Infarction). *Circulation.* 2004;110:282–92.
6. Ashley E, Myers J, Froelicher V. Exercise testing scores as an example of better decisions through science. *Med Sci Sports Exerc.* 2002;34:1391–8.
7. Balady GJ, Larson MG, Vasan RS, et al. Usefulness of exercise testing in the prediction of coronary disease risk among asymptomatic persons as a function of the Framingham risk score. *Circulation.* 2004;110:1920–5.
8. Balady GJ, Weiner DA, McCabe CH, et al. Value of arm exercise testing in detecting coronary artery disease. *Am J Cardiol.* 1985;55:37–9.
9. Balady GJ, Weiner DA, Rose L, et al. Physiologic responses to arm ergometry exercise relative to age and gender. *J Am Coll Cardiol.*1990;16:130–5.
10. Blair SN, Kohl WH, Barlow CE, et al. Changes in physical fitness and all-cause mortality: a prospective study of healthy and unhealthy men. *JAMA.* 1995;273:1093–8.
11. Blair SN, Kohl HW, Paffenbarger Jr RS, et al. Physical fitness and all-cause mortality: a prospective study of healthy men and women. *JAMA.* 1989;262:2395–2401.
12. Borg G. *Borg's Perceived Exertion and Pain Scales.* Champaign (IL): Human Kinetics; 1998.
13. Brubaker PH, Kaminsky LA, Whaley MH. *Coronary Artery Disease.* Champaign (IL): Human Kinetics; 2002. 182 p.
14. Buchfuhrer MJ, Hansen JE, Robinson TE, et al. Optimizing the exercise protocol for cardiopulmonary assessment. *J Appl Physiol.* 1983;55:1558–64.
15. Budoff MJ, Achenbach S, Blumenthal RS, et al. Assessment of coronary artery disease by cardiac computed tomography: a scientific statement from the American Heart Association Committee on Cardiovascular Imaging and Intervention, Council on Cardiovascular Radiology and Intervention, and Committee on Cardiac Imaging, Council on Clinical Cardiology. *Circulation.* 2006;114: 1761–91.

16. Cheitlin MD, Armstrong WF, Aurigemma GP, et al. ACC/AHA/ASE 2003 guideline update for the clinical application of echocardiography: summary article: a report of the American College of Cardiology/American Heart Association Task Force on Practice Guidelines (ACC/AHA/ASE Committee to Update the 1997 Guidelines for the Clinical Application of Echocardiography). *Circulation.* 2003;108:1146–62.

17. Cole CR, Blackstone EH, Pashkow FJ, et al. Heart-rate recovery immediately after exercise as a predictor of mortality. *N Engl J Med.* 1999;341:1351–7.

18. Dorn J, Naughton J, Imamura D, et al. Results of a multicenter randomized clinical trial of exercise and long-term survival in myocardial infarction patients: the National Exercise and Heart Disease Project (NEHDP). *Circulation.* 1999;100:1764–9.

19. Dubach P, Froelicher VF, Klein J, et al. Exercise-induced hypotension in a male population: criteria, causes, and prognosis. *Circulation.* 1988;78:1380–7.

20. Dutcher JR, Kahn J, Grines C, et al. Comparison of left ventricular ejection fraction and exercise capacity as predictors of two- and five-year mortality following acute myocardial infarction. *Am J Cardiol.* 2007;99:436–41.

21. Falk E, Shah PK, Fuster V. Coronary plaque disruption. *Circulation.* 1995;92:657–67.

22. Franklin BA. Exercise testing, training and arm ergometry. *Sports Med.* 1985;2:100–19.

23. Franklin BA. Fitness: the ultimate marker for risk stratification and health outcomes? *Prev Cardiol.* 2007;10:42–5.

24. Franklin BA, Gordon NF. *Contemporary Diagnosis and Management in Cardiovascular Exercise.* Newton (PA): Handbooks in Health Care Co; 2005.

25. Franklin BA, Gordon S, Timmis GC, et al. Is direct physician supervision of exercise stress testing routinely necessary? *Chest.* 1997;111:262–5.

26. Gibbons RJ, Abrams J, Chatterjee K, et al. ACC/AHA 2002 guideline updated for the management of patients with chronic stable angina—summary article: a report of the American College of Cardiology/American Heart Association Task Force on Practice Guidelines (Committee on the Management of Patients with Chronic Stable Angina). *Circulation.* 2003;107:149–58.

27. Gibbons RJ, Balady GJ, Bricker JT, et al. Pretest likelihood of atherosclerotic cardiovascular disease (CVD). ACC/AHA 2002 Guideline Update for Exercise Testing; a report of the American College of Cardiology/American Heart Association Task Force on Practice Guidelines; Committee on Exercise Testing, 2002. *Circulation.* 2002;106(14):1883–92.

28. Hambrecht RP, Schuler GC, Muth T, et al. Greater diagnostic sensitivity of treadmill versus cycle exercise testing of asymptomatic men with coronary artery disease. *Am J Cardiol.* 1992;70:141–6.

29. Hesse B, Morise A, Pothier CE, et al. Can we reliably predict long-term mortality after exercise testing? An external validation. *Am Heart J.* 2005;150:307–14.

30. Hollingsworth V, Bendick P, Franklin B, et al. Validity of arm ergometer blood pressures immediately after exercise. *Am J Cardiol.* 1990;65:1358–60.

31. Kaminsky LA, Whaley MH. Evaluation of a new standardized ramp protocol: the BSU/Bruce ramp protocol. *J Cardiopulm Rehabil.* 1998;18:438–44.

32. Kavanagh T, Mertens DJ, Hamm LF, et al. Peak oxygen intake and cardiac mortality in women referred for cardiac rehabilitation. *J Am Coll Cardiol.* 2003;42:2139–43.

33. Kavanagh T, Mertens DJ, Hamm LF, et al. Prediction of long term prognosis in 12,169 men referred for cardiac rehabilitation. *Circulation.* 2002;106:666–71.

34. Klocke FJ, Baird MG, Lorell BH, et al. ACC/AHA/ASNC guidelines for the clinical use of cardiac radionuclide imaging—executive summary: a report of the American College of Cardiology/American Heart Association Task Force on Practice Guidelines (ACC/AHA/ASNC Committee to Revise the 1995 Guidelines for the Clinical Use of Cardiac Radionuclide Imaging). *Circulation.* 2003;108:1404–18.

35. Knight JA, Laubach Jr CA, Butcher RJ, et al. Supervision of clinical exercise testing by exercise physiologists. *Am J Cardiol.* 1995;75:390–1.

36. Lachterman B, Lehmann KG, Abrahamson D, et al. "Recovery only" ST-segment depression and the predictive accuracy of the exercise test. *Ann Intern Med.* 1990;112:11–6.

37. Lewis WR, Amsterdam EA. Evaluation of the patient with 'rule out myocardial infarction.' *Arch Intern Med.* 1996;156:41–5.

38. Mark DB, Shaw L, Harrell Jr FE, et al. Prognostic value of a treadmill exercise score in outpatients with suspected coronary artery disease. *N Engl J Med.* 1991;325:849–53.

39. Mason RE, Likar I. A new system of multiple-lead exercise electrocardiography. *Am Heart J.* 1996;71:196–205.

40. Milliken JA, Abdollah H, Burggraf GW. False-positive treadmill exercise tests due to computer signal averaging. *Am J Cardiol.*1990;65:946–48.
41. Morris CK, Myers J, Froelicher VF, et al. Nomogram based on metabolic equivalents and age for assessing aerobic exercise capacity in men. *J Am Coll Cardiol.* 1993;22:175–82.
42. Myers J, Buchanan N, Smith D, et al. Individualized ramp treadmill. Observations on a new protocol. *Chest.* 1992;101:236S–41S.
43. Myers J, Buchanan N, Walsh D, et al. Comparison of the ramp versus standard exercise protocols. *J Am Coll Cardiol.*1991;17:1334–42.
44. Myers J, Prakash M, Froelicher V, et al. Exercise capacity and mortality among men referred for exercise testing. *N Engl J Med.* 2002;346:793–801.
45. Myers JN. Perception of chest pain during exercise testing in patients with coronary artery disease. *Med Sci Sports Exerc.* 1994;26:1082–6.
46. Orenstein DM, Curtis SE, Nixon PA, et al. Accuracy of three pulse oximeters during exercise and hypoxemia in patients with cystic fibrosis. *Chest.* 1993;104:1187–90.
47. Pollock ML, Wilmore JH, Fox SM. *Exercise in Health and Disease: Evaluation and Prescription for Prevention and Rehabilitation.* Philadelphia (PA): WB Saunders; 1990.
48. Ries AL, Farrow JT, Clausen JL. Accuracy of two ear oximeters at rest and during exercise in pulmonary patients. *Am Rev Respir Dis.* 1985;132:685–9.
49. Rodgers GP, Ayanian JZ, Balady G, et al. American College of Cardiology/American Heart Association Clinical Competence Statement on Stress Testing: A Report of the American College of Cardiology/American Heart Association/American College of Physicians–American Society of Internal Medicine Task Force on Clinical Competence. *Circulation.* 2000;102:1726–38.
50. Sheldahl LM, Wilke NA, Tristani FE. Evaluation and training for resumption of occupational and leisure-time physical activities in patients after a major cardiac event. *Med Exerc Nutr Health.* 1995;4:273–89.
51. Shetler K, Marcus R, Froelicher VF, et al. Heart rate recovery: validation and methodologic issues. *J Am Coll Cardiol.* 2001;38:1980–7.
52. Vanhees L, Fagard R, Thijs L, et al. Prognostic significance of peak exercise capacity in patients with coronary artery disease. *J Am Coll Cardiol.* 1994;23:358–63.
53. Wilke NA, Sheldahl LM, Dougherty SM, et al. Baltimore Therapeutic Equipment work simulator: energy expenditure of work activities in cardiac patients. *Arch Phys Med Rehabil.* 1993;74:419–24.
54. Wilson PW, D'Agostino RB, Levy D, et al. Prediction of coronary heart disease using risk factor categories. *Circulation.* 1998;97:1837–47.
55. Zeballos RJ, Weisman IM. Reliability of noninvasive oximetry in black subjects during exercise and hypoxia. *Am Rev Respir Dis.* 1991;144:1240–4.

Interpretation of Clinical Exercise Test Data

This chapter addresses the interpretation and clinical significance of exercise test results, with specific reference to hemodynamic, electrocardiographic (ECG), and gas exchange and ventilatory responses. The diagnostic and prognostic value of the exercise test will be discussed along with screening for atherosclerotic cardiovascular disease (CVD).

EXERCISE TESTING AS A SCREENING TOOL FOR CORONARY ARTERY DISEASE

The probability of a patient having CVD cannot be estimated accurately from the exercise test result and the diagnostic characteristics of the test alone. It also depends on the likelihood of having disease before the test is administered. Bayes' theorem states that the posttest probability of having disease is determined by the disease probability *before* the test and the probability that the test will provide a true result. The probability of a patient having disease before the test is related, most importantly, to the presence of symptoms (particularly chest pain characteristics), but also to the patient's age, sex, and the presence of major risk factors for cardiovascular disease.

Exercise testing in individuals with known CVD (prior myocardial infarction, angiographically documented coronary stenoses, and/or prior coronary revascularization) is not regularly used for diagnostic purposes. However, the description of symptoms can be most helpful among individuals in whom the diagnosis is in question. Typical or definite angina (substernal chest discomfort that may radiate to the back, jaw, or arms; symptoms provoked by exertion or emotional stress and relieved by rest and/or nitroglycerin) makes the pretest probability so high that the test result does not dramatically change the likelihood of underlying CVD. Atypical angina (chest discomfort that lacks one of the mentioned characteristics of typical angina) generally indicates an intermediate pretest likelihood of CVD in men older than 30 years and women older than 50 years (see Table 5.1).

The use of exercise testing in screening asymptomatic individuals, particularly among individuals without diabetes or other risk factors for CVD, is problematic in view of the low to very low pretest likelihood of CVD (Table 5.1). A recent American Heart Association Scientific Statement on Exercise Testing in

Asymptomatic Adults (23) confirmed earlier recommendations (17,41) that there is insufficient evidence to support exercise testing as a routine screening modality in asymptomatic individuals. Such testing can have potential adverse consequences (e.g., psychological, work and insurance status, costs for subsequent testing) by misclassifying a large percentage of those without CVD as having disease. Testing in asymptomatic persons *with multiple risk factors* has shown promise for effectively stratifying risk (15), but has not been strongly recommended based on available data (17,23,29). It is likewise difficult to choose a chronologic age beyond which exercise testing becomes valuable as a screening tool before beginning an exercise program because physiologic age often differs from chronologic age. In general, the guidelines presented in Figure 2.4 are recommended if the exercise is more strenuous than brisk walking. The potential ramifications resulting from mass screening must be considered and the results of such testing must be applied using predictive modeling and Bayesian analyses. Test results should be considered as probability statements and not as absolutes.

INTERPRETATION OF RESPONSES TO GRADED EXERCISE TESTING

Before interpreting clinical test data, it is important to consider the purpose of the test (e.g., diagnostic or prognostic) and individual clinical characteristics that may influence the exercise test or its interpretation. Medical conditions influencing test interpretation include orthopedic limitations, pulmonary disease, obesity, neurologic disorders, and deconditioning. Medication effects (Appendix A) and resting ECG abnormalities also must be considered, especially resting ST-segment changes secondary to conduction defects, left ventricular hypertrophy, and other factors that may contribute to spurious ST-segment depression.

Although total body and myocardial oxygen consumption are directly related, the relationship between these variables can be altered by exercise training, drugs, and disease. For example, exercise-induced myocardial ischemia may cause left ventricular dysfunction, exercise intolerance, and a hypotensive blood pressure (BP) response. Although the severity of symptomatic ischemia is inversely related to exercise capacity, left ventricular ejection fraction does not correlate well with exercise tolerance (28,34).

Responses to exercise tests are useful in evaluating the need for and effectiveness of various types of therapeutic interventions. The following variables are important to quantify accurately when assessing the therapeutic, diagnostic, and prognostic applications of the test. Each is described in the following sections and summarized in Box 6.1:

- Hemodynamics: assessed by the heart rate (HR) and systolic BP (SBP)/diastolic BP (DBP) responses
- ECG waveforms: particularly ST-segment displacement and supraventricular and ventricular dysrhythmias
- Limiting clinical signs or symptoms
- Gas exchange and ventilatory responses (e.g., $\dot{V}O_{2max}$, $\dot{V}E$, and $\dot{V}E/\dot{V}CO_2$ slope)

BOX 6.1	Electrocardiographic, Cardiorespiratory, and Hemodynamic Responses to Exercise Testing and Their Clinical Significance

VARIABLE	CLINICAL SIGNIFICANCE
ST-segment depression (ST $\downarrow$)	An abnormal ECG response is defined as $\geq$1.0 mm of horizontal or downsloping ST $\downarrow$ 60–80 msec beyond the J point, suggesting myocardial ischemia.
ST-segment elevation (ST $\uparrow$)	ST $\uparrow$ in leads displaying a previous Q wave MI almost always reflects an aneurysm or wall-motion abnormality. In the absence of significant Q waves, exercise-induced ST $\uparrow$ often is associated with a fixed high-grade coronary stenosis.
Supraventricular dysrhythmias	Isolated atrial ectopic beats or short runs of SVT commonly occur during exercise testing and do not appear to have any diagnostic or prognostic significance for CVD.
Ventricular dysrhythmias	The suppression of resting ventricular dysrhythmias during exercise *does not* exclude the presence of underlying CVD; conversely, PVCs that increase in frequency, complexity, or both do not necessarily signify underlying ischemic heart disease. Complex ventricular ectopy, including paired or multiform PVCs, and runs of ventricular tachycardia ($\geq$3 successive beats) are likely to be associated with significant CVD and/or a poor prognosis if they occur in conjunction with signs and/or symptoms of myocardial ischemia or in patients with a history of sudden cardiac death, cardiomyopathy, or valvular heart disease. Frequent ventricular ectopy during recovery has been found to be a better predictor of mortality than ventricular ectopy that occurs only during exercise.
Heart rate (HR)	The normal HR response to progressive exercise is a relatively linear increase, corresponding to 10 ± 2 beats $\cdot$ MET^{-1} for inactive subjects. Chronotropic incompetence may be signified by: 1. A peak exercise HR that is >2 SD ($\approx$20 beats $\cdot$ min^{-1}) below the age-predicted maximal HR or an inability to achieve >85% of the age-predicted maximal HR for subjects who are limited by volitional fatigue and are not taking β-blockers $>$

> Box 6.1, continued

VARIABLE	CLINICAL SIGNIFICANCE
	2. A chronotropic index (CI) <0.8 (8,9); where CI is calculated as the percentage of heart rate reserve to percent metabolic reserve achieved at any test stage
Heart rate recovery (HRR)	An abnormal (slowed) HRR is associated with a poor prognosis. HRR has frequently been defined as a decrease ≤12 beats/min at 1 min (walking in recovery), or ≤22 beats/min at 2 min (supine position in recovery).
Systolic blood pressure (SBP)	The normal response to exercise is a progressive increase in SBP, typically 10 ± 2 mm Hg · MET^{-1}, with a possible plateau at peak exercise. Exercise testing should be discontinued with SBP values of >250 mm Hg. Exertional hypotension (SBP that fails to rise or falls [>10 mm Hg]) may signify myocardial ischemia and/or LV dysfunction. Maximal exercise SBP of <140 mm Hg suggests a poor prognosis.
Diastolic blood pressure (DBP)	The normal response to exercise is no change or a decrease in DBP. A DBP of >115 mm Hg is considered an endpoint for exercise testing.
Anginal symptoms	Can be graded on a scale of 1 to 4, corresponding to perceptible but mild, moderate, moderately severe, and severe, respectively. A rating of 3 (moderately severe) generally should be used as an endpoint for exercise testing.
Aerobic fitness	Average values of $\dot{V}O_{2max}$ expressed as METs, expected in healthy sedentary men and women, can be predicted from the following regressions (43): men = (57.8-0.445 [age])/3.5; women = (41.2-0.343 [age])/3.5. Also, see Table 4.8 for age-specific $\dot{V}O_{2max}$ norms.

ECG, electrocardiographic; MI, myocardial infarction; SVT, supraventricular tachycardia; CVD, coronary artery disease; PVC, premature ventricular contraction; HR, heart rate; MET, metabolic equivalent; CI, chronotropic index; SD, standard deviation; LV, left ventricular; HRR, heart rate recover; SBP, systolic blood pressure; DBP, diastolic blood pressure; $\dot{V}O_{2max}$, maximal oxygen uptake.

HEART RATE RESPONSE

Maximal heart rate (HR_{max}) may be predicted from age using any of several published equations (27). The relationship between age and HR_{max} for a large sample of subjects is well established; however, interindividual variability is high (standard deviation, 10–12 beats$\cdot$min^{-1}). As a result, there is potential for considerable error in the use of methods that extrapolate submaximal test data to an age-predicted HR_{max}. Aerobic capacity, anthropometric measures such as height and weight, and body composition do not independently influence HR_{max}. The inability to appropriately increase HR during exercise (chronotropic incompetence) is associated with the presence of heart disease and increased mortality (13,20,25). A delayed decrease in HR early in recovery after a symptom-limited maximal exercise test (e.g., <12 beats/min decrease after the first minute in recovery) is also a powerful predictor of overall mortality (20).

Achievement of age-predicted HR_{max} should not be used as an absolute test endpoint or as an indication that effort has been maximal because of its high intersubject variability. The clinical indications for stopping an exercise test are presented in Box 5.2. Good judgment on the part of the physician and/or supervising staff remains the most important criterion for terminating an exercise test.

BLOOD PRESSURE RESPONSE

The normal BP response to dynamic upright exercise consists of a progressive increase in SBP, no change or a slight decrease in DBP, and a widening of the pulse pressure. The following are key points concerning interpretation of the BP response to progressive dynamic exercise:

- A drop in SBP (>10 mm Hg decrease in SBP despite an increase in workload), or failure of SBP to increase with increased workload, is considered an abnormal test response. Exercise-induced decreases in SBP (exertional hypotension) may occur in patients with CVD, valvular heart disease, cardiomyopathies, and serious dysrhythmias. Occasionally, patients without clinically significant heart disease demonstrate exertional hypotension caused by antihypertensive therapy, prolonged strenuous exercise, and vasovagal responses. However, exertional hypotension has been shown to correlate with myocardial ischemia, left ventricular dysfunction, and an increased risk of subsequent cardiac events (11,18). In some cases this response is improved after coronary bypass surgery. Studies have linked an excessive exercise-induced rise in DBP with underlying CVD, but these observations are not as well documented as those for exercise-induced changes in SBP. However, a DBP >115 mm Hg is considered a criterion for termination of graded exercise testing and exercise training.
- The normal postexercise response is a progressive decline in SBP. During passive recovery in an upright posture, SBP may decrease abruptly because of peripheral pooling (and usually normalizes on resuming the supine position). SBP may remain below pretest resting values for several hours after the test. DBP also may drop during the postexercise period.

- In patients on vasodilators, calcium channel blockers, angiotensin-converting enzyme inhibitors, and α- and β-adrenergic blockers, the BP response to exercise is variably attenuated and cannot be accurately predicted in the absence of clinical test data.
- Although HR_{max} is comparable for men and women, men generally have higher SBPs ($\sim 20 \pm 5$ mm Hg) during maximal treadmill testing. However, the sex difference is no longer apparent after 70 years of age. A SBP >250 mm Hg or a DBP >115 mm Hg has empirically been used as a reason for test termination.
- The rate-pressure product, or *double product* (SBP $\times$ HR) is an indicator of myocardial oxygen demand (19). Signs and symptoms of ischemia generally occur at a reproducible double product.

ELECTROCARDIOGRAPH WAVEFORMS

Appendix C provides information to aid in the interpretation of resting and exercise electrocardiograms. Additional information is provided here with respect to common exercise-induced changes in ECG variables. The normal ECG response to exercise includes the following:

- Minor and insignificant changes in P-wave morphology
- Superimposition of the P and T waves of successive beats
- Increases in septal Q-wave amplitude
- Slight decreases in R-wave amplitude
- Increases in T-wave amplitude (although wide variability exists among subjects)
- Minimal shortening of the QRS duration
- Depression of the J point
- Rate-related shortening of the QT interval

However, some changes in ECG wave morphology may be indicative of underlying pathology. For example, although QRS duration tends to decrease slightly with exercise (and increasing HR) in normal subjects, it may increase in patients with either angina or left ventricular dysfunction. Exercise-induced P-wave changes are rarely seen and are of questionable significance. Many factors affect R-wave amplitude; consequently, such changes during exercise have no independent predictive power (33).

ST-Segment Displacement

ST-segment changes are widely accepted criteria for myocardial ischemia and injury. The interpretation of ST segments may be affected by the resting ECG configuration (e.g., bundle-branch blocks, left ventricular hypertrophy) and pharmacologic agents (e.g., digitalis therapy). There may be J-point depression and tall peaked T waves at high exercise intensities and during recovery in normal subjects (37). Depression of the J point that leads to marked ST-segment upsloping is caused by competition between normal repolarization and delayed terminal depolarization forces rather than by ischemia (30). Exercise-induced myocardial ischemia may be manifested by different types of ST-segment changes on the ECG, as shown in Figure 6.1.

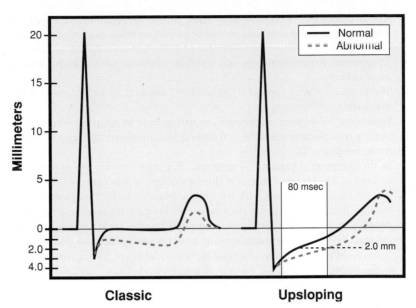

FIGURE 6.1. ST-segment changes during exercise. Classic ST-segment depression (first complex) is defined as a horizontal or downsloping ST segment that is ≥1.0 mm below the baseline 60–80 msec past the J point. Slowly upsloping ST-segment depression (second complex) should be considered a borderline response, and added emphasis should be placed on other clinical and exercise variables.

ST-Segment Elevation

- ST-segment elevation (early repolarization) may be seen in the normal resting ECG. Increasing HR usually causes these elevated ST segments to return to the isoelectric line.
- Exercise-induced ST-segment elevation in leads with Q waves consistent with a prior myocardial infarction may be indicative of wall-motion abnormalities, ischemia, or both (6).
- Exercise-induced ST-segment elevation on an otherwise normal ECG (except in aVR or V_{1-2}) generally indicates significant myocardial ischemia and localizes the ischemia to a specific area of myocardium (36). This response may also be associated with ventricular arrhythmias and myocardial injury.

ST-Segment Depression

- ST-segment depression (depression of the J point and the slope at 80 msec past the J point) is the most common manifestation of exercise-induced myocardial ischemia.
- Horizontal or downsloping ST-segment depression is more indicative of myocardial ischemia than is upsloping depression.
- The standard criterion for a positive test is ≥1.0 mm (0.1 mV) of horizontal or downsloping ST segment at the J point extending for 60 to 80 msec.

- Slowly upsloping ST-segment depression should be considered a borderline response, and added emphasis should be placed on other clinical and exercise variables.
- ST-segment depression does not localize ischemia to a specific area of myocardium.
- The more leads with (apparent) ischemic ST-segment shifts, the more severe the disease.
- Significant ST-segment depression occurring only in recovery likely represents a true positive response and should be considered an important diagnostic finding (23).
- In the presence of baseline ST abnormalities ≥ 1.0 mm on the resting ECG, additional ST-segment depression during exercise is less specific for myocardial ischemia. In patients with left bundle-branch block, ST-segment abnormalities that develop during exercise are uninterpretable with respect to evidence of myocardial ischemia (43). In right bundle-branch block, exercise-induced ST-segment depression in the anterior precordial leads (V_1, V_2, and V_3) should not be used to diagnose ischemia; however, ST-segment changes in the lateral leads (V_4, V_5, and V_6) or inferior leads (II, III, and aVF) may be indicative of ischemia (43).
- Adjustment of the ST-segment relative to the HR may provide additional diagnostic information. The ST/HR index is the ratio of the maximal ST-segment change (measured in mV) to the maximal change in HR from rest to peak exercise (measured in beats $\cdot$ min^{-1}). An ST/HR index of ≥ 1.6 is defined as abnormal. The ST/HR slope reflects the maximal slope relating the amount of the ST-segment depression (measured in mV) to HR (measured in beats $\cdot$ min^{-1}) during exercise. An ST/HR slope of >2.4 mV $\cdot$ beats^{-1} $\cdot$ min^{-1} is defined as abnormal. Several studies have addressed the diagnostic value of these ST/HR variables (16,24,31,38), but the findings have been inconsistent and preclude a recommendation regarding their utility.

ST-Segment Normalization or Absence of Change

- Ischemia may be manifested by normalization of resting ST-segments. ECG abnormalities at rest, including T-wave inversion and ST-segment depression, may return to normal during anginal symptoms and during exercise in some patients (26).

Dysrhythmias

Exercise-associated dysrhythmias occur in healthy subjects as well as patients with cardiac disease. Increased sympathetic drive and changes in extracellular and intracellular electrolytes, pH, and oxygen tension contribute to disturbances in myocardial and conducting tissue automaticity and reentry, which are major mechanisms of dysrhythmias.

Supraventricular Dysrhythmias

Isolated premature atrial contractions are common and require no special precautions. Atrial flutter or atrial fibrillation may occur in organic heart disease or may reflect endocrine, metabolic, or drug effects. Sustained supraventricular tachycardia occasionally is induced by exercise and may require pharmacologic treatment or electroconversion if discontinuation of exercise fails to abolish the rhythm. Patients who experience paroxysmal atrial tachycardia may be evaluated by repeating the exercise test after appropriate treatment.

Ventricular Dysrhythmias

Isolated premature ventricular complexes or contractions (PVCs) occur during exercise in 30% to 40% of healthy subjects and in 50% to 60% of patients with CVD. In some individuals, graded exercise induces PVCs, whereas in others, it reduces their occurrence. The clinical significance of exercise-induced PVCs remains a matter of debate. The suppression of PVCs that are present at rest with exercise testing does not exclude the presence of CVD, and PVCs that increase in frequency, complexity, or both do not necessarily signify underlying ischemic heart disease (5,14). Serious forms of ventricular ectopy, including paired or multiform PVCs or runs of ventricular tachycardia ($\geq$3 PVCs in succession), are likely to be associated with significant CVD, a poor prognosis, or both, if they occur in conjunction with signs or symptoms of myocardial ischemia, or in patients with a history of resuscitated sudden cardiac death, cardiomyopathy, or valvular heart disease. In healthy individuals, however, some studies have shown that exercise-induced PVCs are associated with a higher mortality, whereas other studies report that no such association exists (5,14).

Criteria for terminating exercise tests based on ventricular ectopy include sustained ventricular tachycardia, multifocal PVCs, and short runs of ventricular tachycardia. The decision to terminate an exercise test should also be influenced by simultaneous evidence of myocardial ischemia and/or adverse signs or symptoms (see Box 5.2).

LIMITING SIGNS AND SYMPTOMS

Although patients with exercise-induced ST-segment depression can be asymptomatic, when concomitant angina occurs, the likelihood that the ECG changes result from CVD is significantly increased (42). In addition, angina pectoris *without* ischemic ECG changes may be as predictive of CVD as ST-segment changes alone (10). Both are currently considered independent variables that identify patients at increased risk for subsequent coronary events.

In the absence of untoward signs or symptoms, patients generally should be encouraged to give their best effort so that maximal exercise tolerance can be determined. However, the determination of what constitutes "maximal" effort, although important for interpreting test results, can be difficult. Various criteria have been used to confirm that a maximal effort has been elicited during graded exercise testing. However, all of the following criteria for maximal effort can be subjective and are therefore flawed:

- Failure of HR to increase with further increases in exercise intensity.
- A plateau in oxygen uptake (or failure to increase oxygen uptake by 150 mL · min^{-1}) with increased workload (39). This criterion has fallen into disfavor because a

plateau is inconsistently seen during continuous graded exercise tests and is confused by various definitions and how data are sampled during exercise (35).

- A respiratory exchange ratio >1.1; however, there is considerable interindividual variability in this response.
- Various postexercise venous lactic acid concentrations (e.g., 8–10 mmol · L^{-1}) have been used; however, there is also significant interindividual variability in this response.
- A rating of perceived exertion >17 on the 6–20 scale or >9 on the 0–10 scale.

GAS EXCHANGE AND VENTILATORY RESPONSES

Direct measurement of gas exchange and ventilatory responses to exercise provide a more precise assessment of exercise capacity, help to distinguish causes of exercise intolerance, and provide more accurate estimates of prognosis. These responses can be used to assess patient effort during an exercise test, particularly when a reduction in maximal exercise capacity is suspected. Submaximal efforts from the patient can interfere with the interpretation of the test results and subsequent patient management. Maximal or peak oxygen uptake ($\dot{V}O_{2peak}$) provides important information about cardiovascular fitness and is a powerful marker of prognosis. Population-specific nomograms (see Fig. 5.1) and/or population norms (see Table 4.8) may be used to compare $\dot{V}O_{2peak}$ with the expected value for a given age, sex, and activity status (7,12).

Gas exchange and ventilatory responses often are used in clinical settings as an estimation of the point at which lactate accumulation in the blood occurs, sometimes referred to as the *lactate* or *anaerobic threshold*. Several different methods using both gas exchange and ventilatory responses have been proposed for the estimation of this point. These include the ventilatory equivalents method (8,40) and the V-slope method (4). Whichever method is used, it should be remembered that the use of any of these methods provides only an estimation, and the concept of anaerobiosis during exercise is controversial (34). Because exercise beyond the lactate threshold is associated with metabolic acidosis, hyperventilation, and a reduced capacity to perform work, its estimation has evolved into a useful physiologic measurement when evaluating interventions in patients with heart and pulmonary disease as well as studying the limits of performance in healthy individuals.

In addition to estimating when blood lactate values begin to increase, maximal minute ventilation ($\dot{V}E_{max}$) can be used in conjunction with the maximal voluntary ventilation (MVV) to determine if there is a ventilatory limitation to maximal exercise. A comparison between the $\dot{V}E_{max}$ and the MVV can be used when evaluating responses to a graded exercise test. The relationship between these measures, typically referred to as the ventilatory reserve, traditionally has been defined as the percentage of the MVV achieved at maximal exercise (i.e., the $\dot{V}E_{max}$/MVV ratio). In most normal subjects this ratio ranges from 50% to 85% (2). Patients with pulmonary disease typically have values >85%, indicative of a reduced ventilatory reserve and a possible pulmonary limitation to exercise.

DIAGNOSTIC VALUE OF EXERCISE TESTING

The diagnostic value of conventional exercise testing for the detection of CVD is influenced by the principles of conditional probability (Box 6.2). The factors that determine the predictive outcome of exercise testing (and other diagnostic tests) are the sensitivity and specificity of the test procedure and the prevalence of CVD in the population tested. Sensitivity and specificity determine how effective the test is in making correct diagnoses in individuals with and without disease, respectively. Disease prevalence is an important determinant of the predictive value of the test. Moreover, non-ECG criteria (e.g., duration of exercise or maximal metabolic equivalent [MET] level, hemodynamic responses, symptoms of angina or dyspnea) should be considered in the overall interpretation of exercise test results.

SENSITIVITY

Sensitivity refers to the percentage of patients tested with known CVD who demonstrate significant ST-segment (i.e., positive) changes. Exercise ECG sensitivity for the detection of CVD usually is based on subsequent angiographically determined coronary artery stenosis of 70% or more in at least one vessel. A true-positive exercise test reveals horizontal or downsloping ST-segment depression of 1.0 mm or more and correctly identifies a patient with CVD. False-negative test results show no or nondiagnostic ECG changes and fail to identify patients with underlying CVD.

Common factors that contribute to false-negative exercise tests are summarized in Box 6.3. Test sensitivity is decreased by inadequate myocardial stress, drugs that attenuate cardiac demands to exercise or reduce myocardial ischemia (e.g., β-blockers, nitrates, calcium channel–blocking agents), and insufficient ECG lead monitoring. Pre-existing ECG changes, such as left ventricular hypertrophy, left bundle-branch block, or the pre-excitation syndrome (Wolff-Parkinson-White syndrome), limit the ability to interpret exercise-induced

---

BOX 6.2	**Sensitivity, Specificity, and Predictive Value of Diagnostic Graded Exercise Testing**

Sensitivity = TP/(TP + FN) = the percentage of patients with CVD who have a positive test

Specificity = TN/(TN + FP) = the percentage of patients without CVD who have a negative test

Predictive Value (positive test) = TP/(TP + FP) = the percentage of patients with a positive test result who have CVD

Predictive Value (negative test) = TN/(TN + FN) = the percentage of patients with a negative test who do not have CVD

CVD, cardiovascular disease; TP, true positive (positive exercise test and CVD); FP, false positive (positive exercise test and no CVD); TN, true negative (negative exercise test and no CVD); FN, false negative (negative exercise test and CVD).

BOX 6.3   Causes of False-Negative Test Results

- Failure to reach an ischemic threshold
- Monitoring an insufficient number of leads to detect ECG changes
- Failure to recognize non-ECG signs and symptoms that may be associated with underlying CVD (e.g., exertional hypotension)
- Angiographically significant CVD compensated by collateral circulation
- Musculoskeletal limitations to exercise preceding cardiac abnormalities
- Technical or observer error

ST-segment changes as ischemic ECG responses. The exercise test is most accurate for detecting CVD by applying validated multivariate scores (pretest risk markers in addition to ST-segment changes and other exercise test responses) (3).

SPECIFICITY

The *specificity* of exercise tests refers to the percentage of patients without CVD who demonstrate nonsignificant (i.e., negative) ST-segment changes. A true-negative test correctly identifies a person without CVD. Many conditions may cause abnormal exercise ECG responses in the absence of significant obstructive CVD (Box 6.4).

BOX 6.4   Causes of Abnormal ST Changes in the Absence of Obstructive Coronary Artery Disease[a]

- Resting repolarization abnormalities (e.g., left bundle-branch block)
- Cardiac hypertrophy
- Accelerated conduction defects (e.g., Wolff-Parkinson-White syndrome)
- Digitalis
- Nonischemic cardiomyopathy
- Hypokalemia
- Vasoregulatory abnormalities
- Mitral valve prolapse
- Pericardial disorders
- Technical or observer error
- Coronary spasm in the absence of significant coronary artery disease
- Anemia
- Female sex

[a]Selected variables simply may be associated with rather than be causes of abnormal test results.

Reported values for the specificity and sensitivity of exercise ECG testing vary because of differences in patient selection, test protocols, ECG criteria for a positive test, and the angiographic definition of CVD. In studies that controlled for these variables, the pooled results show a sensitivity of 68% and a specificity of 77% (17). Sensitivity, however, is somewhat lower and specificity is higher when workup bias is removed (16,31).

PREDICTIVE VALUE

The predictive value of exercise testing is a measure of how accurately a test result (positive or negative) correctly identifies the presence or absence of CVD in tested patients. For example, the predictive value of a positive test is the percentage of those persons with an abnormal test who have CVD. Nevertheless, a test should not be classified as "negative" unless the patient has attained an adequate level of myocardial stress, generally defined as having achieved 85% or more of predicted HR_{max} during the test. Predictive value cannot be estimated directly from a test's specificity or sensitivity because it depends on the prevalence of disease in the population being tested.

COMPARISON WITH IMAGING STRESS TESTS

Several imaging tests, including echocardiography and nuclear techniques, are often used in association with exercise testing to diagnose CVD. Guidelines are available that describe these techniques and their accuracy for detecting CVD (19,21). Exercise echocardiography has a weighted mean sensitivity of 86%, specificity of 81%, and overall accuracy of 85% for the detection of CVD. Exercise with concomitant nuclear imaging using technetium (Tc99m) agents has shown similar accuracy to those using thallous (thallium) chloride-201 agents in the detection of myocardial ischemia. Exercise nuclear single-photon emission computed tomography (SPECT) imaging has a sensitivity of 87% and specificity of 73% for detecting CVD with ≥50% coronary stenosis (1). The sensitivity and specificity are similar for planar and tomographic nuclear imaging.

PROGNOSTIC APPLICATIONS OF THE EXERCISE TEST

Risk or prognostic evaluation is an important activity in medical practice on which many patient-management decisions are based. In patients with CVD, several clinical factors contribute to patient outcome, including severity and stability of symptoms; left ventricular function; angiographic extent and severity of CVD; electrical stability of the myocardium; and the presence of other comorbid conditions. Unless cardiac catheterization and immediate coronary revascularization are indicated, an exercise test should be performed in persons with known or suspected CVD to assess risk of future cardiac events and to assist in subsequent management decisions. As stated in Chapter 5, data derived from the exercise test are most useful when considered in the context of other clinical information. Important prognostic variables that can be derived from the exercise test are summarized in Box 6.1.

Several multivariate prognostic scores, such as the Veteran's Administration score (32) (validated for the male veteran population) and the Duke nomogram

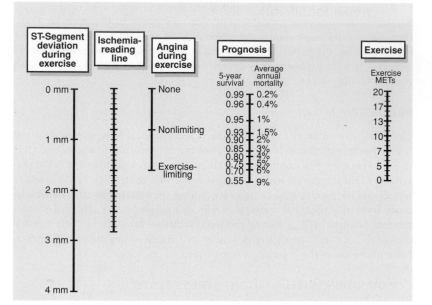

FIGURE 6.2. Duke nomogram uses five steps to estimate prognosis for a given individual from the parameters of the Duke score. First, the observed amount of ST depression is marked on the ST-segment deviation line. Second, the observed degree of angina is marked on the line for angina, and these two points are connected. Third, the point where this line intersects the ischemia reading line is noted. Fourth, the observed exercise tolerance is marked on the line for exercise capacity. Finally, the mark on the ischemia reading line is connected to the mark on the exercise capacity line, and the estimated 5-year survival or average annual mortality rate is read from the point at which this line intersects the prognosis scale.

(28) (validated for the general population, including women) (Fig. 6.2) can be helpful when applied appropriately. The Duke nomogram does not appear to be valid in patients older than age 75 years (22). Patients who recently have suffered an acute myocardial infarction and received thrombolytic therapy and/or have undergone coronary revascularization generally have a low subsequent cardiac event rate. Exercise testing still can provide prognostic information in this population, as well as assist in activity counseling and exercise prescription.

REFERENCES

1. ACCF/ASNC appropriateness criteria for single-photon emission computed tomography perfusion imaging (SPECT MPI): a report of the American College of Cardiology Foundation Quality Strategic Directions Committee Appropriateness Criteria Working Group and the American Society of Nuclear Cardiology endorsed by the American Heart Association. *J Am Coll Cardiol.* 2005;46:1587–605.
2. American Thoracic Society and American College of Chest Physicians. ATS/ACCP Statement on cardiopulmonary exercise testing. *Am J Respir Crit Care Med.* 2003;167:211–77.
3. Ashley E, Myers J, Froelicher VF. Exercise testing scores as an example of better decisions through science. *Med Sci Sports Exerc.* 2002;34:1391–8.

4. Beaver WL, Wasserman K, Whipp BJ. A new method for detecting anaerobic threshold by gas exchange. *J Appl Physiol.* 1986;60:2020–7.

5. Beckerman J, Wu T, Jones S, et al. Exercise test-induced arrhythmias. *Prog Cardiovasc Dis* 2005;47: 285–305,

6. Bruce RA, Fisher LD, Pettinger M, et al. ST segment elevation with exercise: a marker for poor ventricular function and poor prognosis. Coronary Artery Surgery Study (CASS) confirmation of Seattle Heart Watch results. *Circulation.* 1988;77:897–905.

7. Bruce RA, Kusumi F, Hosmer D. Maximal oxygen intake and nomographic assessment of functional aerobic impairment in cardiovascular disease. *Am Heart J.* 1973;85:546–62.

8. Caiozzo VJ, Davis JA, Ellis JF, et al. A comparison of gas exchange indices used to detect the anaerobic threshold. *J Appl Physiol.* 1982;53:1184–9.

9. Cheitlin MD, Armstrong WF, Aurigemma GP, et al. ACC/AHA/ASE 2003 guideline update for the clinical application of echocardiography: summary article: a report of the American College of Cardiology/American Heart Association Task Force on Practice Guidelines (ACC/AHA/ASE Committee to Update the 1997 Guidelines for the Clinical Application of Echocardiography). *Circulation.* 2003; 108:1146–62.

10. Cole JP, Ellestad MH. Significance of chest pain during treadmill exercise: correlation with coronary events. *Am J Cardiol.* 1978;41:227–32.

11. Comess KA, Fenster PE. Clinical implications of the blood pressure response to exercise. *Cardiology.* 1981;68:233–44.

12. Day JR, Rossiter HB, Coats EM, Skasick A, Whipp BJ. The maximally attainable VO_2 during exercise in humans: the peak vs. maximum issue. *J Appl Physiol.* 2003;95:1901–7.

13. Ellestad MH. Chronotropic incompetence: the implications of heart rate response to exercise (compensatory parasympathetic hyperactivity?). *Circulation.* 1996;93:1485–7.

14. Evans CH, Froelcher VF. Some common abnormal responses to exercise testing. In: Evans C, editor. Exercise Testing. *Primary Care.* 2001;28:219–32.

15. Froelicher VF. Screening with the exercise test: time for a guideline change? *Eur Heart J.* 2005;26: 1353–4.

16. Froelicher VF, Lehmann KG, Thomas R, et al. The electrocardiographic exercise test in a population with reduced workup bias: diagnostic performance, computerized interpretation, and multivariable prediction. *Ann Intern Med.* 1998;128:965–74.

17. Gibbons RJ, Balady GJ, Bricker JT, et al. Pretest likelihood of atherosclerotic cardiovascular disease (CVD). ACC/AHA 2002 Guideline Update for Exercise Testing; a report of the American College of Cardiology/American Heart Association Task Force on Practice Guidelines; Committee on Exercise Testing, 2002. *Circulation.* 2002;106(14):1883–92.

18. Irving JB, Bruce RA, DeRouen TA. Variations in and significance of systolic pressure during maximal exercise (treadmill) testing. *Am J Cardiol.* 1977;39:841–8.

19. Kitamura K, Jorgensen CR, Gobel FL, et al. Hemodynamic correlates of myocardial oxygen consumption during upright exercise. *J Appl Physiol.* 1972;32:516–22.

20. Kligfield P, Lauer MS. Exercise electrocardiogram testing: beyond the ST segment. *Circulation.* 2006;114:2070–82.

21. Klocke FJ, Baird MG, Lorell BH, et al. ACC/AHA/ASNC guidelines for the clinical use of cardiac radionuclide imaging—executive summary: report of the American College of Cardiology/American Heart Association Task Force on Practice Guidelines (ACC/AHA/ASNC Committee to Revise the 1995 Guidelines for the Clinical Use of Cardiac Radionuclide Imaging). *J Am Coll Cardiol.* 2003;42:1318–33.

22. Kwok JM, Miller TD, Hodge DO, et al. Prognostic value of the Duke treadmill score in the elderly. *J Am Coll Cardiol.* 2002;39:1475–81.

23. Lachterman B, Lehmann KG, Abrahamson D, et al. "Recovery only" ST segment depression and the predictive accuracy of the exercise test. *Ann Intern Med.* 1990;112:11–6.

24. Lauer MS, Francis GS, Okin PM, et al. Impaired chronotropic response to exercise stress testing as a predictor of mortality. *JAMA* 1999;281:524–9.

25. Lauer MS, Sivarajan-Froelicher E, Williams M, Kligfield P. Exercise testing in asymptomatic adults. A statement for health professionals from the American Heart Association Council on Clinical Cardiology, Subcommittee on Exercise, Cardiac Rehabilitation, and Prevention. *Circulation.* 2005;112: 771–6.

26. Lavie CJ, Oh JK, Mankin HT, et al. Significance of T-wave pseudonormalization during exercise: a radionuclide angiographic study. *Chest.* 1988;94:512–6.

27. Londeree BR, Moeschberger ML. Influence of age and other factors on maximal heart rate. *J Cardiac Rehab*. 1984;4:44–9.

28. Mark DB, Hlatky MA, Harrell FE, et al. Exercise treadmill score for predicting prognosis in coronary artery disease. *Ann Intern Med*. 1987;106:793–800.

29. McKirnan MD, Sullivan M, Jensen D, et al. Treadmill performance and cardiac function in selected patients with coronary heart disease. *J Am Coll Cardiol*. 1984;3:253–61.

30. Mirvis DM, Ramanathan KB, Wilson JL. Regional blood flow correlates of ST segment depression in tachycardia-induced myocardial ischemia. *Circulation*. 1986;73:365–73.

31. Morise AP. Accuracy of heart rate–adjusted ST segments in populations with and without posttest referral bias. *Am Heart J*. 1997;134(4):647–55.

32. Morrow K, Morris CK, Froelicher VF, et al. Prediction of cardiovascular death in men undergoing noninvasive evaluation for coronary artery disease. *Ann Intern Med*. 1993;118:689–95.

33. Myers J, Ahnve S, Froelicher VF, et al. Spatial R wave amplitude changes during exercise: relation with left ventricular ischemia and function. *J Am Coll Cardiol*. 1985;6:603–8.

34. Myers J, Froelicher VF. Hemodynamic determinants of exercise capacity in chronic heart failure. *Ann Intern Med*. 1991;115:377–86.

35. Noakes TD. Maximal oxygen uptake: "classical" versus "contemporary" viewpoints: a rebuttal. *Med Sci Sports Exerc*. 1998;30:1381–98.

36. Nostratian F, Froelicher VF. ST elevation during exercise testing: a review. *Am J Cardiol*. 1989;63:986–8.

37. Okin PM, Kligfield P. Heart rate adjustment of ST segment depression and performance of the exercise electrocardiogram: a critical evaluation. *J Am Coll Cardiol*. 1995;25:1726–35.

38. Taylor HL, Buskirk ER, Henschel A. Maximal oxygen uptake as an objective measure of cardiorespiratory performance. *J Appl Physiol*. 1955;8:73–80.

39. Wasserman K, Whipp BJ, Koyl SN, et al. Anaerobic threshold and respiratory gas exchange during exercise. *J Appl Physiol*. 1973;35:236–43.

40. Weiner DA, McCabe CH, Cutler SS, et al. Decrease in systolic blood pressure during exercise testing: reproducibility, response to coronary bypass surgery and prognostic significance. *Am J Cardiol*. 1982;49:1627–31.

41. Weiner DA, Ryan TJ, McCabe CH, et al. Exercise stress testing: correlations among history of angina, ST-segment response and prevalence of coronary-artery disease in the Coronary Artery Surgery Study (CASS). *N Engl J Med*. 1979;301:230–5.

42. Whinnery JE, Froelicher VF, Longo MR, et al. The electrocardiographic response to maximal treadmill exercise of asymptomatic men with right bundle branch block. *Chest*. 1977;71:335–40.

43. Whinnery JE, Froelicher VF, Stewart AJ, et al. The electrocardiographic response to maximal treadmill exercise of asymptomatic men with left bundle branch block. *Am Heart J*. 1977;94:316–24.

Exercise Prescription

General Principles of Exercise Prescription

An exercise training program is best designed to meet individual health and physical fitness goals. The principles of exercise prescription presented in this chapter are intended to assist exercise and health/fitness professionals in the development of an *individually* tailored exercise prescription. These principles are based on the application of scientific evidence on the physiologic, psychological, and health benefits of exercise training. These principles of exercise prescription are intended as guidelines for the apparently healthy adult. There will be situations in which these principles do not apply because of individual characteristics such as health status, physical ability, and age, or athletic and performance goals. In these cases it is recommended that the exercise or health/fitness professional make accommodations to the exercise prescription as indicated in other chapters of these guidelines. Guidelines for clinical populations and healthy people with special considerations are found in Chapters 8 through 10.

EXERCISE MODE (TYPE)

A variety of exercises to improve the components of physical fitness is recommended for all adults (5,8). The health-related components of physical fitness include cardiovascular (aerobic) fitness, muscular strength and endurance, flexibility, and body composition. Exercises that improve neuromuscular fitness, such as balance and agility, are also recommended, particularly for older adults and very deconditioned persons (31).

Overuse injuries (i.e., tissue damage resulting from repetitive demand over time termed *cumulative trauma disorders*) are of particular concern to middle-aged and older adults. To avoid the potential for overuse syndromes, an assortment of exercise modalities is recommended (8). Adherence to an exercise program may be improved by introducing a varied program of exercise, although there is no clear evidence that variety improves adherence (22). Bone health is of great importance to younger and older adults (Chapters 8 and 10), particularly among women. The American College of Sports Medicine (ACSM) recommends loading exercises (i.e., weight-bearing and resistance exercise) to maintain bone health (6). This recommendation should be considered when designing an exercise program for adults, while balancing the risk of musculoskeletal injury (5,6,31).

TABLE 7.1. GENERAL EXERCISE RECOMMENDATIONS FOR HEALTHY ADULTS

WEEKLY FREQUENCY (d · wk^{-1} devoted to an exercise program)	DO THESE TYPES OF EXERCISES
At least 5 d · wk^{-1}	Moderate intensity (40% to <60% $\dot{V}O_2R$) aerobic (cardiovascular endurance) activities, weight-bearing exercise, flexibility exercise
At least 3 d · wk^{-1}	Vigorous intensity (≥60% $\dot{V}O_2R$) aerobic activities, weight-bearing exercise, flexibility exercise
3–5 d · wk^{-1}	A combination of moderate- and vigorous-intensity aerobic activities, weight-bearing exercise, flexibility exercise
2–3 d · wk^{-1}	Muscular strength and endurance, resistance exercise, calisthenics, balance and agility exercise

When choosing the exercise modalities to be included in an exercise program, the individual's goals, physical ability, health status, and available equipment should be considered. Depending on these considerations, the exercise prescription may not include exercises to improve all components of physical fitness. Table 7.1 provides general recommendations for the types of exercises to be included in a health/fitness exercise training program for apparently healthy adults based on a combination of the frequency and intensity of exercise. Specific recommendations for the exercise prescription to improve health/fitness follow in the sections below.

COMPONENTS OF THE EXERCISE TRAINING SESSION

A single exercise session should include the following phases:

- Warm-up
- Stretching
- Conditioning or sports-related exercise
- Cool-down

The warm-up phase consists of a minimum of 5 to 10 minutes of low- [i.e., <40% $\dot{V}O_2R$ (oxygen uptake reserve)] to moderate- (i.e., 40% to <60% $\dot{V}O_2R$) intensity cardiovascular (aerobic) and muscular endurance activity designed to increase body temperature and reduce the potential for after-exercise muscle soreness or what many describe as muscle stiffness. The warm-up phase is a transitional phase that allows the body to adjust to the changing physiologic, biomechanical, and bioenergetic demands placed on it during the conditioning or sports phase of the exercise session. The stretching phase is distinct from the warm-up and cool-down phases and may be performed following the warm-up or cool-down phase.

BOX 7.1   Components of the Exercise Training Session

- Warm-up: At least 5 to 10 minutes of low- (<40% $\dot{V}O_2R$) to moderate- (40%–<60% $\dot{V}O_2R$) intensity cardiovascular and muscular endurance activities
- Conditioning: 20 to 60 minutes of aerobic, resistance, neuromuscular, and/or sport activities (exercise bouts of 10 minutes are acceptable if the individual accumulates at least 20 to 60 min · d^{-1} of daily exercise)
- Cool-down: At least 5 to 10 minutes of low- (<40% $\dot{V}O_2R$) to moderate- (40%–<60% $\dot{V}O_2R$) intensity cardiovascular and muscular endurance activities
- Stretching: At least 10 minutes of stretching exercises performed after the warm-up or cool-down phase

Note: These recommendations are consistent with the United States Department of Health & Human Services Physical Activity Guidelines for Americans, available at http://www.health.gov/PAGuidelines/pdf/paguide.pdf (October 7, 2008).

The conditioning phase includes aerobic, resistance, and/or sports-related exercise. Specifics about the FITT principle (*Frequency, Intensity, Time* [duration] and *Type* [mode]) of aerobic and resistance exercise are discussed in subsequent sections of this chapter. The conditioning phase is followed by a cooldown period involving cardiovascular (aerobic) and muscular endurance activity of low to moderate intensity lasting at least 5 to 10 minutes. The purpose of the cool-down period is to allow for a gradual recovery of HR (heart rate) and BP (blood pressure) and removal of metabolic end products from the muscles used during the more intense exercise conditioning phase. Box 7.1 summarizes the components of the exercise training sessions.

AEROBIC (CARDIOVASCULAR ENDURANCE) EXERCISE

QUANTITY OF EXERCISE: HOW MUCH EXERCISE IS ENOUGH FOR HEALTH/FITNESS BENEFITS?

The quantity or volume of exercise is a function of the frequency, intensity, and duration (time) of the exercise performed. There is a dose-response relationship for the volume of exercise necessary for health/fitness benefits. Even small increases in caloric expenditure with physical activity may improve health/fitness outcomes, with sedentary persons accruing the most benefit (8,19). The minimum and maximum amount (dose) of exercise remains to be more precisely quantified for health/fitness benefits. However, some exercise is generally preferable to physical inactivity.

Frequency of Exercise

Although the total volume of physical activity is a key factor in attaining health/fitness benefits, the frequency of physical activity (i.e., the number of days per week dedicated to an exercise program) is important as well. Health/fitness benefits occur in some people with as little as one to two exercise sessions per week performed at moderate to vigorous intensity ($\geq$60% $\dot{V}O_2R$) (23,27). However, this minimal frequency of physical activity cannot be recommended for the general adult population because of the higher risk of musculoskeletal injury and adverse cardiovascular events in persons who are not physically active on a regular basis (3).

The U.S. Surgeon General (47) and other U.S. government agencies (23,46) recommend physical activity on most days of the week, operationally defined as $\geq$5 $d \cdot wk^{-1}$; whereas ACSM (8) recommends 3–5 $d \cdot wk^{-1}$. There is an attenuation of the magnitude of improvement in physical fitness with exercise frequencies >3 $d \cdot wk^{-1}$ and a plateau in improvement (9) with exercise done $\geq$5 $d \cdot wk^{-1}$. Vigorous intensity exercise performed >5 $d \cdot wk^{-1}$ may increase the incidence of injury, so this amount of physical activity is not generally recommended for most adults. However, if a variety of exercise modes placing different impact stresses on the body (e.g., running and cycling) or using different muscle groups (e.g., swimming and running) are included in the exercise program, daily vigorous intensity physical activity may be recommended for some individuals. Alternatively, a weekly combination of 3–5 $d \cdot wk^{-1}$ of moderate and vigorous intensity exercise may be recommended for most adults.

Frequency: Moderate intensity aerobic exercise done at least 5 $d \cdot wk^{-1}$, or vigorous intensity aerobic exercise done at least 3 $d \cdot wk^{-1}$, or a weekly combination of 3–5 $d \cdot wk^{-1}$ of moderate and vigorous intensity exercise is recommended for the majority of adults to achieve and maintain health/fitness benefits.

Intensity of Exercise

There is a positive continuum of health/fitness benefits with increasing exercise intensity. A minimum intensity threshold that results in health/fitness benefits exists for most people, with the possible exception of physically deconditioned persons (8,19,26). Exercise of at least moderate intensity (i.e., 40% to <60% $\dot{V}O_2R$ that noticeably increases HR and breathing) is recommended as the minimum exercise intensity for adults to achieve health/fitness benefits (19,47). However, a combination of moderate- and vigorous-intensity ($\geq$60% $\dot{V}O_2R$ that results in substantial increases in HR and breathing) exercise is ideal for the attainment of improvements in health/fitness in most adults (19).

A discussion concerning exercise intensity cannot be complete without understanding the prediction of maximal heart rate when a graded exercise test to maximal capacity has not been completed on the subject or patient. Historically, the formula "220 – age" has been used to predict maximal heart rate in both men and women. It is simple to use but comes with a high degree of variability (underestimating HR_{max} for both sexes younger than the age of 40 years and overestimating HR_{max} for both sexes older than 40 years). Recently, more accurate predictors of maximal heart rate have been introduced (15,28,42). The following formula of Gellish et al. (15) represents the most accurate. The practitioner must decide if ease of use or accuracy is more important when deciding which age-predicted maximal heart rate equation to use.

$$HR_{max} = 206.9 - (0.67 \times age)$$

BOX 7.2	Summary of Methods for Prescribing Exercise Intensity Using Heart Rate (HR), Oxygen Uptake ($\dot{V}O_2$), and Metabolic Equivalents (METs)

- HR reserve (HRR) method: Target HR (THR) = [($HR_{max} - HR_{rest}$) × % intensity desired] + HR_{rest}
- $\dot{V}O_2$ reserve ($\dot{V}O_2$R) method: Target $\dot{V}O_2R^a$ = [($\dot{V}O_{2max} - \dot{V}O_{2rest}$) × % intensity desired] + $\dot{V}O_{2rest}$
- Peak HR method: Target HR = $HR_{max}^{\ b}$ × % intensity desired
- Peak $\dot{V}O_2$ method: Target $\dot{V}O_2^a$ = $\dot{V}O_{2max}^c$ × % intensity desired
- Peak MET × (% MET) method: Target MET^a = [($\dot{V}O_{2max}^c$)/ 3.5 mL·kg^{-1}·min^{-1}]^c × % intensity desired

[a]Activities at the target $\dot{V}O_2$ and MET can be determined using a compendium of physical activity (8,9) or metabolic calculations (6) (Table 7.2).

[b]HR_{max} is estimated by 220 − age or some other prediction equation.

[c]$\dot{V}O_{2max}$ is estimated by maximal or submaximal exercise testing.

Various methods are used to quantify exercise intensity, including HR reserve (HRR), $\dot{V}O_2$R, perceived exertion (i.e., RPE [ratings of perceived exertion]) (4,32), OMNI (37,38,48), talk test (33), affective valence (13), absolute energy expenditure per minute (kcal·min^{-1}), percent age-predicted maximum HR (HR_{max}), percent oxygen update ($\dot{V}O_2$), and METs (metabolic equivalents) (Chapter 4). Each of these methods for prescribing exercise intensity may result in health/fitness improvements when properly applied. Their use for exercise prescription is recommended depending on preference and/or circumstance.

HRR and $\dot{V}O_2$R reflect the rate of energy expenditure during physical activity more accurately than the other exercise intensity prescription methods (41). For this reason, these are the preferred methods for prescribing exercise intensity whenever possible. However, accurate measurement of resting HR (HR_{rest}) and HR_{max} or $\dot{V}O_2$ is not always feasible for the determination of HRR and $\dot{V}O_2$R. In these situations, percent age-predicted HR_{max} or estimated maximum oxygen update ($\dot{V}O_{2max}$) may be more practical when direct measurements obtained from exercise testing are not available.

A summary of methods for calculating exercise intensity using HR, $\dot{V}O_2$, and METs are presented in Box 7.2. Intensity of exercise training is usually determined as a range, so the calculation using the formulae presented in Box 7.2 will need to be repeated two times: once for the lower limit of the desired intensity range and once for the upper limit of the desired intensity range (see examples of these calculations in Fig. 7.2). The prescribed exercise intensity range for an individual should be determined by taking a variety of factors into consideration, including age, habitual physical activity level, physical fitness level, and health status. Table 7.4 provides for discussion of the FITT principle and further recommendations for prescribing exercise intensity. In some individuals with cognitive or developmental impairment, assigning two points in a range may be confusing and even hazardous. In these cases, the exercise or health/fitness professional is urged to use the low to midpoint of the recommended range or to calculate a single safe HR or MET level.

When using $\dot{V}O_2$ or METs to prescribe exercise, the health/fitness professional can identify activities within the desired $\dot{V}O_2$ or MET range by using a compendium of physical activities (1,2) or metabolic calculations (9) (Table 7.2 and Fig. 7.2). A direct method of exercise prescription using the relationship between HR and $\dot{V}O_2$ may be used when HR and $\dot{V}O_2$ are measured during an exercise test (Fig. 7.1). This method may be particularly useful when prescribing exercise in persons taking medications such as β-blockers or who have a chronic condition, such as diabetes mellitus or atherosclerotic cardiovascular disease (CVD), that alters the HR response to exercise.

Examples illustrating the use of several methods of prescribing exercise intensity are found in Figure 7.2. The reader is directed to other ACSM publications (e.g., references 9,10) for further explanation and examples using these additional methods of exercise prescription.

Perceived exertion using either RPE (11,32) (See Table 4.7), or the OMNI (37,38,48) scales is recommended as either a primary or adjunct measure of exercise intensity (24). The talk test (33) and measures of affective valence (13) such as the Feeling Scale (17) may also be useful measures of perceived exertion; however, further research is needed before they can be recommended as primary tools for the estimation of exercise intensity. For this reason, the talk test and affective valence are recommended as adjunct measures of exercise intensity.

There are no studies available comparing all exercise intensity prescription methods simultaneously. Thus, the various methods described in this chapter to quantify exercise intensity may not necessarily be equivalent to each other.

Intensity: A combination of moderate- (i.e., 40% to <60% $\dot{V}O_2R$ that noticeably increases HR and breathing) and vigorous- (i.e., ≥60% $\dot{V}O_2R$ that substantially increases HR and breathing) intensity exercise is recommended for most adults. Exercise intensity may be estimated using HRR, $\dot{V}O_2R$, percent age-predicted HR_{max}, percent estimated $\dot{V}O_{2max}$, and perceived exertion.

Exercise Quantity and Duration (Time)

Exercise duration is prescribed as a measure of amount of time physical activity is performed (i.e., per session, day, or week) or by the total caloric expenditure. Step counts obtained on a pedometer may also be used to determine the quantity of exercise and/or physical activity. The quantity of physical activity may be performed continuously (i.e., one session) or intermittently and accumulated over the course of a day through one or more sessions of physical activity of at least 10 minutes in duration (19,47).

There is a dose-response relationship between total calories expended per week in physical activity and exercise and health/fitness benefits (19,47). The evidence indicates that accumulating at least 1,000 kcal of physical activity per

TABLE 7.2. METABOLIC CALCULATIONS FOR THE ESTIMATION OF ENERGY EXPENDITURE [$\dot{V}O_2$ (mL · kg^{-1} · min^{-1})] DURING COMMON PHYSICAL ACTIVITIES

	SUM THESE COMPONENTS			
ACTIVITY	RESTING COMPONENT	HORIZONTAL COMPONENT	VERTICAL COMPONENT/ RESISTANCE COMPONENT	LIMITATIONS
Walking	3.5	0.1 × speed[a]	1.8 × speed[a] × grade[b]	Most accurate for speeds of 1.9–3.7 mph (50–100 m · min^{-1})
Running	3.5	0.2 × speed[a]	0.9 × speed[a] × grade[b]	Most accurate for speeds >5 mph (134 m · min^{-1})
Stepping	3.5	0.2 × steps per min	1.33 × (1.8 × step height[c] × steps per min)	Most accurate for stepping rates of 12–30 steps per min
Leg cycling	3.5	3.5	(1.8 × work rate[d])/ body mass[e]	Most accurate for work rates of 300–1,200 kg · m · min^{-1} (50–200 W)
Arm cycling	3.5		(3 × work rate[d])/body mass[e]	Most accurate for work rates between 150–750 kg · m · min^{-1} (25–125 W)

[a]Speed in m · min^{-1}.

[b]Grade is percent grade expressed in decimal format (e.g., 10% = 0.10).

[c]Step height in m.

Multiply by the following conversion factors:
lb to kg: 0.454
in to cm: 2.54
ft to m: 0.3048
mi to km: 1.609
mph to m · min^{-1}: 26.8
kg · m · min^{-1} to W: 0.164
W to kg · m · min^{-1}: 6.12
$\dot{V}O_{2max}$ L · min^{-1} to kcal · min^{-1}: 4.9
$\dot{V}O_{2max}$ mL · kg^{-1} · min^{-1} to MET: 3.5

[d]Work rate in kilogram meters per minute (kg · m · min^{-1}) is calculated as resistance (kg) × distance per revolution of flywheel × pedal frequency per minute. Note: Distance per revolution is 6 m for Monark leg ergometer, 3 m for the Tunturi and BodyGuard ergometers, and 2.4 m for Monark arm ergometer.

[e]Body mass in kg.

Adapted from American College of Sports Medicine. *ACSM's Guidelines for Exercise Testing and Prescription.* 7th ed. Philadelphia (PA): Lippincott Williams & Wilkins; 2005. p. 289.

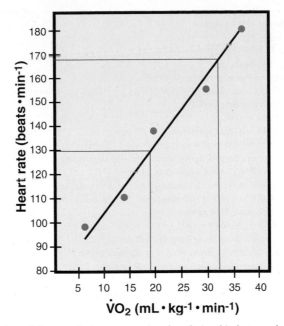

FIGURE 7.1. Prescribing exercise heart rate using the relationship between heart rate and $\dot{V}O_2$. A line of best fit has been drawn through the data points on this plot of HR and $\dot{V}O_2$ during a hypothetical exercise test in which $\dot{V}O_{2max}$ was observed to be 38 $mL \cdot kg^{-1} \cdot min^{-1}$ and HR_{max} was 184 beats $\cdot min^{-1}$. A target HR range was determined by finding the HR that corresponds to 50% and 85% $\dot{V}O_{2max}$. For this individual, 50% $\dot{V}O_{2max}$ was ~19 $mL \cdot kg^{-1} \cdot min^{-1}$, and 85% $\dot{V}O_{2max}$ was ~32 $mL \cdot kg^{-1} \cdot min^{-1}$. The corresponding THR range is 130 to 168 beats $\cdot min^{-1}$. (Adapted from American College of Sports Medicine. *ACSM's Guidelines for Exercise Testing and Prescription*. 7th ed. Philadelphia (PA): Lippincott Williams & Wilkins; 2005. 145 p.)

week consistently results in health/fitness benefits (19). This caloric expenditure is also the minimum level recommended in the Surgeon General's Report (47) and by ACSM and the American Heart Association (AHA) (8). Thus, 1,000 kcal·wk^{-1} is the recommended minimum quantity of physical activity and exercise for most healthy adults. This quantity of physical activity is approximately equal to 150 min · wk^{-1} or 30 min · d^{-1} of exercise (27). Pedometer step counts are also useful to assess the quantity of exercise (44). Moderate-intensity walking for 30 min · d^{-1} equates to 3,000 to 4,000 steps per day (44). Attainment of 10,000 or more steps per day has been suggested as the goal for classification as being physically active, although this recommendation needs further study before such a universal recommendation can be made (45).

For some individuals with health or practical considerations or poor physical fitness, a quantity of physical activity <1,000 kcal · wk^{-1} may result

(*text continues on page 163*)

Heart Rate Reserve (HRR) Method
　Available test data:
　　　HR_{rest}: 70 beats $\cdot$ min^{-1}
　　　HR_{max}: 180 beats $\cdot$ min^{-1}
　Desired exercise intensity range: 50%–60%
　Formula: Target Heart Rate (THR) = [(HR_{max} − HR_{rest}) × % intensity] + HR_{rest}
　　　1) Calculation of HRR:
　　　　$HRR = (HR_{max} - HR_{rest})$
　　　　$HRR - (180$ beats $\cdot$ min^{-1} − 70 beats $\cdot$ mm^{-1}) = 110 beats $\cdot$ min^{-1}
　　　2) Determination of exercise intensity as %HRR:
　　　　Convert desired %HRR into a decimal by dividing by 100
　　　　%HRR = desired intensity × HRR
　　　　%HRR = 0.5 × 110 beats $\cdot$ min^{-1} = 55 beats $\cdot$ min^{-1}
　　　　%HRR = 0.6 × 110 beats $\cdot$ min^{-1} = 66 beats $\cdot$ min^{-1}
　　　3) Determine THR range:
　　　　THR= (%HRR) + HR_{rest}
　　　　To determine lower limit of THR range:
　　　　　THR = 55 beats $\cdot$ min^{-1} + 70 beats $\cdot$ min^{-1} = 125 beats $\cdot$ min^{-1}
　　　　To determine upper limit of THR range:
　　　　　THR = 66 beats $\cdot$ min^{-1} + 70 beats $\cdot$ min^{-1} = 136 beats $\cdot$ min^{-1}
　　　　THR range: 125 beats $\cdot$ min^{-1} to 136 beats $\cdot$ min^{-1}

$\dot{V}O_2$ *Reserve ($\dot{V}O_2R$) Method*
　Available test data:
　　　$\dot{V}O_{2max}$: 30 mL $\cdot$ kg^{-1} $\cdot$ min^{-1}
　　　$\dot{V}O_{2rest}$: 3.5 mL $\cdot$ kg^{-1} $\cdot$ min^{-1}

　Desired exercise intensity range: 50%–60%
　Formula: Target $\dot{V}O_2$ = [($\dot{V}O_{2max}$ − $\dot{V}O_{2rest}$) × % intensity] + $\dot{V}O_{2rest}$
　　　1) Calculation of $\dot{V}O_2R$:
　　　　$\dot{V}O_2R = \dot{V}O_{2max} - \dot{V}O_{2rest}$
　　　　$\dot{V}O_2R = 30$ mL $\cdot$ kg^{-1} $\cdot$ min^{-1} − 3.5 mL $\cdot$ kg^{-1} $\cdot$ min^{-1}
　　　　$\dot{V}O_2R = 26.5$ mL $\cdot$ kg^{-1} $\cdot$ min^{-1}
　　　2) Determination of exercise intensity as % $\dot{V}O_2R$:
　　　　Convert desired intensity (%$\dot{V}O_2R$) into a decimal by dividing by 100
　　　　%$\dot{V}O_2R$ = desired intensity × %$\dot{V}O_2R$
　　　　Calculate %$\dot{V}O_2R$:
　　　　%$\dot{V}O_2R$ = 0.5 × 26.5 mL $\cdot$ kg^{-1} $\cdot$ min^{-1} = 13.3 mL $\cdot$ kg^{-1} $\cdot$ min^{-1}
　　　　%$\dot{V}O_2R$ = 0.6 × 26.5 mL $\cdot$ kg^{-1} $\cdot$ min^{-1} = 15.9 mL $\cdot$ kg^{-1} $\cdot$ min^{-1}
　　　3) Determine target $\dot{V}O_2R$ range:
　　　　(%$\dot{V}O_2R$) + $\dot{V}O_{2rest}$
　　　　To determine the lower target $\dot{V}O_2$ range:
　　　　　Target $\dot{V}O_2$ − 13.3 mL $\cdot$ kg^{-1} $\cdot$ min^{-1} + 3.5 mL $\cdot$ kg^{-1} $\cdot$ min^{-1}=
　　　　　16.8 mL $\cdot$ kg^{-1} $\cdot$ min^{-1}
　　　　To determine upper target $\dot{V}O_2$ range:
　　　　　Target $\dot{V}O_2$ = 15.9 mL $\cdot$ kg^{-1} $\cdot$ min^{-1} + 3.5 mL $\cdot$ kg^{-1} $\cdot$ min^{-1} =
　　　　　19.4 mL $\cdot$ kg^{-1} $\cdot$ min^{-1}
　　　　Target $\dot{V}O_2$ range: 16.8 mL $\cdot$ kg^{-1} $\cdot$ min^{-1} to 19.4 mL $\cdot$ kg^{-1} $\cdot$ min^{-1}

FIGURE 7.2. Examples of the application of various methods for prescribing exercise intensity (9,10). (continued)

4) Determine MET target range (optional):

1 MET = 3.5 mL·kg^{-1}·min^{-1}

Calculate lower MET target:

1 MET/3.5 mL·kg^{-1}·min^{-1} = × MET/16.8 mL·kg^{-1}·min^{-1}

× MET =16.8 mL·kg^{-1}·min^{-1}/3.5 mL·kg^{-1}·min^{-1} = 4.8 MET

Calculate upper MET target:

1 MET/3.5 mL·kg^{-1}·min^{-1} = × MET/19.4 mL·kg^{-1}·min^{-1}

× MET = 19.4 mL·kg^{-1}·min^{-1}/3.5 mL·kg^{-1}·min^{-1} = 5.5 MET

5) Identify physical activities requiring energy expenditure within the target range from compendium of physical activities (8,9) or by using metabolic calculations shown in Table 7.2 or references (6,7). Also see examples of use of metabolic equations below.

%HR$_{max}$ *(Measured or Estimated) Method:*

Available data:

A man 45 yr of age

Desired exercise intensity: 70%–80%

Formula: THR = HR$_{max}$ × desired %

Calculate estimated HR$_{max}$ (if measured HR$_{max}$ not available):

HR$_{max}$ = 220 − age

HR$_{max}$ = 220–45 = 175 beats·min^{-1}

1) Determine THR range:

THR = Desired % × HR$_{max}$

Convert desired %HR$_{max}$ into a decimal by dividing by 100

Determine lower limit of THR range:

THR = 175 beats·min^{-1} × 0.70 = 123 beats·min^{-1}

Determine upper limit of THR range:

THR = 175 beats·min^{-1} × 0.80 = 140 beats·min^{-1}

THR range: 123 beats·min^{-1} to 140 beats·min^{-1}

%$\dot{V}O_{2max}$ *(Measured or Estimated) Method*

Available data:

A woman 45 yr of age

Estimated $\dot{V}O_{2max}$: 30 mL·kg^{-1}·min^{-1}

Desired $\dot{V}O_2$ range: 50%–60%

Formula: $\dot{V}O_{2max}$ × desired %

Determine target $\dot{V}O_2$ range:

Target $\dot{V}O_2$ = Desired % × $\dot{V}O_{2max}$

Convert desired intensity (%$\dot{V}O_2$) into a decimal by dividing by 100

Determine lower limit of target $\dot{V}O_{2max}$ range

Target $\dot{V}O_2$ = 0.50 × 30 mL·kg^{-1}·min^{-1} = 15 mL·kg^{-1}·min^{-1}

Determine upper limit of target $\dot{V}O_{2max}$ range:

Target $\dot{V}O_2$ = 0.60 × 30 mL·kg^{-1}·min^{-1} = 18 mL·kg^{-1}·min^{-1}

Target $\dot{V}O_2$ range: 15 mL·kg^{-1}·min^{-1} to 18 mL·kg^{-1}·min^{-1}

1) Determine MET target range (optional):

1 MET = 3.5 mL·kg^{-1}·min^{-1}

Calculate lower MET target:

1 MET/3.5 mL·kg^{-1}·min^{-1} × MET/16.8 mL·kg^{-1}·min^{-1}

× MET =16.8 mL·kg^{-1}·min^{-1}/3.5 mL·kg^{-1}·min^{-1} = 4.8 METs

FIGURE 7.2. *Continued.*

Calculate upper MET target:

$$1 \text{ MET}/3.5 \text{ mL}\cdot\text{kg}^{-1}\cdot\text{min}^{1} = \text{X MET}/19.5 \text{ mL}\cdot\text{kg}^{-1}\cdot\text{min}^{-1}$$
$$\text{X MET} = 19.5 \text{ mL}\cdot\text{kg}^{-1}\cdot\text{min}^{-1}/3.5 \text{ mL}\cdot\text{kg}^{-1}\cdot\text{min}^{-1} = 5.6 \text{ METs}$$

2) Identify physical activities requiring energy expenditure within the target range from compendium of physical activities (9,19) or by using metabolic calculations shown in Table 7.2 and reference (6,7). See examples of use of metabolic equations below.

Using metabolic calculations (6) (Table 7.2) to determine running speed on a treadmill
Available data:

A man 32 yr of age
Weight: 130 lb (59 Kg)
Height: 70 in (177.8 cm)
$\dot{V}O_{2max}$: 54 mL·kg^{-1}·min^{-1}

Desired treadmill grade: 2.5%
Desired exercise intensity: 80%
Formula: $\dot{V}O_2 = 3.5 + (0.2 \times \text{speed}) + (0.9 \times \text{speed}) \times \text{\% grade})$

1. Determine target $\dot{V}O_2$
   Target $\dot{V}O_2$ = desired % × $\dot{V}O_{2max}$
   Target $\dot{V}O_2$ = 0.80 × 54 mL·kg^{-1}·min^{-1} = 43.2 mL·kg^{-1}·min^{-1}
2. Determine treadmill speed:
   $\dot{V}O_2 = 3.5 + (0.2 \times \text{speed}) + (0.9 \times \text{speed} \times \text{\% grade})$
   43.2 mL·kg^{-1}·min^{-1} = 3.5 + (0.2 × speed) + (0.9 × speed × 0.025)
   39.7 = (0.2 × speed) + (0.9 × speed × 0.025)
   39.7 = (0.2 × speed) + (0.0225 × speed)
   39.7 = 0.2225 × speed
   175.6 m·min^{-1} = speed
   Speed on treadmill: 10.5 km·hr^{-1} (6.5 mph)

Using metabolic calculations (6) (Table 7.2) to determine % grade during walking on a treadmill
Available data:

A man 54 yr of age who is moderately physically active
Weight: 190 lb (86.4 kg)
Height: 70 in (177.8 cm)
Desired walking speed: 2.5 mph (4 km·hr^{-1}; 67 m·min^{-1})
Desired MET: 5 METs
Formula: $\dot{V}O_2 = 3.5 + (0.1 \times \text{speed}) + (1.8 \times \text{speed} \times \text{\% grade})$

1. Determine target $\dot{V}O_2$:
   Target $\dot{V}O_2$ = MET × 3.5 mL·kg^{-1}·min^{-1}
   Target $\dot{V}O_2$ = 5 × 3.5 mL·kg^{-1}·min^{-1} = 17.5 mL·kg^{-1}·min^{-1}
2. Determine treadmill grade:
   $\dot{V}O_2 = 3.5 + (0.1 \times \text{speed}) + (1.8 \times \text{speed} \times \text{\% grade})$
   17.5 mL·kg^{-1}·min^{-1} = 3.5 + (0.1 × 67 m·sec^{-1}) + (1.8 × 67 m·sec^{-1} × % grade)
   14 = (0.1 × 67 m·sec^{-1}) + (1.8 × 67 m·sec^{-1} × % grade)
   14 = 6.7 + (120.6 × % grade)
   7.3 = 120.6 × % grade
   0.06 = % grade
   % grade = 6%

FIGURE 7.2. *Continued.*

Using metabolic calculations (6) (Table 7.2) to determine target work rate (kg · m · min⁻¹) on a Monarch leg cycle ergometer

Available data:

    A woman 42 yr of age

    Weight: 190 lb (86.4 kg)

    Height: 70 in (177.8 cm)

Desired $\dot{V}O_2$: 18 kg · m · min^1

Formula: $\dot{V}O_2 = 7.0 + (1.8 \times \text{work rate})/\text{body mass}$

    1. Calculate work rate on cycle ergometer:

        $\dot{V}O_2 = 7.0 + (1.8 \times \text{work rate})/\text{body mass})$

        18 mL · kg^{-1} · min^{-1} = 7.0 + (1.8 $\times$ work rate)/86.4 kg

        11 = (1.8 $\times$ work rate)/86.4

        950.4 = 1.8 $\times$ work rate

        528 = work rate

        Work rate = 528 kg · m^1 · min = 86.6 W

FIGURE 7.2. *Continued.*

in improved health/fitness outcomes and may be appropriate to prescribe (27). For most adults, however, a larger quantity of exercise (i.e., $\geq$2,000 kcal · wk^{-1}) results in greater health/fitness benefits and may be necessary for promoting and sustaining weight loss (4). This quantity of exercise is equal to about 250–300 min · wk^{-1} or 50–60 min · d^{-1} or more of physical activity and exercise (4). See Chapter 10 on exercise prescription recommendations for promoting and sustaining weight loss for additional information.

The maximum safe volume of exercise is not known. Recommendations for quantities of exercise exceeding ~3,500–4,000 kcal · wk^{-1} need to be weighed carefully against the probability of overuse injury, although further investigation is needed to establish the maximum safe dose of exercise.

Time: Moderate-intensity exercise performed for at least 30 minutes on $\geq$5 d · wk^{-1} to a total of at least 150 minutes, or vigorous intensity aerobic exercise done for at least 20–25 minutes on $\geq$3 d · wk^{-1} to total 75 minutes, or at least 20 to 30 minutes of moderate and vigorous intensity exercise on 3–5 d · wk ^{1} is recommended for most adults. To promote or maintain weight loss, 50–60 min · d^{-1} to total 300 minutes moderate, 150 minutes vigorous or an equivalent combination of daily exercise is recommended. Performance of intermittent exercise of at least 10 minutes in duration to accumulate the minimum duration recommendations above is an effective alternative to continuous exercise. Total caloric expenditure and step counts may be used as surrogate measures of exercise duration. A minimum caloric expenditure of 1,000 kcal · wk^{-1} of physical activity and exercise and at least 3,000 to 4,000 steps per day of moderate to vigorous intensity walking is recommended.

AEROBIC (CARDIOVASCULAR) EXERCISE MODE (TYPE)

Rhythmic, aerobic type exercises involving large muscle groups are recommended for improving cardiovascular fitness. The modes of physical activity that result in improvement and maintenance of cardiovascular fitness are found in

TABLE 7.3. AEROBIC (CARDIOVASCULAR ENDURANCE) EXERCISES TO IMPROVE PHYSICAL FITNESS

EXERCISE GROUP	EXERCISE DESCRIPTION	RECOMMENDED FOR	EXAMPLES
A	Endurance activities requiring minimal skill or physical fitness to perform	All adults	Walking, leisurely cycling, aqua-aerobics, slow dancing
B	Vigorous-intensity endurance activities requiring minimal skill	Adults with a regular exercise program and/or at least average physical fitness	Jogging, running, rowing, aerobics, spinning, elliptical exercise, stepping exercise, fast dancing
C	Endurance activities requiring skill to perform	Adults with acquired skill and/or at least average physical fitness levels	Swimming, cross-country skiing, skating
D	Recreational sports	Adults with a regular exercise program and at least average physical fitness	Racquet sports, basketball, soccer, down-hill skiing, hiking

Adapted from American College of Sports Medicine. *ACSM's Guidelines for Exercise Testing and Prescription.* 7th ed. Philadelphia (PA): Lippincott Williams & Wilkins; 2005. p. 140.

Table 7.3. The health/fitness professional should keep in mind the principle of specificity of training when selecting the exercise modalities to be included in the exercise prescription. This principle states that the physiologic adaptations to exercise are specific to the type of exercise performed (7,8).

Exercises of type A are recommended for all adults as they require little skill to perform, and the intensity of these exercises is easily modified to accommodate individual physical fitness levels. Type B exercises are typically performed at a vigorous intensity and, therefore, are recommended for persons who exercise regularly or who are at least of average physical fitness. Type C exercises require skill to perform. They are recommended for persons who are able to perform these exercises safely, have already acquired the skill and degree of physical fitness to perform the skill, and possess adequate physical fitness to learn the skills. Type D exercises are recreational sports that may improve physical fitness, but which are generally recommended for most adults as ancillary physical activities that are performed in addition to recommended physical activities to achieve or maintain health/fitness benefits. Type D physical activities are recommended only for persons who possess adequate physical fitness to perform the sport; however, many of these sports may be modified to accommodate persons of lower physical fitness levels.

Type: Rhythmic, aerobic (cardiovascular endurance) exercise of at least moderate intensity that involves large muscle groups and requires little skill to perform is recommended for all adults to improve health/fitness. Other exercise and sports requiring skill to perform or higher levels of fitness are recommended only for individuals possessing adequate skill and fitness to perform the activity.

THE COMPONENTS OF THE AEROBIC (CARDIOVASCULAR ENDURANCE) EXERCISE PRESCRIPTION: THE FITT PRINCIPLE OR *F*REQUENCY, *I*NTENSITY, *T*IME, AND *T*YPE OF EXERCISE

The FITT principle of exercise prescription features an individually tailored exercise program that includes specification of the Frequency (F), Intensity (I), Time or duration (T), and Type or mode (T) of exercise to be performed. The exact composition of FITT will vary depending on the characteristics and goals of the individual. The FITT exercise prescription will need to be revised according to the individual response, need, limitation, and adaptation to exercise as well as evolution of the goals and objectives of the exercise program. Table 7.4 shows the FITT recommendations for aerobic exercise. The FITT framework will be used throughout these *Guidelines*.

RATE OF PROGRESSION

The recommended rate of progression in an exercise program depends on the individual's health status, exercise tolerance, and exercise program goals. Progression may consist of increasing any of the components of the FITT framework as tolerated by the individual. During the initial phase of the exercise program, increasing exercise duration (i.e., minutes per session) is recommended. An increase in exercise duration per session of 5 to 10 minutes every 1 to 2 weeks over the first 4 to 6 weeks of an exercise training program is reasonable for the average adult (8). After the individual has been exercising regularly for one month or more, the frequency, intensity, and/or time of exercise is gradually adjusted upward over the next 4 to 8 months—or longer for older adults and very deconditioned persons—to meet the recommended quantity and quality of exercise presented in these *Guidelines*. Any progression in the FITT exercise prescription should be made gradually, avoiding large increases in any of the FITT components to minimize risks of muscular soreness and injury. Following any adjustments in the exercise prescription, the individual should be monitored for any adverse effects of the increased volume, and downward adjustments should be made if the exercise is not well tolerated (8).

MUSCULAR FITNESS

An essential component of any exercise training program is resistance training. A resistance-training program usually takes the form of weight lifting, but also may include other exercise devices. There are many types of resistance-training

TABLE 7.4. RECOMMENDED FITT FRAMEWORK FOR THE FREQUENCY, INTENSITY AND TIME OF AEROBIC EXERCISE FOR APPARENTLY HEALTHY ADULTS[a]

HABITUAL PHYSICAL ACTIVITY/ EXERCISE LEVEL	PHYSICAL FITNESS CLASSIFICATION[c]	FREQUENCY		INTENSITY[b]			TIME		
		kcal·wk[-1]	d·wk[-1]	HRR/$\dot{V}O_2R$	% HR$_{max}$	PERCEPTION OF EFFORT[d]	TOTAL DURATION PER DAY (min)	TOTAL DAILY STEPS DURING EXERCISE[e]	WEEKLY DURATION (min)
Sedentary/no habitual activity/exercise/extremely deconditioned	Poor	500–1,000	3–5	30%–45%	57%–67%	Light–moderate	20–30	3,000–3,500	60–150
Minimal physical activity/no exercise/moderately–highly deconditioned	Poor–fair	1,000–1,500	3–5	40%–55%	64%–74%	Light–moderate	30–60	3,000–4,000	150–200
Sporadic physical activity/no or suboptimal exercise/moderately to mildly deconditioned	Fair–average	1,500–2,000	3–5	55%–70%	74%–84%	Moderate–hard	30–90	≥3,000–4,000	200–300

| Habitual physical activity/regular moderate to vigorous intensity exercise | Average–good | >2,000 | 3–5 | 65%–80% | 80%–91% | Moderate–hard | 30–90 | ≥3,000–4,000 | 200–300 |
| High amounts of habitual activity/regular vigorous intensity exercise | >Good–excellent | >2,000 | 3–5 | 70%–85% | 84%–94% | Somewhat hard–hard | 30–90 | ≥3,000–4,000 | 200–300 |

kcal, kilocalories; $\dot{V}O_2R$, oxygen uptake reserve; HRR, heart rate reserve; %HR$_{max}$, % age-predicted maximal heart rate.

[a]See Table 7.1 for exercise type (T).

[b]The various methods to quantify exercise intensity in this table may not necessarily be equivalent to each other.

[c]Fitness classification based on normative fitness data categorized by $\dot{V}O_{2max}$.

[d]Perception of effort using the ratings of perceived exertion (RPE) (11,32), OMNI (37,38,48), talk test (33), or feeling scale (17).

[e]Total steps based on step counts from a pedometer.

Note: These recommendations are consistent with the United States Department of Health & Human Services Physical Activity Guidelines for Americans, available at http://www.health.gov/PAGuidelines/pdf/paguide.pdf (October 7, 2008).

equipment available including free weights, machines with stacked weights or pneumatic resistance, and rubber bands that can be effective in developing muscular fitness and mass as long as properly used. When correctly performed, resistance training improves all components of muscular fitness, including strength, endurance, and power. Although muscular power is important for athletic events such as the shot put or javelin throw, the other areas of muscular fitness—strength and endurance—are of greater importance in a general training regimen focusing on health/fitness outcomes. Indeed, goals of a health-related resistance-training program should be to (a) make activities of daily living (e.g., stair climbing and carrying bags of groceries) less stressful physiologically; and (b) effectively manage, attenuate, and even prevent chronic diseases such as osteoporosis, type 2 diabetes mellitus, and obesity. For these reasons, resistance training becomes more rather than less important with age (6,7,31).

FREQUENCY OF RESISTANCE EXERCISE

For general muscular fitness, particularly among those who are untrained or recreationally trained (i.e., not engaged in a formal training program), an individual should resistance train each major muscle group (i.e., the muscle groups of the chest, shoulders, upper and lower back, abdomen, hips, and legs) 2–3 $d \cdot wk^{-1}$ with at least 48 hours separating the exercise training sessions for the same muscle group (7). Depending on the individual's daily schedule, all muscle groups to be trained may be done so in the same session (i.e., whole body), or each session may "split" the body into selected muscle groups so that only a few of them are trained in any one session (7). For example, muscles of the lower body may be trained on Mondays and Thursdays, and upper body muscles may be trained on Tuesdays and Fridays. This "split" weight training routine entails 4 $d \cdot wk^{-1}$ to train each muscle group twice weekly; however, each session is of shorter duration than a whole-body session used to train all muscle groups of the body. Both methods are effective as long as each muscle group is trained 2–3 $d \cdot wk^{-1}$. Having these different resistance-training options provides the individual with more flexibility in scheduling which may help to improve the likelihood of incorporating a resistance-training regimen into his/her daily schedule.

Frequency: Resistance training of each major muscle group 2–3 $d \cdot wk^{-1}$ with at least 48 hours separating the exercise training sessions for the same muscle group is recommended for all adults.

TYPES OF RESISTANCE EXERCISES

Resistance-training regimens should include multijoint or compound exercises—such as the bench press, leg press, and dips—that affect more than one muscle group. These exercises should focus on the major muscle groups of the chest, shoulders, upper and lower back, abdomen, hips, and legs. Examples of multijoint exercises include the chest press, shoulder press, pull-down, dips, lower-back extension, abdominal crunch/curl-up, and leg press. Single-joint exercises targeting major muscle groups, such as biceps curls, triceps extensions, quadriceps extensions, leg curls, and calf raises, can also be included in a resistance-training program (7).

To avoid creating muscle imbalances that may lead to injury, train opposing muscle groups (i.e., agonists and antagonists), such as the lower back and abdomen or the quadriceps and hamstring muscles (7). Examples of these types of resistance exercises are lower-back extensions and abdominal crunches to target the muscles in the lower back and abdomen, and leg presses and leg curls to exercise the quadriceps and hamstring muscles.

Type: Multijoint exercises affecting more than one muscle group and targeting agonist and antagonist muscle groups are recommended for all adults. Single-joint exercises targeting major muscle groups may also be included in a resistance-training program.

VOLUME OF RESISTANCE EXERCISE (REPETITIONS AND SETS)

Each muscle group should be trained for a total of two to four sets. These sets may be derived from the same exercise or from a combination of exercises affecting the same muscle group (7). For example, the pectoral muscles of the chest region may be trained either with four sets of bench presses or with two sets of bench presses and two sets of dips. A reasonable rest interval between sets is 2 to 3 minutes. Using different exercises to train the same muscle group adds variety, may prevent long-term mental "staleness," and may improve adherence to the training program, although evidence that these factors improve adherence is lacking (7).

Four sets per muscle group is more effective than two sets (7,35); however, even a single set per exercise will significantly improve muscular strength, particularly among the novice (8,49). By completing one set of two different exercises that affect the same muscle group, the muscle has executed two sets. For example, bench presses and dips affect the pectoralis muscles of the chest, so that by completing one set of each, the muscle group has performed a total of two sets. Moreover, compound exercises, such as the bench press and dips, also train the triceps muscle group. From a practical standpoint of program adherence, each individual should carefully assess his/her own daily schedule, time demands, and level of commitment to determine how many sets per muscle should be performed during resistance-training sessions. Of paramount importance is the adoption of a resistance-training program that will be realistically maintained over the long term.

The resistance-training intensity and number of repetitions performed with each set are inversely related. That is, the greater the intensity or resistance, the fewer the number of repetitions that will need to be completed. To improve muscular strength, mass, and—to some extent—endurance, a resistance exercise that allows a person to complete 8 to 12 repetitions per set should be selected. This translates to a resistance that is ~60% to 80% of the individual's one repetition maximum (1-RM) or the greatest amount of weight lifted for a single repetition. For example, if an individual's 1-RM in the shoulder press is 100 lb (45.5 kg), then when performing that exercise during the training sessions, he/she should choose a resistance between 60 and 80 lb (27–36 kg). If a person performs multiple sets per exercise, the number of repetitions completed before fatigue occurs will be at or close to 12 repetitions with the first set and will decline to about 8 repetitions during the last set for that exercise. Each set should be performed to the point of muscle fatigue but not failure, because exerting muscles to the point of failure increases the likelihood of injury or debilitating residual muscle soreness, particularly among novices (7).

If the objective of the resistance-training program is mainly to improve muscular endurance rather than strength and mass, a higher number of repetitions, perhaps 15 to 25, should be performed per set along with shorter rest intervals and fewer sets (i.e., one or two sets per muscle group) (7). This regimen necessitates a lower intensity or resistance typically of no more than 50% 1-RM. Similarly, older and very deconditioned individuals, who are more susceptible to musculotendinous injury, should begin a resistance-training program conducting more repetitions (i.e., 10–15) at a moderate RPE of 5 to 6 on a 10-point scale (5,31). Subsequent to a period of adaptation to resistance training and improved musculotendinous conditioning, older individuals may choose to follow guidelines for younger adults (i.e., higher intensity with 8 to 12 repetitions per set) (7,8).

Repetitions and sets: Adults should train each muscle group for a total of 2 to 4 sets with 8 to 12 repetitions per set with a rest interval of 2 to 3 minutes between sets to improve muscular fitness. For older adults and very deconditioned persons, one or more sets of 10 to 15 repetitions of moderate intensity (i.e., 60%–70% 1-RM) resistance exercise are recommended.

RESISTANCE EXERCISE TECHNIQUE

Each resistance exercise should be performed with proper technique, regardless of training status or age. Proper technique ensures optimal health/fitness gains and minimizes the chance of injury. Individuals who are naïve to resistance training should receive instruction on proper technique from a qualified health/fitness professional (e.g., ACSM Certified Health Fitness Specialist or ACSM Certified Personal Trainer[SM]) on each exercise used during resistance-training sessions. In addition to proper body positioning and breathing (i.e., exhalation during lifting phase and inhalation during lowering phase), instruction should emphasize that all exercises use a full range of motion conducted in a deliberate, controlled manner with each repetition including concentric and eccentric muscle action during the lifting and lowering phases, respectively. However, it is not recommended that resistance training be composed exclusively of eccentric or lengthening contractions conducted at very high intensities (e.g., >100% 1-RM) because of the significant chance of injury and severe muscle soreness (7).

Technique: All individuals should receive professional instruction in proper resistance-training techniques. Proper resistance exercise techniques employ controlled movements through the full range of motion and involve concentric and eccentric muscle actions.

PROGRESSION/MAINTENANCE

As muscles adapt to a resistance exercise training program, the participant should continue to subject them to overload or greater stimuli to continue to increase muscular strength and mass. This "progressive overload" principle may be performed in several ways. The most common approach is to increase the amount of resistance lifted during training. For example, if an individual is using 100 lb (45.5 kg) of resistance for a given exercise, and his/her muscles have adapted to the point to which 12 repetitions are easily performed, then the resistance should be increased so that no more than 12 repetitions are completed without significant muscle fatigue and difficulty in completing the last repetition of that set. Other ways to progressively overload muscles include performing more sets per muscle group and increasing the number of days per week the muscle groups are trained (7).

On the other hand, if the individual has attained the desired levels of muscular strength and mass, and he/she seeks to simply maintain that level of muscular fitness, it is not necessary to progressively increase the training stimulus. That is, increasing the overload by adding resistance, sets, or training sessions per week is not required during a maintenance resistance training program. Muscular strength may be maintained by training muscle groups as little as $1 \ d \cdot wk^{-1}$ as long as the training intensity or the resistance lifted is held constant (7).

The guidelines described in this chapter for resistance training are most appropriate for an overall or general physical fitness program that includes but does not necessarily emphasize muscle development. The recommendations are summarized in Box 7.3. A more rigorous training program must be employed if one's goal is to maximally increase muscular strength and mass, particularly among competitive athletes in sports such as football and bodybuilding. If the reader is interested in more than health/fitness and general outcomes or instead desires to maximally develop muscular strength and mass, he/she is referred to the ACSM position stand on progression models in resistance training for healthy adults for additional information (7).

FLEXIBILITY EXERCISE (STRETCHING)

Stretching exercise is recommended for inclusion in an exercise training program for all adults (5,8,31). Box 7.4 summarizes the recommendations for stretching. Stretching exercises improve range of motion and physical function, which are factors particularly important in countering the loss in range of motion with aging (8,18,31). Regular stretching exercise improves range of motion, although there is little effect observed acutely or immediately except as can be attributed to muscle-warming activities (18,39,43).

The acute effects of stretching on exercise and sport performance have been and are currently debatable. Some studies report decrements in muscle contraction velocity, force, and power, whereas others show an improvement or no change (40,43). Evidence suggests that the effects of stretching exercise on muscle performance are dependent on the type of stretching (i.e., static vs. dynamic) and muscular activity (i.e., concentric vs. eccentric muscle action) performed. It appears that static stretching may have significant detrimental effects on muscular strength and endurance, whereas dynamic stretching improves performance, although this has not been a universal finding (50).

BOX 7.3 **Resistance-Training Guidelines for Healthy Adults**

- Each major muscle group (chest, shoulders, abdomen, back, hips, legs, arms) should be trained with two to four sets. These sets may be of the same exercise or from different exercises affecting the same muscle group.
- The resistance-training program should feature exercises (total of 8–10) that are multijoint or compound exercises that involve more than one muscle group.
- Each major muscle group should be trained 2–3 $d \cdot wk^{-1}$. This recommendation may be accomplished either with two to three whole-body sessions of longer duration per week or with a greater number of shorter sessions using a split-body (lower body/upper body) approach, when only selected muscle groups are trained each session. In the split routine, two sessions performed on alternate days are required to train all muscle groups once with a total of four sessions needed to train all muscle groups 2 $d \cdot wk^{-1}$. Regardless of the approach used, any single muscle group should be rested at least 48 hours between sessions.
- A resistance that allows 8 to 12 repetitions to be performed each set should be selected. With each set the muscle should feel fatigued but should not be brought to failure. Maximal strength (1-RM) should be periodically assessed for each exercise so that a proper resistance (60%–80% 1-RM) is selected to enable 8 to 12 repetitions per set during training sessions.
- Older individuals should begin a resistance-training program at a lower intensity (e.g., 5–6 on the 10-point rating of perceived exertion scale) that permits 10 to 15 repetitions per set. Once properly conditioned, older individuals may prefer to increase the resistance and perform 8 to 12 repetitions with each set.
- Each exercise should be performed with proper technique and include both lifting (concentric contractions) and lowering (eccentric contractions) phases of the repetition. Each repetition should be completed in a controlled, deliberate fashion throughout the full range of motion.
- While performing repetitions, maintain a regular breathing pattern that typically involves exhaling during the lifting phase and inhaling during the lowering phase.
- If continued gains in muscular fitness and mass are desired, the individual will have to progressively overload his/her muscles to present a greater training stimulus (i.e., the progressive overload principle). This principle is achieved by using a greater resistance or more weight, performing more repetitions per set but not >12 repetitions, or training muscle groups more frequently.
- In contrast, if the individual is satisfied with the muscular fitness improvements made, a maintenance program may be adopted. During maintenance training, there is no need to progressively overload muscles; rather, the same regimen of sets, repetitions, resistance, and frequency is performed. In fact, assuming the intensity (i.e., resistance) remains the same, muscular fitness may be maintained by training muscle groups only 1 $d \cdot wk^{-1}$.

BOX 7.4   Summary of Key Points about Stretching

- Stretching exercise is most effective when the muscles are warm.
- Stretching should be performed before and/or after the conditioning phase.
- Stretching following exercise may be preferable for sports for which muscular strength, power, and endurance are important for performance.
- Stretching may not prevent injury.
- Stretching should be performed at least 2–3 d·wk^{-1}.
- Static, dynamic or ballistic, proprioceptive neuromuscular facilitation (PNF), and dynamic range of motion techniques improve flexibility.
- Stretching exercises should involve the major muscle tendon groups of the body.
- ≥4 repetitions per muscle group is recommended.
- Ballistic stretching may be considered particularly for persons whose sports activities involve ballistic movements.
- Static stretches should be held for 15 to 60 seconds.
- A 6-second contraction followed by a 10- to 30-second assisted stretch is recommended for PNF techniques.

Stretching exercise is widely recommended for injury prevention despite the fact that there is minimal scientific evidence to demonstrate its efficacy in doing so [14]. The limited evidence seems to suggest that stretching may be beneficial in preventing injury only in certain types of exercise, such as gymnastics, in which flexibility is an important part of performance; there may be little or no benefit in preventing injury during rhythmic, aerobic activities [16]. Stretching does not seem to reduce muscle soreness [20].

There is no conclusive evidence available at this time to support a universal recommendation to discontinue stretching before exercise [43]. However, for sport activities where muscular strength, power, and endurance are important for performance, it is recommended that stretching be performed following activity rather than during the warm-up period [43]. For adults exercising for overall physical fitness and athletes performing activities in which flexibility is important, stretching following a warm-up is still recommended because of the potential for injury prevention, and stretching following the conditioning exercise phase is recommended as a reasonable practice.

A stretching exercise program of at least 10 minutes in duration involving the major muscle tendon groups of the body (i.e., neck, shoulders, upper and lower back, pelvis, hips, and legs) with four or more repetitions per muscle group performed for a minimum of 2–3 d·wk^{-1} is recommended for most adults [8,31]. Static, dynamic (i.e., ballistic), proprioceptive neuromuscular facilitation (PNF), and dynamic range of motion techniques improve flexibility and are recommended (8). Ballistic stretching is often avoided by many health/fitness professionals because of concerns about increased injury, but there is no evidence that properly performed ballistic stretching results in injury (8). In particular, ballistic stretching may be considered for persons whose sports activities involve ballistic movements. Static stretches should be held for 15 to 60 seconds (36). A 6-second contraction followed by a 10- to 30-second assisted stretch is recommended for PNF techniques (8).

Stretching: A stretching exercise program of at least 10 minutes in duration involving the major muscle tendon groups of the body with four or more repetitions per muscle group performed on a minimum of $2–3 \; d \cdot wk^{-1}$ is recommended for most adults. Stretching exercises should be performed to the limits of discomfort within the range of motion, but no further. This will be perceived as the point of mild tightness without discomfort.

NEUROMUSCULAR EXERCISE

Neuromuscular training is recommended as part of an exercise program, particularly for older persons who are at increased risk of falling (31). Neuromuscular training includes balance, agility, and proprioceptive training. Exercise involving balance and agility, such as tai chi, is effective in reducing falls and is recommended as part of a comprehensive program of physical fitness and fall prevention in older adults (Chapter 8) (31). There are few studies evaluating the benefits of balance and agility exercise in younger adults so that definitive recommendations for neuromuscular exercise for this age group cannot be made at this time. However, there is limited evidence showing that a comprehensive exercise training program that includes neuromuscular training, balance, and agility exercise may reduce anterior cruciate injury in female athletes (21). Although evidence for specific benefits has been shown only in older adults who are frequent fallers or who have functional impairments, it is likely that all adults may gain benefits from these types of exercise, especially if participating in sports and occupational activities requiring agility and balance.

Neuromuscular exercise: Neuromuscular exercise done at least $2–3 \; d \cdot wk^{-1}$ is recommended for older adults who are frequent fallers or with mobility impairments and suggested for all adults, such as tai chi, Pilates, and yoga.

EXERCISE PROGRAM SUPERVISION

The health/fitness professional may determine the level of supervision that is optimal for an individual by evaluating information derived from the pre-exercise screening, medical evaluation, and exercise testing. Methods for pre-exercise screening and risk stratification are discussed in Chapters 2 and 3. Individualized exercise instruction by a certified exercise professional such as an

TABLE 7.5. GENERAL GUIDELINES FOR EXERCISE PROGRAM SUPERVISION

	LEVEL OF SUPERVISION[a]		
	UNSUPERVISED	PROFESSIONALLY SUPERVISED	CLINICALLY SUPERVISED
Health status	Low risk[a]	Moderate risk[b] or high risk[b] with stable disease[c] and regular physical activity habit	High risk[b]
Functional capacity	>7 METs	>7 METs	<7 METs

MET, metabolic equivalent.

[a]Supervision:
- Professional supervision refers to a health/fitness professional possessing a combination of academic training and certification equivalent to the ACSM Certified Health Fitness Specialist or higher.
- Clinical supervision refers to a health/fitness professional possessing a combination of advanced college training and certification equivalent to the ACSM Registered Clinical Exercise Physiologist® and ACSM Certified Clinical Exercise Specialist® or higher.

[b]Risk status:

Low risk	Asymptomatic men and women who have ≤1 risk factor from Table 2.3
Moderate risk	Asymptomatic men and women who have ≥2 risk factors from Table 2.3
High risk	Individuals who have one or more signs and symptoms listed in Table 2.2 or known cardiovascular, pulmonary, or metabolic disease

[c]Stable disease refers to stable CVD, well-controlled metabolic or pulmonary disease, and other stable chronic diseases or conditions for which professional supervision is adequate to ensure safety.

Adapted from American College of Sports Medicine. *ACSM's Guidelines for Exercise Testing and Prescription.* 7th ed. Philadelphia (PA): Lippincott Williams & Wilkins; 2005. p. 163.

ACSM Certified Personal Trainer[SM] or ACSM Certified Health Fitness Specialist® is recommended for most sedentary adults initiating a new exercise program. Individuals who have or are at high risk of CVD or who have a chronic disease or health condition that may be exacerbated by exercise should be supervised by a well-trained exercise professional, such as an ACSM Registered Clinical Exercise Physiologist® or ACSM Certified Clinical Exercise Specialist®, until the individual exercise can be performed safely without supervision by a clinical professional. Table 7.5 presents general guidelines for exercise program supervision.

STRATEGIES FOR IMPROVING EXERCISE ADOPTION AND MAINTENANCE

Substantial public health efforts have been directed to promote increased physical activity, and the prevalence of sedentary behavior has begun to decline (12). However, the prevalence of physical inactivity remains too high. Some interventions based on behavior-change theory have been successful in helping individuals to adopt an exercise program over the short term (22,30). Behavioral interventions to increase physical activity have shown little, modest, or inconsistent effects on increasing long-term maintenance of regular physical activity (22,30). Attrition rates for structured exercise programs range from 9% to 87% (30).

Individualized lifestyle physical activity programs may be an effective alternative to improve adherence to exercise for some individuals (30). Tailoring physical activity interventions to the individual using behavioral theory improves the effectiveness of physical activity programs (22,29,30). Effective physical activity interventions include (a) increasing social support and self-efficacy (i.e., self-confidence in performing physical activity), (b) reducing barriers to exercise, (c) using informational prompts, and (d) making social and physical environmental changes. Recommendations given by a healthcare provider may be an effective motivator to increase physical activity.

Evaluation of the client's readiness to change and motivation for exercise is helpful as this evaluation assists the health/fitness professional in tailoring communications to the individual. Assessment tools for self-motivation and stage of change are shown in Figures 7.3 and 7.4, respectively. Practical recommendations to enhance exercise program adherence are shown in Box 7.5. The Five-A's model for physical activity counseling is shown in Box 7.6. The Five-A's model provides a simple and effective framework for tailoring counseling for health-behavior change according to the client's stage of change (34).

A B C D E
5 4 3 2 1   1. I get discouraged easily.
5 4 3 2 1   2. I don't work any harder than I have to.
1 2 3 4 5   3. I seldom if ever let myself down.
5 4 3 2 1   4. I'm just not the goal-setting type.
1 2 3 4 5   5. I'm good at keeping promises, especially the ones I make myself.
5 4 3 2 1   6. I don't impose much structure on my activities.
1 2 3 4 5   7. I have a very hard-driving, aggressive personality

Directions: Circle the number beneath the letter corresponding to the alternative that best describes how characteristic the statement is when applied to you. The alternatives are:
  A. *extremely* uncharacteristic of me.
  B. *somewhat* uncharacteristic of me.
  C. neither characteristic nor uncharacteristic of me.
  D. *somewhat* characteristic of me.
  E. *extremely* characteristic of me.

Scoring: Add together the seven numbers you circled. A score ≤24 suggests dropout-prone behavior. The lower the self-motivation score, the greater the likelihood toward exercise noncompliance. If the score suggests dropout proneness, it should be viewed as an incentive to remain active, rather than a self-fulfilling prophecy to quit exercising.

FIGURE 7.3. Self-Motivation Assessment Scale. (Adapted from Falls HB, Baylor AM, Dishman RK. *Essentials of Fitness*. Philadelphia (PA): Saunders College; 1980, Appendix A-13. Copyright Rod K. Dishman 1978.)

PHYSICAL ACTIVITY STAGES OF CHANGE

Instructions: For each question below, please fill in the circle Yes or No. Please be
sure to follow the instructions carefully.

	Yes	No
1. I am currently physically active	Ⓨ	Ⓝ
2. I intend to become more physically active in the next 6 months.	Ⓨ	Ⓝ

For activity to be regular, it must add up to a total of 30 or more minutes per day and
be done at least 5 days per week. For example, you could take one 30-minute walk
or three 10-minute walks each day.

	Yes	No
3. I currently engage in regular physical activity.	Ⓨ	Ⓝ
4. I have been regularly physically active for the past 6 months.	Ⓨ	Ⓝ

	ITEM			
Stage	1	2	3	4
Precontemplation	No	No	—	—
Contemplation	No	Yes	—	—
Preparation	Yes	—	No	—
Action	Yes	—	Yes	No
Maintenance	Yes	—	Yes	Yes

FIGURE 7.4. Assessing physical activity stages of change. (Used with permission from
Marcus BH, Forsyth LH. *Motivating People to be Physically Active.* Champaign (IL): Human
Kinetics; 2003. 21–22 p.)

**BOX 7.5   Practical Recommendations to Enhance
Exercise Adherence**

- Obtain healthcare provider support of the exercise program.
- Clarify individual needs to establish the motive for exercise.
- Identify individualized, attainable goals and objectives for exercise.
- Identify safe, convenient, and well-maintained facilities for exercise.
- Identify social support for exercise.
- Identify environmental supports and reminders for exercise.
- Identify motivational exercise outcomes for self-monitoring of exercise
  progress and achievements, such as exercise logs and step counters. ➤

> **Box 7.5. continued**

- Emphasize and monitor the acute or immediate effects of exercise (i.e., reduced blood pressure, blood glucose, and need for certain medications).
- Emphasize variety and enjoyment in the exercise program.
- Establish a regular schedule of exercise.
- Provide qualified, personable, and enthusiastic exercise professionals.
- Minimize muscle soreness and injury by participation in exercise of moderate intensity, particularly in the early phase of exercise adoption.

Adapted from American College of Sports Medicine. *ACSM's Guidelines for Exercise Testing and Prescription*. 7th ed. Philadelphia (PA): Lippincott Williams & Wilkins; 2005. 167 p.

BOX 7.6	Client-Centered Physical Activity Counseling (Five-A's Model)

ADDRESS AGENDA (FOR INDIVIDUALS IN ALL STAGES OF CHANGE)
- Attend to client's agenda (e.g., "Why did you come to see me today?").
- Express desire to talk about a health behavior (e.g., "I'd like to talk with you about your physical activity.").

ASSESS (FOR INDIVIDUALS IN ALL STAGES OF CHANGE)
- Readiness for change (e.g., "Have you considered changing your exercise habits?")
- Knowledge of risks/problems (e.g., "Do you think there are any risks of exercise?")
- History of risk-related symptoms/illnesses (e.g., "You are concerned about getting too tired if you exercise. Has fatigue been a problem for you?")
- Fears/concerns (e.g., "Do you have any concerns about increasing your physical activity?")
- Feelings about the health behavior (e.g., "How do you feel about exercising more?")
- History of addressing health behavior (e.g., "Have you ever tried to exercise in the past?")
- History of problems during previous attempts to change (e.g., "Tell me about what happened when you were exercising previously. Did you have any problems?") >

> Box 7.6. continued

- History of problems that may interfere with change (e.g., "Is there any reason why you can't begin to exercise now?")
- Reasons for wanting to change behavior (e.g., "Why do you want to start exercising?")
- Reasons for maintaining risk behavior (e.g., "Why do you want to keep things as they are and not exercise?")

ADVISE (FOR INDIVIDUALS IN ALL STAGES OF CHANGE)
- Tell client you strongly advise behavioral change (e.g., "As your exercise professional, I'd strongly recommend that you begin a program of exercise to improve your health.").
- Personalize risk (e.g., "You are worried about having a heart attack. Remaining inactive doubles your risk of having a heart attack.").
- Personalize immediate and long-term benefits of change (e.g., "Exercise will help you to control your high blood pressure and greatly reduce your risk of developing heart disease.").

ASSIST (FOR INDIVIDUALS IN ALL STAGES OF CHANGE)
- Use verbal and nonverbal relationship/facilitation skills. (Use open-ended questions. Avoid prescriptive statements, such as "You should . . . " Make direct eye contact; lean toward the client, etc.)
- Correct misunderstandings; provide information (e.g., "You want to lose 10 pounds [4.5 kg] in 6 weeks by exercising more. That is not a realistic or healthy goal. Exercise will help you over the long term to maintain a weight loss, but it will have only a small effect, if any, in the short term.").
- Address feelings/provide support (e.g., "I understand you are nervous about starting to exercise. It is hard to get started, but I am confident you can do it.").
- Address barriers to change (e.g., "You mentioned that you have a tight schedule. Let's look at your schedule to see if we can identify some time when you can fit in a short walk.").
- Identify potential resources and support (e.g., "Is your spouse interested in exercising with you? Is there a gym or park near your home?").

ASSIST: (FOR INDIVIDUALS IN PREPARATION OR
ACTION STAGES)
- Describe options available for change (e.g., "Based on what you have told me, it seems your choices are to join an exercise class at the Y or to begin walking during your lunch break.").
- Negotiate selection among options (e.g., "Which of these options do you think would be best for you?") >

> Box 7.6. continued

- Provide resources/materials (e.g., "Here is a tip sheet with some simple steps to help you with your walking program.").
- Teach skills/recommend behavior strategies (e.g., "It is hard to begin an exercise program. One thing that can help is to put exercise on your calendar and treat it as an appointment.").
- Refer, when appropriate (e.g., "I think you would enjoy going to a yoga class at _____.").
- Consider a written contract (e.g., "Many people find a written contract to be helpful in staying on track with their exercise plans. Is it OK with you if we try that?").
- Identify barriers and solve problems (e.g., "People usually run into challenges that make it hard to exercise. What do you think may be a problem for you? Let's think about strategies to overcome these challenges.").
- Encourage use of supports, coping strategies (e.g., "Bad weather often makes it difficult to walk outside. Can you think of an alternate place to walk? How about another kind of exercise for bad weather days?").

ARRANGE FOLLOW-UP (FOR INDIVIDUALS IN ALL STAGES OF CHANGE)
- Reaffirm plan (e.g., "Now let's be sure we both understand our plan. You plan to visit three gyms near your house to check out the facilities and exercise classes. Is that correct?").
- Schedule follow-up appointment or phone call (e.g., "Let's check in with each other in 2 weeks to see how things are going. Can you give me a call in 2 weeks?").

Reprinted from Pinto BM, Goldstein MG, Marcus BH. Activity counseling by primary care physicians. *Prev Med.* 1998;27:506–13 with permission from Elsevier.

REFERENCES

1. Ainsworth BE, Haskell WL, Leon AS, Jacobs DR, Montoye HJ, Sallis JF, Paffenbarger RS. Compendium of physical activities: classification of energy costs of human physical activities. *Med Sci Sports Exerc.* 1993;25:71–80.
2. Ainsworth BE, Haskell WL, Whitt MC, et al. Compendium of physical activities: an update of activity codes and MET intensities. *Med Sci Sports Exerc.* 2000;32:S498–S504.
3. Almeida SA, Williams KM, Shaffer RA, Brodine SK. Epidemiological patterns of musculoskeletal injuries and physical training. *Med Sci Sports Exerc.* 1999;31:1176–82.
4. American College of Sports Medicine. Position Stand. Appropriate intervention strategies for weight loss and prevention of weight regain for adults. *Med Sci Sports Exerc.* 2001;33:2145–56.
5. American College of Sports Medicine. Position Stand. Exercise and physical activity for older adults. *Med Sci Sports Exerc.* 1998;30(6):992–1008.
6. American College of Sports Medicine. Position Stand. Physical activity and bone health. *Med Sci Sports Exerc.* 2004;36:1985–96.

7. American College of Sports Medicine. Position Stand. Progression models in resistance training for healthy adults. *Med Sci Sports Exerc*. 2002;34:364–80.

8. American College of Sports Medicine. Position Stand. The recommended quantity and quality of exercise for developing and maintaining cardiorespiratory and muscular fitness, and flexibility in healthy adults. *Med Sci Sports Exerc*. 1998;30:975–91.

9. American College of Sports Medicine. *ACSM's Metabolic Calculations Handbook*. Philadelphia (PA): Lippincott Williams & Wilkins; 2006.

10. American College of Sports Medicine. *ACSM's Resource Manual for the Guidelines for Exercise Testing and Prescription*. 6th ed. Philadelphia (PA): Lippincott Williams & Wilkins; 2009.

11. Borg GA. Perceived exertion. *Exerc Sport Sci Rev*. 1974;2:131–53.

12. Centers for Disease Control and Prevention. Trends in leisure-time physical inactivity by age, sex, and race/ethnicity—United States, 1994–2004. *MMWR Morb Mortal Wkly Rep* 2005;54:991–4.

13. Ekkekakis P, Hall EE, Petruzzello SJ. Practical markers of the transition from aerobic to anaerobic metabolism during exercise: rationale and a case for affect-based exercise prescription. *Prev Med*. 2004;38:149–59.

14. Fradkin AJ, Gabbe BJ, Cameron PA. Does warming up prevent injury in sport? The evidence from randomised controlled trials. *J Sci Med Sport*. 2006;9:214–20.

15. Gellish, RL, Goslin BR, Olson RE, McDonald A, Russi GD, Moudgil VK. *Med Sci Sport Exer*. 2007;39(5):822–9.

16. Gremion G. Is stretching for sports performance still useful? A review of the literature. *Rev Med Suisse*. 2005;1:1830–4.

17. Hardy CJ, Rejeski WJ. Not what, but how one feels: the measurement of affect during exercise. *J Sport Exerc Psychol*. 1989;11:304–17.

18. Harvey L, Herbert R, Crosbie J. Does stretching induce lasting increases in joint ROM? A systematic review. *Physiother Res Int*. 2002;7:1–13.

19. Haskell WL, Minn LI, Pate RR, et al. Physical activity and public health: updated recommendations from the American College of Sports Medicine and the American Heart Association. *Med Sci Sports Exer*. 2007;39(8):1423–34.

20. Herbert RD, Gabriel M. Effects of stretching before and after exercising on muscle soreness and risk of injury: systematic review. *BMJ*. 2002;325:468.

21. Hewett TE, Myer GD, Ford KR. Reducing knee and anterior cruciate ligament injuries among female athletes: a systematic review of neuromuscular training interventions. *J Knee Surg*. 2005;18:82–8.

22. Hillsdon M, Foster C, Thorogood M. Interventions for promoting physical activity (rev.). *Cochrane Database Sys Rev*. CD003180, 2005.

23. Institute of Medicine. *Dietary Reference Intakes for Energy, Carbohydrate, Fiber, Fat, Fatty Acids, Cholesterol, Protein, and Amino Acids*. Washington, DC: The National Academies Press, 2005. p. 880–935.

24. Irving BA, Rutkowski J, Brock DW, Davis CK, Barrett EJ, Gaesser GA, Weltman A. Comparison of Borg- and OMNI-RPE as markers of the blood lactate response to exercise. *Med Sci Sports Exerc*. 2006;38:1348–52.

25. Kohl HW, Lee IM, Vuori IM, Wheeler FW, Bauman A, Sallis JF. Physical act and public health: the emergence of a subdiscipline—report from the International Congress on Physical Activity and Public Health, April 17–21, 2006, Atlanta, GA. *J Phys Act Health*. 2006;3:344–64

26. Lee IM, Rexrode KM, Cook NR, Manson JE, Buring JE. Physical activity and coronary heart disease in women: is "no pain, no gain" passe? *JAMA*. 2001;285:1447–54.

27. Lee IM, Skerrett PJ. Physical activity and all-cause mortality: what is the dose-response relation? *Med Sci Sports Exerc*. 2001;33:S459–71 and S493–454.

28. Londeree BR, Moeschberger ML. Effect of age and other factors on maximal heart rate. *Res Q Exerc Sport*. 1982;53:297–304.

29. Marcus BH, Forsyth LH. *Motivating People to be Physically Active*. Champaign (IL): Human Kinetics; 2003.

30. Marcus BH, Williams DM, Dubbert PM, et al. Physical activity intervention studies: what we know and what we need to know: a scientific statement from the American Heart Association Council on Nutrition, Physical Activity, and Metabolism (Subcommittee on Physical Activity); Council on Cardiovascular Disease in the Young; and the Interdisciplinary Working Group on Quality of Care and Outcomes Research. *Circulation*. 2006;114:2739–52.

31. Nelson ME, Rejeski WJ, Blair SN, et al. Physical activity and public health in older adults: recommendation from the American College of Sports Medicine and the American Heart Association. *Med Sci Sports Exerc.* 2007;39(8):1435–45.

32. Noble BJ, Borg GA, Jacobs I, Ceci R, Kaiser P. A category-ratio perceived exertion scale: relationship to blood and muscle lactates and heart rate. *Med Sci Sports Exerc.* 1983;15:523–8.

33. Persinger R, Foster C, Gibson M, Fater DC, Porcari JP. Consistency of the talk test for exercise prescription. *Med Sci Sports Exerc.* 2004;36:1632–6.

34. Pinto BM, Goldstein MG, Marcus BH. Activity counseling by primary care physicians. *Prev Med.* 1998;27:506–13.

35. Rhea MR, Alvar BA, Burkett LN, Ball SD. A meta-analysis to determine the dose response for strength development. *Med Sci Sports Exerc.* 2003;35:456–64.

36. Roberts JM, Wilson K. Effect of stretching duration on active and passive range of motion in the lower extremity. *Br J Sports Med.* 1999;33:259–63.

37. Robertson RJ, Goss FL, Dube J, Rutkowski J, Dupain M, Brennan C, Andreacci J. Validation of the adult OMNI scale of perceived exertion for cycle ergometer exercise. *Med Sci Sports Exerc.* 2004;36:102–8.

38. Robertson RJ, Goss FL, Rutkowski J, et al. Concurrent validation of the OMNI perceived exertion scale for resistance exercise. *Med Sci Sports Exerc.* 2003;35:333–41.

39. Shrier I. Does stretching improve performance? A systematic and critical review of the literature. *Clin J Sport Med.* 2004;14:267–73.

40. Shrier I. Flexibility versus stretching. *Br J Sports Med.* 2001;35:364.

41. Swain DP, Leutholtz BC. Heart rate reserve is equivalent to %VO$_2$ reserve, not to %VO$_{2max}$. *Med Sci Sports Exerc.* 1997;29:410–4.

42. Tanaka HK, Monahan KD, Seals DR. Age-predicted maximal heart rate revisited. *J Am Coll Cardiol.* 2001;37:153–6.

43. Thacker SB, Gilchrist J, Stroup DF, Kimsey CD. The impact of stretching on sports injury risk: a systematic review of the literature. *Med Sci Sports Exerc.* 2004;36:371–8.

44. Tudor-Locke C, Bassett DR. How many steps/day are enough? Preliminary pedometer indices for public health. *Sports Med.* 2004;34:1–8.

45. Tudor-Locke C, Williams JE, Reis JP, Pluto D. Utility of pedometers for assessing physical activity: convergent validity. *Sports Med.* 2002;32:795–808.

46. U.S. Department of Health and Human Services and the Department of Agriculture. *Dietary Guidelines for Americans 2005.* Washington, DC: U.S. Government Printing Office, 2005. p.19–22.

47. U.S. Department of Health and Human Services. Physical activity and health: a report of the Surgeon General. Atlanta, GA: U.S. Department of Health and Human Services, Centers for Disease Control and Prevention, and National Center for Chronic Disease Prevention and Health Promotion, 1996.

48. Utter AC, Robertson RJ, Green JM, Suminski R, McAnulty SR, Nieman DC. Validation of the adult OMNI scale of perceived exertion for walking/running exercise. *Med Sci Sports Exerc.* 2004;36:1776–80.

49. Wolfe BL, LeMura LM, Cole PJ. Quantitative analysis of single- vs. multiple-set programs in resistance training. *J Strength Cond Res.* 2004;18:35–47.

50. Yamaguchi T, Ishii K. Effects of static stretching for 30 seconds and dynamic stretching on leg extension power. *J Strength Cond Res.* 2005;19:677–83.

Exercise Prescription for Healthy Populations and Special Considerations

PREGNANCY

The acute physiologic responses to exercise are generally increased during pregnancy compared with pregnancy levels (Table 8.1). Healthy, pregnant women without exercise contraindications (Box 8.1) are encouraged to exercise throughout the pregnancy. Regular exercise during pregnancy provides health/fitness benefits to the mother and child (1,12). Exercise may also reduce the risk of developing conditions associated with pregnancy, such as pregnancy-induced hypertension and gestational diabetes mellitus (12,28). The American College of Sports Medicine (ACSM) endorses guidelines (24) regarding exercise in pregnancy and the postpartum period set forth by the American College of Obstetricians and Gynecologists (1,7), the Joint Committee of the Society of Obstetricians and Gynecologists of Canada (11), and the Canadian Society for Exercise Physiology (CSEP) (11). These guidelines outline the importance of exercise during pregnancy and also provide guidance on exercise prescription and contraindications to beginning and continuing exercise during pregnancy. The CSEP Physical Activity Readiness Medical Examination, termed the *PARmed-X for Pregnancy,* should be used for the health screening of pregnant women before their participation in exercise programs (Fig. 8.1).

EXERCISE TESTING

Maximal exercise testing should not be performed on pregnant women unless medically necessary (1,7,11). If a maximal exercise test is warranted, the test should be performed with physician supervision. Submaximal exercise testing (i.e., <75% heart rate reserve [HRR]) may be performed to predict maximum oxygen uptake ($\dot{V}O_{2max}$) to develop a more precise exercise prescription (Chapter 4). A women who has been sedentary before pregnancy or who has a medical condition (Box 8.1) should receive clearance from her physician before beginning an exercise program.

TABLE 8.1. PHYSIOLOGIC RESPONSES TO ACUTE EXERCISE DURING PREGNANCY COMPARED WITH PREPREGNANCY

Oxygen uptake (during weight-dependent exercise) $\dot{V}O_2$	Increase
Heart rate	Increase
Stroke volume	Increase
Cardiac output	Increase
Tidal volume	Increase
Minute ventilation ($\dot{V}E$)	Increase
Ventilatory equivalent for oxygen ($\dot{V}E/\dot{V}O_2$)	Increase
Ventilatory equivalent for carbon dioxide ($\dot{V}E/\dot{V}CO_2$)	Increase
Systolic blood pressure (SBP)	No change/Decrease
Diastolic blood pressure (DBP)	No change/Decrease

Adapted from Wolfe LA. Differences between children and adults for exercise testing and prescription. In: Skinner JS, editor. *Exercise Testing and Exercise Prescription for Special Cases*. 2nd ed. Philadelphia (PA): Lippincott Williams & Wilkins; 2005. p. 377–91.

EXERCISE PRESCRIPTION

The recommended exercise prescription for pregnant women is generally consistent with recommendations for the general adult population (Chapter 7). However, it is important to monitor and adjust exercise prescriptions according to the woman's symptoms, discomforts, and abilities during pregnancy and be aware of contraindications for exercising during pregnancy (Box 8.1).

Frequency: At least three—and preferably all—days of the week.

Intensity: Moderate intensity (40%–60% $\dot{V}O_2$ reserve [$\dot{V}O_2R$]). Because of heart rate (HR) variability during pregnancy, consider using the rating of perceived exertion (RPE) (12–14 on a scale of 6–20) or the "talk test" (being able to maintain a conversation during activity) to monitor exercise intensity. HR ranges that correspond to moderate-intensity exercise have also been developed for pregnant women based on age (11).

AGE (YEARS)	HEART RATE RANGE (Beats · min^{-1})
<20	140–155
20–29	135–150
30–39	130–145
>40	125–140

Time: At least 15 min · d^{-1} gradually increasing to at least 30 min · d^{-1} of accumulated moderate-intensity physical activity to total 150 minutes per week.

Type: Dynamic, rhythmic physical activities that use the large muscle groups, such as walking and cycling.

BOX 8.1 Contraindications for Exercising during Pregnancy

Relative
- Severe anemia
- Unevaluated maternal cardiac dysrhythmia
- Chronic bronchitis
- Poorly controlled type 1 diabetes mellitus
- Extreme morbid obesity
- Extreme underweight
- History of extremely sedentary lifestyle
- Intrauterine growth restriction in current pregnancy
- Poorly controlled hypertension
- Orthopedic limitations
- Poorly controlled seizure disorder
- Poorly controlled hyperthyroidism
- Heavy smoker

Absolute
- Hemodynamically significant heart disease
- Restrictive lung disease
- Incompetent cervix/cerclage
- Multiple gestation at risk for premature labor
- Persistent second- or third-trimester bleeding
- Placenta previa after 26 weeks of gestation
- Premature labor during the current pregnancy
- Ruptured membranes
- Preeclampsia/pregnancy-induced hypertension

Reprinted with permission from American College of Obstetricians and Gynecologists. Exercise during pregnancy and the postpartum period. ACOG Committee Opinion No. 267. *Obstet Gynecol*. 2002;99:171-3.

SPECIAL CONSIDERATIONS

- Pregnant women who have been sedentary or have a medical condition should gradually increase activity to meet the recommended levels above.
- Pregnant women who are morbidly obese and/or have gestational diabetes mellitus or hypertension should consult their physician before beginning an exercise program and have their exercise prescriptions adjusted to their medical condition, symptoms, and functional capacity.
- Pregnant women should avoid contact sports and sports/activities that may cause loss of balance or trauma to the mother or fetus. Examples of sports/activities to avoid include soccer, basketball, ice hockey, horseback riding, and vigorous-intensity racquet sports.

Physical Activity Readiness
Medical Examination for
Pregnancy (2002)

PARmed-X for PREGNANCY
PHYSICAL ACTIVITY READINESS MEDICAL EXAMINATION

PARmed-X for PREGNANCY is a guideline for health screening prior to participation in a prenatal fitness class or other exercise.

Healthy women with uncomplicated pregnancies can integrate physical activity into their daily living and can participate without significant risks either to themselves or to their unborn child. Postulated benefits of such programs include improved aerobic and muscular fitness, promotion of appropriate weight gain, and facilitation of labour. Regular exercise may also help to prevent gestational glucose intolerance and pregnancy-induced hypertension.

The safety of prenatal exercise programs depends on an adequate level of maternal-fetal physiological reserve. PARmed-X for PREGNANCY is a convenient checklist and prescription for use by health care providers to evaluate pregnant patients who want to enter a prenatal fitness program and for ongoing medical surveillance of exercising pregnant patients.

Instructions for use of the 4-page PARmed-X for PREGNANCY are the following:

1. The patient should fill out the section on PATIENT INFORMATION and the PRE-EXERCISE HEALTH CHECKLIST (PART 1, 2, 3, and 4 on p. 1) and give the form to the health care provider monitoring her pregnancy.

2. The health care provider should check the information provided by the patient for accuracy and fill out SECTION C on CONTRAINDICATIONS (p. 2) based on current medical information.

3. If no exercise contraindications exist, the HEALTH EVALUATION FORM (p. 3) should be completed, signed by the health care provider, and given by the patient to her prenatal fitness professional.

In addition to prudent medical care, participation in appropriate types, intensities and amounts of exercise is recommended to increase the likelihood of a beneficial pregnancy outcome. PARmed-X for PREGNANCY provides recommendations for individualized exercise prescription (p. 3) and program safety (p. 4).

NOTE: Sections A and B should be completed by the patient before the appointment with the health care provider.

A PATIENT INFORMATION

NAME

ADDRESS

TELEPHONE_____ BIRTHDATE _____ HEALTH INSURANCE No. _____

NAME OF
PRENATAL FITNESS PROFESSIONAL_____

PRENATAL FITNESS
PROFESSIONAL?S PHONE NUMBER_____

B PRE-EXERCISE HEALTH CHECKLIST

PART 1: GENERAL HEALTH STATUS

In the past, have you experienced (check YES or NO):

	YES	NO
1. Miscarriage in an earlier pregnancy?	❑	❑
2. Other pregnancy complications?	❑	❑
3. I have completed a PAR-Q within the last 30 days.	❑	❑

If you answered YES to question 1 or 2, please explain:

Number of previous pregnancies? _____

PART 2: STATUS OF CURRENT PREGNANCY

Due Date: _____

During this pregnancy, have you experienced:

	YES	NO
1. Marked fatigue?	❑	❑
2. Bleeding from the vagina ("spotting")?	❑	❑
3. Unexplained faintness or dizziness?	❑	❑
4. Unexplained abdominal pain?	❑	❑
5. Sudden swelling of ankles, hands or face?	❑	❑
6. Persistent headaches or problems with headaches?	❑	❑
7. Swelling, pain or redness in the calf of one leg?	❑	❑
8. Absence of fetal movement after 6th month?	❑	❑
9. Failure to gain weight after 5th month?	❑	❑

If you answered YES to any of the above questions, please explain:

PART 3: ACTIVITY HABITS DURING THE PAST MONTH

1. List only regular fitness/recreational activities:

INTENSITY	FREQUENCY (times/week)			TIME (minutes/day)		
	1-2	2-4	4+	<20	20-40	40+
Heavy	—	—	—	—	—	—
Medium	—	—	—	—	—	—
Light	—	—	—	—	—	—

2. Does your regular occupation (job/home) activity involve:

	YES	NO
Heavy Lifting?	❑	❑
Frequent walking/stair climbing?	❑	❑
Occasional walking (>once/hr)?	❑	❑
Prolonged standing?	❑	❑
Mainly sitting?	❑	❑
Normal daily activity?	❑	❑
3. Do you currently smoke tobacco?*	❑	❑
4. Do you consume alcohol?*	❑	❑

PART 4: PHYSICAL ACTIVITY INTENTIONS

What physical activity do you intend to do?

Is this a change from what you currently do?   ❑ YES   ❑ NO

*NOTE: PREGNANT WOMEN ARE STRONGLY ADVISED NOT TO SMOKE OR CONSUME ALCOHOL DURING PREGNANCY AND DURING LACTATION.

CSEP / SCPE
© Canadian Society for Exercise Physiology
Société canadienne de physiologie de l'exercice

Supported by: 🍁 Health Canada Santé Canada

FIGURE 8.1. Physical Activity Readiness (PARmedX) for Pregnancy. (Source: Physical Activity Readiness Medical Examination for Pregnancy [PARmed-X for Pregnancy] © 2002. Reprinted with permission of the Canadian Society for Exercise Physiology. www.csep.ca.) (continued)

- Exercise should be terminated should any of the following occur: vaginal bleeding, dyspnea before exertion, dizziness, headache, chest pain, muscle weakness, calf pain or swelling, preterm labor, decreased fetal movement, and amniotic fluid leakage (1). In the case of calf pain and swelling, thrombophlebitis should be ruled out.

Physical Activity Readiness
Medical Examination for
Pregnancy (2002)

PARmed-X for PREGNANCY   PHYSICAL ACTIVITY READINESS MEDICAL EXAMINATION

C CONTRAINDICATIONS TO EXERCISE: to be completed by your health care provider		
Absolute Contraindications	**Relative Contraindications**	

Absolute Contraindications

Does the patient have:

	YES	NO
1. Ruptured membranes, premature labour?	☐	☐
2. Persistent second or third trimester bleeding/placenta previa?	☐	☐
3. Pregnancy-induced hypertension or pre-eclampsia?	☐	☐
4. Incompetent cervix?	☐	☐
5. Evidence of intrauterine growth restriction?	☐	☐
6. High-order pregnancy (e.g., triplets)?	☐	☐
7. Uncontrolled Type I diabetes, hypertension or thyroid disease, other serious cardiovascular, respiratory or systemic disorder?	☐	☐

Relative Contraindications

Does the patient have:

	YES	NO
1. History of spontaneous abortion or premature labour in previous pregnancies?	☐	☐
2. Mild/moderate cardiovascular or respiratory disease (e.g., chronic hypertension, asthma)?	☐	☐
3. Anemia or iron deficiency? (Hb < 100 g/L)?	☐	☐
4. Malnutrition or eating disorder (anorexia, bulimia)?	☐	☐
5. Twin pregnancy after 28th week?	☐	☐
6. Other significant medical condition?	☐	☐

Please specify: _____

NOTE: Risk may exceed benefits of regular physical activity. The decision to be physically active or not should be made with qualified medical advice.

PHYSICAL ACTIVITY RECOMMENDATION: ☐ Recommended/Approved   ☐ Contraindicated

FIGURE 8.1. *Continued.*

- Pregnant women should avoid exercising in the supine position after the first trimester to ensure that venous obstruction does not occur.
- Pregnant women should avoid performing the Valsalva maneuver during exercise.
- Pregnant women should exercise in a thermoneutral environment and be well hydrated to avoid heat stress. See this chapter and the ACSM position stands on exercising in the heat (4) and fluid replacement (2) for additional information.
- During pregnancy, the metabolic demand increases by ~ 300 kcal $\cdot$ d^{-1}. Women should increase caloric intake to meet the caloric costs of pregnancy and exercise.
- Pregnant women may participate in a strength-training program that incorporates all major muscle groups with a resistance that permits multiple repetitions (i.e., 12–15 repetitions) to be performed to a point of moderate fatigue. Isometric muscle actions and the Valsalva maneuver should be avoided, as should the supine position after the first trimester.
- Generally, exercise in the postpartum period may begin ~ 4 to 6 weeks after delivery. Deconditioning typically occurs during the initial postpartum period, so women should gradually increase physical activity levels until prepregnancy physical fitness levels are achieved.

CHILDREN AND ADOLESCENTS

Most children (defined as <13 years) participate in adequate amounts of physical activity. However, recent trends show physical activity levels decreasing through adolescence (defined as 13–18 years or Tanner stage 5), such that the majority of adolescents are not participating in sufficient amounts of physical activity to meet recommended guidelines (20,32). Children and adolescents require special consideration when exercising as a result of growth and the immaturity of their physiologic regulatory systems at rest and during exercise (20). Cardiovascular disease (CVD) risk factors that are present in youth have a tendency to track into adulthood. Youth who are overweight tend to have a higher prevalence of CVD risk factors than their normal weight peers. Physical activity also has a positive influence on academic performance and self-esteem. Because of the health benefits of habitual physical activity, it is important that children are physically active and that they continue this behavior through adolescence into adulthood (33).

EXERCISE TESTING

Generally the adult guidelines for standard exercise testing apply to children and adolescents (Chapter 5). However, the physiologic responses during exercise differ from those of adults (Table 8.2) so that the following issues should be considered (27,34).

- Exercise testing for clinical or health/fitness purposes is generally not indicated for children or adolescents unless there is a health concern.
- The exercise testing protocol should be based on the reason the test is being performed and the functional capability of the child or adolescent.
- Children and adolescents should be familiarized with the test protocol and procedure before testing to minimize stress and maximize the potential for a successful test.
- Both treadmill and cycle ergometers should be available for testing. Treadmills tend to elicit a higher peak oxygen uptake ($\dot{V}O_{2\ peak}$) and maximum heart rate (HR_{max}). Cycle ergometers provide less risk for injury but need to be correctly sized for the child or adolescent.

TABLE 8.2. PHYSIOLOGIC RESPONSES TO ACUTE EXERCISE OF CHILDREN COMPARED WITH ADULTS

VARIABLE	RESPONSE
Absolute oxygen uptake ($\dot{V}O_2$ [L·min^{-1}])	Lower
Relative oxygen uptake ($\dot{V}O_2$ [mL·kg^{-1}min^{-1}])	Higher
Heart rate	Higher
Cardiac output	Lower
Stroke volume	Lower
Systolic blood pressure	Lower
Diastolic blood pressure	Lower
Respiratory rate	Higher
Tidal volume	Lower
Minute ventilation ($\dot{V}E$)	Lower
Respiratory exchange ratio	Lower

Adapted from Hebestreit HU, Bar-Or O. Differences between children and adults for exercise testing and prescription. In: Skinner JS, editor. *Exercise Testing and Exercise Prescription for Special Cases*. Philadelphia (PA): Lippincott Williams & Wilkins; 2005. p. 68–84; and Strong WB, Malina RM, Blimke CJR, et al. Evidence based physical activity for school-age youth. *J Pediatrics*. 2005;146:732–7.

- Compared with adults, children and adolescents are mentally and psychologically immature and may require extra motivation and support during the exercise test.

In addition, health/fitness testing may be performed outside of the clinical setting. In these types of settings, the FITNESSGRAM test battery may be used to assess the components of health-related fitness in youth (21).

EXERCISE PRESCRIPTION

The exercise prescription guidelines outlined below for children and adolescents establish the minimal amount of physical activity needed to achieve the various components of health-related fitness (32).

Frequency: At least 3–4 d · wk^{-1} and preferably daily.

Intensity: Moderate (physical activity that noticeably increases breathing, sweating, and HR) to vigorous (physical activity that substantially increases breathing, sweating, and HR) intensity.

Time: 30 min · d^{-1} of moderate and 30 min · d^{-1} of vigorous intensity to total 60 min · d^{-1} of accumulated physical activity.

Type: A variety of activities that are enjoyable and developmentally appropriate for the child or adolescent; these may include walking, active play/games, dance, sports, and muscle- and bone-strengthening activities.

SPECIAL CONSIDERATIONS

- Children and adolescents may safely participate in strength-training activities provided that they receive proper instruction and supervision. Generally, adult guidelines for resistance training may be applied. Eight to 15 repetitions of an exercise should be performed to the point of moderate fatigue with good mechanical form before the resistance is increased.
- Because of immature thermoregulatory systems, youth should exercise in thermoneutral environments and be properly hydrated. See this chapter and the ACSM position stands on exercising in the heat (4) and fluid replacement (2) for additional information.
- Children and adolescents who are overweight or physically inactive may not be able to achieve 60 min · d^{-1} of physical activity. Therefore, gradually increase the frequency and time of physical activity to achieve this goal.
- Children and adolescents with diseases or disabilities such as asthma, diabetes mellitus, obesity, cystic fibrosis, and cerebral palsy should have their exercise prescriptions tailored to their condition, symptoms, and functional capacity. See Chapter 10 for additional information on exercise recommendations for these diseases and conditions.
- Efforts should be made to decrease sedentary activities (i.e., television watching, surfing the Internet, and playing video games) and increase activities that promote lifelong activity and fitness (i.e., walking and cycling).

OLDER ADULT

The term *older adult* (defined as people ≥65 years and people 50–64 years with clinically significant conditions or physical limitations that affect movement, physical fitness, or physical activity) represents a diverse spectrum of ages and physiologic capabilities (31). Because physiologic aging does not occur uniformly across the population, individuals of similar chronological age may differ dramatically in their response to exercise. In addition, it is difficult to distinguish the effects of aging on physiologic function from the effects of deconditioning or disease. Health status is often a better indicator of ability to engage in physical activity than chronological age. Individuals with chronic disease should be under the care of a health care provider who can guide them with their exercise program.

Overwhelming evidence exists that supports the benefits of physical activity in (a) slowing physiologic changes of aging that impair exercise capacity; (b) optimizing age-related changes in body composition; (c) promoting psychological and cognitive well-being; (d) managing chronic diseases; (e) reducing the risks of physical disability; and (f) increasing longevity (14). Despite these benefits, older adults are the least physically active of all age groups. Although recent trends indicate a slight improvement in reported physical activity, only about 21% of people aged 65 years and older engage in regular physical activity. The percentage of reported physical activity decreases with advancing age, with fewer than 10% of individuals older than age 85 years engaging in regular physical activity (13).

To safely administer an exercise test and develop a sound exercise prescription requires knowledge of the effects of aging on physiologic function at rest and during exercise. Table 8.3 provides a list of age-related changes on key physio-

TABLE 8.3. EFFECTS OF AGING ON SELECTED PHYSIOLOGIC AND HEALTH-RELATED VARIABLES

VARIABLE	CHANGE
HR_{rest} (resting heart rate)	Unchanged
HR_{max} (maximum heart rate)	Lower
$\dot{Q}_{max}$ (maximum cardiac output)	Lower
Resting and exercise BP (blood pressure)	Higher
$\dot{V}O_2R_{max}$ (maximum oxygen uptake reserve) ($L \cdot min^{-1}$ and $mL \cdot kg^{-1} \cdot min^{-1}$)	Lower
Residual volume	Higher
Vital capacity	Lower
Reaction time	Slower
Muscular strength	Lower
Flexibility	Lower
Bone mass	Lower
Fat-free body mass	Lower
% Body fat	Higher
Glucose tolerance	Lower
Recovery time	Longer

Adapted from Skinner JS. Aging for exercise testing and prescription. In: Skinner JS, editor. *Exercise Testing and Exercise Prescription for Special Cases.* 2nd ed. Philadelphia (PA): Lippincott Williams & Wilkins; 2005. p. 85–99.

logic variables. Underlying disease and medication use may alter the expected response to acute exercise.

EXERCISE TESTING

Most older adults do not require an exercise test prior to initiating a moderate physical activity program. For older adults with risk factors as defined in Table 2.3, a person is considered at moderate risk for adverse responses to exercise and is advised to undergo medical examination and exercise testing before initiating vigorous-intensity exercise. Exercise testing may require subtle differences in protocol, methodology, and dosage. The following list details the special considerations for testing older adults (31).

- The initial workload should be low (i.e., ≤3 metabolic equivalents [METs] and workload increments should be small (i.e., 0.5–1.0 MET) for those with low work capacities. The Naughton treadmill protocol is a good example of such a protocol (See Table 5.3).
- A cycle ergometer may be preferable to a treadmill for those with poor balance, poor neuromuscular coordination, impaired vision, impaired gait patterns, weight-bearing limitations, and/or foot problems. However, local muscle fatigue may be a factor for premature test termination when using a cycle ergometer.
- Adding a treadmill handrail support may be required because of reduced balance, decreased muscular strength, poor neuromuscular coordination, and fear. However, handrail support for gait abnormalities will reduce the accuracy of estimating peak MET capacity based on the exercise duration or peak workload achieved.
- Treadmill workload may need to be adapted according to walking ability by increasing grade rather than speed.
- For those who have difficulty adjusting to the exercise protocol, the initial stage may need to be extended, the test restarted, or the test repeated. In these situations, also consider an intermittent protocol (Chapter 5).
- Exercise-induced dysrhythmias are more frequent in older adults than in people in other age groups.
- Prescribed medications are common and may influence the electrocardiographic and hemodynamic responses to exercise (Appendix A: Common Medications).
- The exercise electrocardiogram (ECG) has higher sensitivity (i.e., ~84%) and lower specificity (i.e., ~70%) than in younger age groups (i.e., <50% sensitivity and >80% specificity). The higher rate of false-positive outcomes may be related to the greater frequency of left ventricular hypertrophy (LVH) and the presence of conduction disturbances among older than younger adults (17).

There are no specific exercise test termination criteria for older adults beyond those presented for all adults in Chapter 5. The increased prevalence of cardiovascular, metabolic, and orthopedic problems among older adults increases the likelihood of an early test termination. In addition, many older adults exceed the age-predicted HR_{max} during a maximal exercise test.

Exercise Testing for the Oldest Segment of the Population

The oldest segment of the population (≥75 years and individuals with mobility limitations) most likely has one or more chronic medical conditions. The likelihood of physical limitations also increases with age. The approach described above is not applicable for the oldest segment of the population and for individuals with mobility limitations because (a) a prerequisite exercise test may be perceived as a barrier to physical activity promotion; (b) exercise testing is advocated before initiation of vigorous-intensity exercise, but relatively few individuals in the oldest segment of the population are capable or likely to participate in vigorous-intensity exercise, especially upon initiation of an exercise program; (c) the distinction between moderate- and vigorous-intensity exercise among older adults is difficult—e.g., a moderate walking pace for one person may be near the upper limit of capacity for an older, unfit adult with multiple chronic conditions; and (d) there is a paucity of evidence of increased mortality or cardiovascular event risk during exercise or exercise testing in this segment of the population. Therefore, the following recommendations are made for the aging population.

- In lieu of an exercise test, a thorough medical history and physical examination should serve to determine cardiac contraindications to exercise.
- Individuals with CVD symptoms or diagnosed disease can be stratified and treated according to standard guidelines (Chapter 2).
- Individuals free from CVD symptoms and disease should be able to initiate a low-intensity (≤3 METs) exercise program without undue risk (18).

EXERCISE PRESCRIPTION

The general principles of exercise prescription (Chapter 7) apply to adults of all ages. The relative adaptations to exercise and the percentage of improvement in the components of physical fitness among older adults are comparable with those reported in younger adults. Low functional capacity, muscle weakness, and deconditioning are more common in older adults than in any other age group and contribute to loss of independence. An exercise prescription should include aerobic, muscle strengthening, and flexibility exercises. Individuals who are frequent fallers or have mobility problems should also perform specific exercises to improve balance, agility, and proprioceptive training in addition to the other components of health-related physical fitness. However, age should not be a barrier to physical activity promotion because positive improvements are attainable at any age.

For exercise prescription, an important distinction between older adults and their younger counterparts should be made relative to intensity. For apparently healthy adults, moderate- and vigorous-intensity physical activities are defined relative to METs, with moderate-intensity activities defined as 3 to 6 METs and vigorous-intensity activities as <6 METs. In contrast, for older adults, activities should be defined relative to an individual's fitness within the context of perceived physical exertion using a 10-point scale, on which zero is considered an effort equivalent to sitting and 10 is considered an all-out effort, a moderate-intensity activity is defined as 5 or 6, and a vigorous-intensity activity as a 7 or 8. A moderate-intensity activity should produce a noticeable increase in HR and breathing, whereas a vigorous-intensity activity should produce a large increase in HR or breathing (26).

Aerobic Activity

To promote and maintain health, older adults should adhere to the following prescription for aerobic activities. When older adults cannot do these recommended amounts of physical activity because of chronic conditions, they should be as physically active as their abilities and conditions allow.

Frequency: A minimum of 5 $d \cdot wk^{-1}$ for moderate-intensity activities or 3 $d \cdot wk^{-1}$ for vigorous-intensity activities, or some combination of moderate- and vigorous-intensity exercise 3–5 $d \cdot wk^{-1}$.

Intensity: On a scale of 0 to 10 for level of physical exertion, 5 to 6 for moderate intensity, and 7 to 8 for vigorous intensity (26).

Time: For moderate intensity activities, accumulate at least 30 or up to 60 (for greater benefit) min/day in bouts of at least 10 minutes each to total 150–300 min/wk or at least 20–30 min/day of more vigorous-intensity activities to total 75–100 min/wk or an equivalent combination of moderate and vigorous activity.

Type: Any modality that does not impose excessive orthopedic stress; walking is the most common type of activity. Aquatic exercise and stationary-cycle exercise may be advantageous for those with limited tolerance for weight-bearing activity.

Muscle-Strengthening Activity

Frequency: At least 2 $d \cdot wk^{-1}$.

Intensity: Between moderate (5–6) and vigorous (7–8) intensity on a scale of 0 to 10 (26).

Type: Progressive weight-training program or weight-bearing calisthenics (8–10 exercises involving the major muscle groups of 10–15 repetitions each), stair climbing, and other strengthening activities that use the major muscle groups.

Flexibility Activity

Frequency: At least 2 $d \cdot wk^{-1}$.

Intensity: Moderate (5–6) intensity on a scale of 0 to 10 (26).

Type: Any activities that maintain or increase flexibility using sustained stretches for each major muscle group and static rather than ballistic movements.

Balance Exercises for Frequent Fallers or Individuals with Mobility Problems

There are no specific recommendations for exercises that incorporate balance training into an exercise prescription. However, neuromuscular training, which combines balance, agility, and proprioceptive training, is effective in reducing and preventing falls if performed 2–3 $d \cdot wk^{-1}$. General recommendations include using (a) progressively difficult postures that gradually reduce the base of support (e.g., two-legged stand, semitandem stand, tandem stand, and one-legged stand); (b) dynamic movements that perturb the center of gravity (e.g., tandem walk and circle turns); (c) stressing postural muscle groups (e.g., heel stands and toe stands); (d) reducing sensory input (e.g., standing with eyes closed); and (e) tai chi. Supervision of these activities may be warranted (3).

SPECIAL CONSIDERATIONS

There are numerous considerations that should be taken into account to maximize the effective development of an exercise program, including the following.

- Intensity and duration of physical activity should be low at the beginning in particular for older adults who are highly deconditioned, functionally limited, or have chronic conditions that affect their ability to perform physical tasks.
- Progression of activities should be individualized and tailored to tolerance and preference; a conservative approach may be necessary for the most deconditioned and physically limited older adults.
- For strength training involving use of weight-lifting machines, initial training sessions should be supervised and monitored by personnel who are sensitive to the special needs of older adults (Chapter 7).
- In the early stages of an exercise program, muscle-strengthening activities may need to precede aerobic-training activities among very frail individuals.
- Older adults should gradually exceed the recommended minimum amounts of physical activity and attempt continued progression if they desire to improve their fitness.
- If chronic conditions preclude activity at the recommended minimum amount, older adults should perform physical activities as tolerated so as to avoid being sedentary.
- Older adults should consider exceeding the recommended minimum amounts of physical activity to improve management of chronic conditions for which a higher level of physical activity is known to confer a therapeutic benefit.
- Incorporation of behavioral strategies, such as social support, self-efficacy, the ability to make healthy choices, and perceived safety, all may enhance participation in a regular exercise program.
- The health/fitness professional should also provide regular feedback, positive reinforcement, and other behavioral/programmatic strategies to enhance adherence.

In summary, all older adults should be guided in the development of a personalized exercise or physical activity plan that meets their needs and personal preferences.

ENVIRONMENTAL CONSIDERATIONS

EXERCISE IN HOT ENVIRONMENTS

Active muscles not only generate metabolic heat, but also stimulate sweat glands to secrete water and electrolytes onto the skin. Concurrently, the smooth muscle within skin blood vessels dilates, increasing blood flow to the skin. The evaporation of sweat cools the skin, and skin blood flow carries heat from the body's core to the air. When the amount of metabolic heat exceeds heat loss, hyper-thermia (i e , elevated internal body temperature) may develop. The cardiovas-cular system is essential for temperature regulation. Acclimatized individuals are most successful in regulating body heat.

Counteracting Dehydration

Dehydration to between 3% and 5% loss of body weight may be tolerated without a loss of maximal strength. However, sustained or repeated exercise that lasts longer than a few minutes deteriorates when moderate to severe dehydration exists (i.e., loss of ≥6% of body weight). The greater the dehydration, the greater the aerobic exercise performance decrement. Acute dehydration degrades endurance performance, regardless of whole-body hyperthermia or environmen-tal temperature; and endurance capacity (i.e., time to exhaustion) is reduced more in a hot environment than in a temperate or cold one. The simplest way to main-tain normal hydration status is to measure body weight before and after exercise. Sweat rate ($L \cdot h^{-1}$ or $q \cdot h^{-1}$) provides a fluid replacement guide. Active individ-uals should drink at least 1 pint of fluid for each pound of body weight lost. See the ACSM position stand on fluid replacement (2) for additional information.

Medical Considerations: Exertional Heat Illnesses

Heat illnesses range from muscle cramps to life-threatening hyperthermia and are described in Table 8.4. Dehydration may be either a direct (i.e., heat exhaus-tion and heat cramps) or indirect (i.e., heatstroke) factor in heat illness (6,8).

Heat exhaustion is the most common form of heat illness. It is defined as the inability to continue exercise in the heat and is characterized by prominent fatigue and progressive weakness without severe hyperthermia. Oral fluids are preferred for rehydration in patients who are conscious, able to swallow, and not losing fluid (i.e., vomiting or diarrhea). Intravenous fluid administration facilitates recovery in those unable to ingest oral fluids or who have severe dehydration.

Exertional heatstroke is caused by hyperthermia (i.e., a core temperature eleva-tion of >40°C, >104°F) and is associated with central nervous system distur-bances and multiple organ system failure. It is a life-threatening medical emergency that requires immediate and effective whole-body cooling with cold-water and ice-water immersion therapy. The greatest risk for heatstroke exists during high-intensity exercise when the ambient wet bulb globe temperature (WBGT) exceeds 28°C (82°F). Inadequate physical fitness, excess adiposity, improper clothing, protec-tive pads, incomplete heat acclimatization, illness, or medications also increase risk.

Heat cramps usually occur in large abdominal or limb muscles during participa-tion in the sports of American football, tennis, or distance running. Muscle fatigue, water loss, and significant sweat sodium are contributing factors. Heat cramps respond well to rest, prolonged stretching, dietary sodium chloride (i.e., one-eighth to one-fourth teaspoon of table salt or one to two salt tablets added to 300–500 mL of fluid, bullion broth, or salty snacks), or intravenous normal saline fluid.

Heat syncope occurs more often among unfit, sedentary, and nonacclimatized individuals. It is caused by standing erect for a long period of time or at the ces-sation of strenuous, prolonged, upright exercise because maximal cutaneous ves-

TABLE 8.4. A COMPARISON OF THE SIGNS AND SYMPTOMS OF
ILLNESSES THAT OCCUR IN HOT ENVIRONMENTS

DISORDER	PROMINENT SIGNS AND SYMPTOMS	MENTAL STATUS CHANGES	CORE TEMPERATURE ELEVATION
Exertional heatstroke	Disorientation, dizziness, irrational behavior, apathy, headache, nausea, vomiting, hyperventilation, wet skin	Marked (disoriented, unresponsive)	Marked (>40.0°C)
Exertional heat exhaustion	Low blood pressure, elevated heart and respiratory rates, wet and pale skin, headache, weakness, dizziness, decreased muscle coordination, chills, nausea, vomiting, diarrhea	Little or none, agitated	None to moderate (37°C–40°C)
Heat syncope	Heart rate and breathing rates slow; pale skin; patient may experience sensations of weakness, tunnel vision, vertigo, or nausea before syncope	Brief fainting episode	Little or none
Exertional heat cramps	Begins as feeble, localized, wandering spasms that may progress to debilitating cramps	None	Moderate (37°C–40°C)

Adapted from American College of Sports Medicine Position Stand. Exertional heat illness during training and competition. *Med Sci Sports Exerc.* (2007; 39(3):556–572) and Armstrong LE. Heat and humidity. In: *Performing in Extreme Environments.* Champaign (IL): Human Kinetics Publishers; 2000. p. 15–70.

sel dilation results in a decline of blood pressure (BP) and insufficient oxygen delivery to the brain. See the ACSM position stand on heat illness during exercise for additional information (4).

Exercise Prescription

Health/fitness professionals and clinicians may use standards established by National Institute for Occupational Safety and Health (NIOSH) to define WBGT levels at which the risk of heat injury is increased, but exercise may be performed if preventive steps are taken (25). These steps include required rest breaks between exercise periods.

Individuals whose exercise prescription specifies a target heart rate (THR) should maintain the same exercise HR in the heat. This approach reduces the risk of heat illness during acclimatization. For example, in hot or humid weather, reduced speed or resistance will achieve the THR. As heat acclimatization develops, a progressively higher exercise intensity will be required to elicit the THR. The first exercise session in the heat may last as little as 10 to 15 minutes for safety reasons but can be increased gradually.

Developing a Personalized Plan

Adults and children who are adequately rested, nourished, hydrated, and acclimatized to heat are at less risk for exertional heat illnesses. The following factors should be considered when developing an individualized plan to minimize the effects of hyperthermia and dehydration along with the questions in Box 8.2 (6).

BOX 8.2 | **Questions to Evaluate Readiness to Exercise in a Hot Environment**

Adults should ask the following questions to evaluate readiness to exercise in a hot environment. Corrective action should be taken if any question is answered "no."

1. Have I developed a plan to avoid dehydration and hyperthermia?
2. Have I acclimatized by gradually increasing exercise duration and intensity for 10 to 14 days?
3. Do I limit intense exercise to the cooler hours of the day (early morning)?
4. Do I avoid lengthy warm-up periods on hot/humid days?
5. When training outdoors, do I know where fluids are available, or do I carry water bottles in a belt or backpack?
6. Do I know my sweat rate and the amount of fluid that I should drink to replace body-weight loss?
7. Was my body weight this morning within 1% of my average body weight?
8. Is my 24-hour urine volume plentiful?
9. Is my urine color pale yellow or straw colored?
10. When heat and humidity are high, do I reduce my expectations, my exercise pace, the distance, and/or the duration of my workout or race?
11. Do I wear loose-fitting, porous, lightweight clothing?
12. Do I know the signs and symptoms of heat exhaustion, exertional heatstroke, heat syncope, and heat cramps (Table 8.4)?
13. Do I exercise with a partner and provide feedback about his/her physical appearance?
14. Do I consume adequate salt in my diet?
15. Do I avoid or reduce exercise in the heat if I experience sleep loss, infectious illness, fever, diarrhea, vomiting, carbohydrate depletion, some medications, alcohol, or drug abuse?

Adapted from Armstrong LE. Heat and humidity. In: *Performing in Extreme Environments*. Champaign (IL): Human Kinetics Publishers; 2000: p. 15–70.

Monitor the environment: Use the WBGT index to determine appropriate action.

Modify activity in extreme environments: Enable access to ample fluid, provide longer and/or more rest breaks to facilitate heat dissipation, and shorten or delay playing times. Consider heat acclimatization status, fitness, nutrition, sleep deprivation, and age of participants; intensity, duration, and time of day for exercise; availability of fluids; and playing-surface heat reflection (i.e., grass versus asphalt). Allow at least 3 hours, and preferably 6 hours, of recovery and rehydration time between exercise sessions.

Heat acclimatization: Increase exercise heat stress gradually across 10 to 14 days to stimulate adaptations to warmer ambient temperatures. These adaptations include decreased rectal temperature, HR, RPE, increased exercise tolerance time, increased sweating rate, and a reduction in sweat salt. Acclimatization results in (a) improved heat transfer from the body's core to the external environment; (b) improved cardiovascular function; (c) more effective sweating; and (d) improved exercise performance and heat tolerance.

Clothing: Clothes that have a high wicking capacity may assist in evaporative heat loss. Athletes should remove as much clothing and equipment (especially head gear) as possible to permit heat loss and reduce the risks of hyperthermia, especially during the initial days of acclimatization.

Education: The training of participants, personal trainers, coaches, and community emergency-response teams enhances the reduction, recognition (Table 8.4), and treatment of heat-related illness. Such programs should emphasize the importance of recognizing signs/symptoms of heat intolerance, being hydrated, fed, rested, and acclimatized to heat.

Organizational Planning

When clients exercise in hot/humid conditions, fitness facilities and organizations should formulate a standardized heat-stress management plan that incorporates the following considerations.

- Screening and surveillance of at-risk participants
- Environmental assessment (i.e., WBGT index) and criteria for modifying or canceling exercise
- Heat acclimatization procedures
- Easy access to fluids
- *Optimized but not maximized* fluid intake that (a) matches the volume of fluid consumed to the volume of sweat lost and (b) limits body weight change to <2% of body weight
- Awareness of the signs and symptoms of heatstroke, heat exhaustion, heat cramps, and heat syncope (Table 8.4)
- Implementation of specific emergency procedures

EXERCISE IN COLD ENVIRONMENTS

People exercise and work in many cold-weather environments (i.e., low temperature, high winds, low solar radiation, and rain/water exposure). For the most part, cold weather is not a barrier to performing physical activity. Many factors—including the environment, clothing, body composition, health status, nutrition, age, and exercise intensity—interact to determine if exercising in the cold elicits additional physiologic strain and injury risk beyond that associated with the same exercise done under temperate conditions. In most cases, exercise in the cold does not increase strain or injury risk. However, there are scenarios (i.e., immersion, rain, and low ambient temperature with wind) in which whole-body or local thermal balance cannot be maintained during exercise-cold stress and that contribute to hypothermia, frostbite, and diminished exercise capability and performance. Furthermore, exercise-cold stress may increase the risk of morbidity and mortality in at risk populations, such as those with ischemic heart disease and asthmatic conditions. Inhalation of cold air may also exacerbate these conditions.

Hypothermia develops when heat loss exceeds heat production, causing the body heat content to decrease (29). The environment, individual characteristics, and clothing all affect the development of hypothermia. Some specific factors that increase the risk of developing hypothermia include immersion, rain, wet clothing, low body fat, older age (i.e., ≥60 years), and hypoglycemia (5).

Medical Considerations: Cold Injuries

Frostbite occurs when tissue temperatures fall below 0°C (32°F) (10,23). Frostbite is most common in exposed skin (i.e., nose, ears, cheeks, and exposed wrists) but also occurs in the hands and feet. Contact frostbite may occur by touching cold objects with bare skin, particularly highly conductive metal or stone, which causes rapid heat loss.

The principal cold-stress determinants for frostbite are air temperature, wind speed, and wetness. Wind exacerbates heat loss by facilitating convective heat loss and reduces the insulative value of clothing. The wind chill temperature index (WCT) (Fig. 8.2) integrates wind speed and air temperature to provide an estimate of the cooling power of the environment. WCT is specific in its correct application and only estimates the danger of cooling for the exposed skin of persons walking at $1.3 \text{ m} \cdot \text{s}^{-1}$ ($3 \text{ mi} \cdot \text{h}^{-1}$). The following considerations include important information about wind and the WCT.

- Wind does not cause an exposed object to become cooler than the ambient temperature.
- Wind speeds obtained from weather reports do not take into account man-made wind (e.g., running and skiing).
- The WCT presents the relative risk of frostbite and predicted times to freezing (Fig. 8.2) of exposed facial skin. Facial skin was chosen because this area of the body is typically not protected.
- Frostbite cannot occur if the air temperature is above 0°C (32°F).
- Wet skin exposed to the wind cools faster. If the skin is wet and exposed to wind, the ambient temperature used for the WCT table should be 10°C lower than the actual ambient temperature (9).
- The risk of frostbite is <5% when the ambient temperature is above −15°C (5°F), but increased safety surveillance of exercisers is warranted when the WCT falls below −27°C (−8°F). In those conditions, frostbite can occur in 30 minutes or less in exposed skin (5).

Wind Speed (mph)   **Air Temperature (°F)**

	40	35	30	25	20	15	10	5	0	-5	-10	-15	-20	-25	-30	-35	-40	-45
5	36	31	25	19	13	7	1	-5	-11	-16	-22	-28	-34	-40	-46	-52	-57	-63
10	34	27	21	15	9	3	-4	-10	-16	-22	-28	-35	-41	-47	-53	-59	-66	-72
15	32	25	19	13	6	0	-7	-13	-19	-26	-32	-39	-45	-51	-58	-64	-71	-77
20	30	24	17	11	4	-2	-9	-15	-22	-29	-35	-42	-48	-55	-61	-68	-74	-81
25	29	23	16	9	3	-4	-11	-17	-24	-31	-37	-44	-51	-58	-64	-71	-78	-84
30	28	22	15	8	1	-5	-12	-19	-26	-33	-39	-46	-53	-60	-67	-73	-80	-87
35	28	21	14	7	0	-7	-14	-21	-27	-34	-41	-48	-55	-62	-69	-76	-82	-89
40	27	20	13	6	-1	-8	-15	-22	-29	-36	-43	-50	-57	-64	-71	-78	-84	-91
45	26	19	12	5	-2	-9	-16	-23	-30	-37	-44	-51	-58	-65	-72	-79	-86	-93
50	26	19	12	4	-3	-10	-17	-24	-31	-38	-45	-52	-60	-67	-74	-81	-88	-95
55	25	18	11	4	-3	-11	-18	-25	-32	-39	-46	-54	-61	-68	-75	-82	-89	-97
60	25	17	10	3	-4	-11	-19	-26	-33	-40	-48	-55	-62	-69	-76	-84	-91	-98

Frostbite Times
☐ Frostbite could occur in 30 min
☐ Frostbite could occur in 10 min
■ Frostbite could occur in 5 min

FIGURE 8.2. Wind chill temperature index in Fahrenheit and frostbite times for exposed facial skin. The Wind Chill Top chart is from the U.S. National Weather Service; the Frostbite Times bottom chart is from the Meteorological Society of Canada/Environment Canada.

Clothing Considerations

Cold-weather clothing protects against hypothermia and frostbite by reducing heat loss through the insulation provided by the clothing and the trapped air within and between clothing layers (5). Typical cold-weather clothing consists of three layers: (a) an inner layer (i.e., lightweight polyester or polypropylene); (b) a middle layer (i.e., polyester fleece or wool), which provides the primary insulation; and (c) an outer layer designed to allow moisture transfer to the air while repelling wind and rain. Recommendations for clothing wear include the following considerations (5).

• Adjust clothing insulation to minimize sweating.
• Use clothing vents to reduce sweat accumulation.
• Do not wear an outer layer unless it is rainy or very windy.
• Reduce clothing insulation as exercise intensity increases.
• Do not impose a single clothing standard on an entire group of exercisers.

Exercise Prescription

Whole-body and facial cooling theoretically lower the threshold for the onset of angina during aerobic exercise. The type and intensity of exercise-cold stress also modifies the risk for the patient with cardiac disease. Activities that involve the upper body or increase metabolism potentially increase risk.

• Shoveling snow raises the HR to 97% HR_{max} and SBP (systolic blood pressure) increases to 200 mm Hg (15).

- Walking in snow that is either packed or soft significantly increases energy requirements and myocardial oxygen demands so that patients with atherosclerotic CVD may have to slow their walking pace.
- Swimming in water colder than 25°C (77°F) may be a threat to patients with CVD because they may not be able to recognize angina symptoms and therefore may place themselves at greater risk (5).

EXERCISE IN HIGH-ALTITUDE ENVIRONMENTS

The progressive decrease in atmospheric pressure associated with ascent to higher altitudes reduces the partial pressure of oxygen in the inspired air, resulting in decreased arterial oxygen levels. Immediate compensatory responses include increased ventilation and cardiac output ($\dot{Q}$), the latter usually through elevated HR (22). For most individuals, the effects of altitude appear at and above 5,000 feet (1,524 m). In this section, *low altitude* refers to locations below 5,000 feet (1,524 m), *moderate altitude* to locations between 5,000 and 8,000 feet (1,524–2,438 m), *high altitude* between 8,000 and 14,000 feet (2,438–4,267 m), and *very high altitude* above 14,000 feet (4,267 m).

Physical performance decreases with increasing altitude above 5,000 feet (1,524 m). In general, the physical performance decrement will be greater as elevation, activity duration, and muscle mass increases, but is lessened with altitude acclimatization. The most common altitude effect on physical-task performance is an increased time for task completion or more frequent rest breaks. With exposure of 1 week or more, altitude acclimatization occurs. The time to complete a task is improved but the time remains longer relative to sea level. The estimated percentage increases in performance time to complete tasks of various durations during initial altitude exposure and after 1 week of altitude acclimatization are given in Table 8.5 (16).

Medical Considerations: Altitude Illnesses

Rapid ascent to high and very high altitude increases individual susceptibility to altitude illness. The primary altitude illnesses are acute mountain sickness (AMS), high-altitude pulmonary edema (HAPE), and high-altitude cerebral edema (HACE). Additionally, many individuals develop a sore throat and bron-

TABLE 8.5. ESTIMATED IMPACT OF INCREASING ALTITUDE ON TIME TO COMPLETE PHYSICAL TASKS AT HIGHER ALTITUDES

	% INCREASE IN TIME TO COMPLETE PHYSICAL TASKS RELATIVE TO SEA LEVEL							
	TASKS <2 MIN		TASKS 2–5 MIN		TASKS 10–30 MIN		TASKS >3 H	
ALTITUDE	INITIAL	>1 WK	INITIAL	>1 WK	INITIAL	>1 WK	INITIAL	>1 WK
Moderate	0	0	2–7	0–2	4–11	1–3	7–18	3–10
High	0–2	0	12–18	5–9	20–45	9–20	40–65	20–45
Very high	2	0	50	25	90	60	200	90

Adapted from Fulco CS, Rock PB, Cymerman A. Maximal and submaximal exercise performance at altitude. *Aviat Space Environ Med.* 1998;69:793–801.

chitis that may produce disabling, severe coughing spasms at high altitudes. Susceptibility to altitude sickness is increased in individuals with a prior history and by prolonged physical exertion early in the altitude exposure.

AMS is the most common form of altitude sickness. AMS is short-lived (i.e., 2–7 days). Symptoms include headache, nausea, fatigue, decreased appetite, and poor sleep, and, in severe cases, poor balance and mild swelling in the hands, feet, or face. AMS develops within the first 24 hours of altitude exposure. Its incidence and severity increases in direct proportion to ascent rate and altitude. The estimated incidence of AMS in unacclimatized individuals rapidly ascending directly to moderate altitudes is 0% to 20%; to high altitudes, 20% to 60%; and to very high altitudes, 50% to 80% (30).

HAPE is a potentially fatal—although not common—illness that occurs in <10% of persons ascending above 12,000 feet (3,658 m). Individuals making repeated ascents and descents above 12,000 ft (3,658 m) and who exercise strenuously early in the exposure have an increased susceptibility to HAPE. The presence of crackles and rales in the lungs may indicate increased susceptibility to developing HAPE. Blue lips and nail beds may be present with HAPE.

HACE is a potentially fatal—although not common—illness that occurs in <2% of persons ascending above 12,000 ft (3,658 m). HACE is an exacerbation of unresolved, severe AMS and most often occurs in people who have AMS symptoms and continue to ascend.

Prevention and Treatment of Altitude Sickness

Altitude acclimatization is the best countermeasure to all altitude sickness. Minimizing sustained physical activity and maintaining adequate hydration and food intake will reduce susceptibility to altitude sickness and facilitate recovery. When moderate to severe symptoms and signs of an altitude-related sickness develop, the preferred treatment is to descend to a lower altitude. Descents of 1,000 to 3,000 feet (305–914 m) with an overnight stay are effective in prevention and recovery of all altitude sickness.

AMS may be significantly diminished or prevented with prophylactic or therapeutic use of acetazolamide (i.e., Diamox). Headaches may be treated with aspirin, acetaminophen, ibuprofen, indomethacin, or naproxen. Oxygen or hyperbaric chamber therapy will usually relieve some symptoms, such as headache, fatigue, and poor sleep. Prochlorperazine may be used to help relieve nausea and vomiting. Dexamethasone may be used if other treatments are not available or effective (19). Treatment of individuals with diagnosed HAPE includes descent, oxygen therapy, and/or hyperbaric bag therapy. Acetazolamide may be helpful (19). Treatment of individuals diagnosed with HACE includes descent, oxygen therapy, and/or hyperbaric bag therapy. Dexamethasone and acetazolamide are also helpful.

Altitude Acclimatization

Altitude acclimatization allows individuals to achieve maximum physical and cognitive performance for the altitude to which they are acclimatized and decreases their susceptibility to altitude sickness. Altitude acclimatization consists of physiologic adaptations that develop in a time-dependent manner during continuous or repeated exposures to moderate or high altitudes. At least partial altitude acclimatization can develop by living at a moderate elevation, termed *staging*, before ascending to a higher target elevation. The goal of staged ascents is to gradually promote development of altitude acclimatization while averting the adverse consequences (e.g., altitude sickness) of rapid ascent to high altitudes.

For individuals ascending from low altitude, the first stage of all staged ascent protocols should be 3 days or more of residence at moderate altitude. At this altitude, individuals will experience small decrements in physical performance and a low incidence of altitude sickness. At any given altitude, almost all of the acclimatization response is attained between 7 and 12 days of residence at that altitude. Short stays of 3 to 7 days at moderate altitudes will decrease susceptibility to altitude sickness at higher altitudes. Longer stays of 9 to 12 days are required to improve physical work performance. The magnitude of the acclimatization response is increased with additional higher staging elevations. The final staging elevation should be as close as possible to the target elevation.

The general staging guideline to follow is: For every day spent above 5,000 feet (1,524 m), an individual is prepared for a subsequent rapid ascent to a higher altitude equal to the number of days at that altitude times 1,000 feet (305 m). For example, if a person stages at 6,000 feet (1,829 m) for 5 days, physical performance will be improved and altitude sickness will be reduced at altitudes to 11,000 feet (3,353 m). This guideline applies to altitudes to 14,000 feet (4,267 m).

Assessing Individual Altitude Acclimatization Status

The best indices of altitude acclimatization are absence of altitude sickness, improved physical performance, and a progressive increase in arterial oxygen saturation (SaO_2). The presence and severity of AMS may be evaluated by the extent of symptoms (i.e., headache, nausea, fatigue, decreased appetite, and poor sleep) and signs (i.e., poor balance and mild swelling in the hands, feet, or face) of AMS. The absence of AMS or its uncomplicated resolution in the first 3 to 4 days following ascent indicates a normal acclimatization response. Submaximal physical performance improves with 1 to 2 weeks of altitude acclimatization. Ability to exercise and work for longer periods of time at a given altitude also improves with acclimatization. An early sign of appropriate adaptation to high altitude is increased urine volume, which generally occurs during the first several days at a given high altitude. Urine volume will continue to increase with additional ascent and decrease with subsequent adaptation.

Measurement of SaO_2 by noninvasive pulse oximetry is a very good indicator of acclimatization. Pulse oximetry should be done under resting conditions. From its nadir on the first day at a given altitude, SaO_2 will progressively increase over the first 3 to 7 days before stabilizing.

Exercise Prescription

During the first few days at high altitudes, individuals should minimize their physical activity to reduce susceptibility to altitude illness. After this period, individuals whose exercise prescription specifies a THR should maintain the same exercise HR at higher altitudes. This approach reduces the risk of altitude illness and excessive physiologic strain. For example, at high altitudes, reduced speed, distance, or resistance will achieve the same THR as at lower altitudes. As altitude acclimatization develops, the THR will be achieved at progressively higher exercise intensity.

Developing a Personalized Plan

Adults and children who are acclimatized to altitude, adequately rested, nourished, and hydrated minimize their risk for developing altitude sickness and maximize their physical performance capabilities for the altitude to which they are acclimatized. The following factors should be considered to further minimize the effects of high altitude.

- **Monitor the environment:** High altitude regions usually are associated with more daily extremes of temperature, humidity, wind, and solar radiation. Follow appropriate guidelines for hot (2) and cold (5) environments.
- **Modify activity at high altitudes:** Consider altitude acclimatization status, fitness, nutrition, sleep quality and quantity, age, exercise duration and intensity, and availability of fluids. Provide longer and/or more rest breaks to facilitate rest and recovery and shorten activity times. Longer-duration activities are affected more by high altitude than shorter-duration activities.
- **Develop an altitude acclimatization plan:** Monitor progress.
- **Clothing:** Individual clothing and equipment need to provide protection over a greater range of temperature and wind conditions.
- **Education:** The training of participants, personal trainers, coaches, and community emergency-response teams enhances the reduction, recognition, and treatment of altitude-related illnesses.

Organizational Planning

When clients exercise in high-altitude locations, fitness facilities and organizations should formulate a standardized management plan that includes the following procedures.

- Screening and surveillance of at-risk participants
- Utilization of altitude acclimatization procedures to minimize the risk of altitude sickness and enhance physical performance
- Consideration of the hazards of mountainous terrain when designing exercise programs and activities
- Awareness of the signs and symptoms of altitude illness
- Develop organizational procedures for emergency medical care of altitude illnesses

REFERENCES

1. American College of Obstetricians and Gynecologists. Exercise during pregnancy and the postpartum period. ACOG Committee Opinion No. 267. *Obstet Gynecol.* 2002;99:171–3.
2. American College of Sports Medicine Position Stand. Exercise and fluid replacement. *Med Sci Sports Exerc.* 2007;39(2):377–90.

3. American College of Sports Medicine Position Stand. Exercise and physical activity for older adults. *Med Sci Sports Exerc.* 1998;30(6):992–1008.

4. American College of Sports Medicine Position Stand. Exertional heat illness during training and competition. *Med Sci Sports Exerc.* 2007;39(3):556–72.

5. American College of Sports Medicine Position Stand. Prevention of cold injuries during exercise. *Med Sci Sports Exerc.* 2006;38:2012–29.

6. Armstrong LE. Heat and humidity. In: *Performing in Extreme Environments.* Champaign (IL): Human Kinetics Publishers; 2000. p. 15–70.

7. Artal R, O'Toole M. Guidelines of the American College of Obstetricians and Gynecologists for exercise during pregnancy and the postpartum period. *Br J Sports Med.* 2003;37:6–12.

8. Binkley HM, Beckett JDJ, Casa D, Kleiner M, Plummer PE. National Athletic Trainer's Association Position Statement: Exertional heat illnesses. *J Athl Train.* 2002;37:329–43.

9. Brajkovic D, Ducharme MB. Facial cold-induced vasodilatation and skin temperature during exposure to cold wind. *Eur J Appl Physiol.* 2006;96:711–21.

10. Danielsson U. Windchill and the risk of tissue freezing. *J Appl Physiol.* 1996;81:2666–73.

11. Davies GA, Wolfe LA, Mottola MF, MacKinnon C. Society of Obstetricians and Gynecologists of Canada, SOGC Clinical Practice Obstetrics Committee. Joint SOGC/CSEP Clinical Practice Guideline: Exercise in pregnancy and the postpartum period. *Can J Appl Physiol.* 2003;28:330–41.

12. Dempsey FC, Butler FL, Williams FA. No need for a pregnant pause: physical activity may reduce the occurrence of gestational diabetes mellitus and preeclampsia. *Exerc Sports Sci Rev.* 2005;33: 141–9.

13. Federal Interagency Forum on Aging-Related Statistics. *Older Americans 2004: Key Indicators of Well-Being.* Washington (DC): U.S. Government Printing Office, 2004.

14. Fiatarone Singh MA. Exercise comes of age: rationale and recommendations for a geriatric exercise prescription. *J Gerontol A Biol Sci Med Sci.* 2002;57:M262–82.

15. Franklin BA, Hogan P, Bonzheim K, Bakalyar D, Terrien E, Gordon S, Timmis GC. Cardiac demands of heavy snow shoveling. *JAMA.* 1995;273:880–2.

16. Fulco CS, Rock PB, Cymerman A. Maximal and submaximal exercise performance at altitude. *Aviat Space Environ Med.* 1998;69:793–801.

17. Gibbons RJ, Balady GJ, Bricker JT, et al. ACC/AHA 2002 guideline update for exercise testing: a report of the American College of Cardiology/American Heart Association Task Force on Practice Guidelines. *Circulation.* 2002;106:1883–92.

18. Gill TM, DiPietro L, Krumholtz HM. Role of exercise stress testing and safety monitoring for older persons starting an exercise program. *JAMA.* 2000;284:342–9.

19. Hackett PH, Roach RC. High-altitude illness. *N Engl J Med.* 2001;345:107–14.

20. Hebestreit HU, Bar-Or O. Differences between children and adults for exercise testing and prescription. In: Skinner JS, editor. *Exercise Testing and Exercise Prescription for Special Cases.* Philadelphia (PA): Lippincott Williams & Wilkins; 2005. p. 68–84.

21. Institute for Aerobics Research. *The Prudential FITNESSGRAM Test Administration Manual.* Dallas (TX): Institute for Aerobics Research; 1994.

22. Mazzeo RS, Fulco CS. Physiological systems and their responses to conditions of hypoxia. In: Tipton CM, Sawka MN, Tate CA, Terjung RL, editors. *ACSM's Advanced Exercise Physiology.* Baltimore (MD): Lippincott Williams & Williams; 2006. p. 564–80.

23. Molnar GW, Hughes AL, Wilson O, Goldman RF. Effect of skin wetting on finger cooling and freezing. *J Appl Physiol.* 1973;205–7.

24. Mottola MF, Davenport MH, Brun CR, Inglis SD, Charlesworth S, Sopper MM. VO_{2max} prediction and exercise prescription for pregnant women. *Med Sci Sports Exerc.* 2006;38:1389–95.

25. National Institute for Occupational Safety and Health. *Working in Hot Environments.* Washington (DC): U.S. Department of Health and Human Services; 1992.

26. Nelson ME, Rejeski WJ, Blair SN, et al. Physical activity and public health in older adults: recommendations from the American College of Sport Medicine. *Med Sci Sports Exerc.* 2007;39(8):1435–45.

27. Paridon SM, Alpert BS, Boas SR, et al. Clinical stress testing in the pediatric age group: a statement from the American Heart Association Council on Cardiovascular Disease in the Young, Committee on Atherosclerosis, Hypertension, and Obesity in Youth. *Circulation* 2006;113:1905–20.

28. Pivarnik JM, Chambliss HO, Clapp JF, et al. Impact of physical activity during pregnancy and postpartum on chronic disease risk. *Med Sci Sports Exerc.* 2006;38:989–1006.

29. Pozos RS, Danzl DF. Human physiological responses to cold stress and hypothermia. In: Pandolf KB, Burr RE, editors. *Textbooks of Military Medicine: Medical Aspects of Harsh Environments,* vol. 1. Falls Church (VA): Office of the Surgeon General, U.S. Army; 2002. p. 351–82.

30. Roach RC, Stepanek J, Hackett PH. Acute mountain sickness and high-altitude cerebral edema. In: Lounsbury DE, Bellamy RF, Zajtchuk R, editors. *Medical Aspects of Harsh Environments*. Washington (DC): Office of the Surgeon General, Borden Institute; 2002. p. 765–93.

31. Skinner JS. Aging for exercise testing and prescription. In: Skinner JS, editor. *Exercise Testing and Exercise Prescription for Special Cases*. 2nd ed. Philadelphia (PA): Lippincott Williams & Wilkins; 2005. p. 85–99.

32. Strong WB, Malina RM, Blimke CJR, et al. Evidence based physical activity for school-age youth. *J Pediatrics*. 2005;146:732–7.

33. U.S. Department of Health and Human Services. Physical activity and health: a report of the Surgeon General. Atlanta (GA): U.S. Department of Health and Human Services, Centers for Disease Control and Prevention, and National Center for Chronic Disease Prevention and Health Promotion; 1996.

34. Wolfe LA. Differences between children and adults for exercise testing and prescription. In: Skinner JS, editor. *Exercise Testing and Exercise Prescription for Special Cases*. 2nd ed. Philadelphia (PA): Lippincott Williams & Wilkins; 2005. p. 377–91.

Exercise Prescription for Patients with Cardiac Disease

The intent of this chapter is to describe the process for developing an exercise prescription for people with cardiovascular disease (see Box 9.1 for definitions of atherosclerotic cardiovascular disease [CVD]). Specifically, this chapter will focus on (a) the structure of inpatient and outpatient cardiac rehabilitation programs; (b) procedures to design a safe and effective exercise prescription for those who have and have not had an exercise test; (c) resistance-training guidelines; and (d) procedures to prepare for returning to work.

INPATIENT REHABILITATION PROGRAMS

Following a documented physician referral, patients hospitalized after a cardiac event or a procedure associated with coronary artery disease (CAD), cardiac valve replacement, or myocardial infarction (MI) should be provided with a program consisting of early assessment and mobilization, identification of and education regarding CVD risk factors, assessment of the patient's level of readiness for physical activity, and comprehensive discharge planning (1). The goals for inpatient rehabilitation programs are as follows:

- Offset the deleterious physiologic and psychological effects of bed rest.
- Provide additional medical surveillance of patients.
- Identify patients with significant cardiovascular, physical, or cognitive impairments that may influence prognosis.
- Enable patients to safely return to activities of daily living within limits imposed by their CVD.
- Prepare the patient and support system at home or in a transitional setting to optimize recovery following acute-care hospital discharge.
- Facilitate patient entry, including physician referral into an outpatient cardiac rehabilitation program.

Before beginning formal physical activity in the inpatient setting, a baseline assessment should be conducted by a healthcare provider who possesses the skills and competencies necessary to assess and document heart and lung sounds, peripheral pulses, and musculoskeletal strength and flexibility (2).

207

BOX 9.1	Manifestations of Atherosclerotic Cardiovascular Disease

- Acute coronary syndromes (ACS)—the manifestation of coronary artery disease (CAD) as angina pectoris, myocardial infarction (MI), or sudden death
- Cardiovascular disease (CVD)—atherosclerotic disease of the arteries of the heart, brain (i.e., stroke), and peripheral vasculature (i.e., peripheral artery disease [PAD])
- Coronary artery disease (CAD)—atherosclerotic disease of the arteries of the heart
- Myocardial ischemia—lack of coronary blood flow with resultant lack of oxygen supply often manifested as angina pectoris
- Myocardial infarction (MI)—death of the muscular tissue of the heart

Initiation and progression of physical activity depends on the findings of the initial assessment and varies with level of risk. Thus, inpatients should be risk stratified as early as possible following their acute cardiac event. The American College of Sports Medicine (ACSM) has found that the American Association of Cardiovascular and Pulmonary Rehabilitation (AACVPR) risk stratification of patients with known CVD is useful because it is based on overall prognosis of the patient potential for rehabilitation (3). The ACSM has adopted this risk stratification for patients with CVD (see Box 2.3).

The indications and contraindications for inpatient and outpatient cardiac rehabilitation are listed in Box 9.2. Exceptions should be considered based on the clinical judgment of the physician and the rehabilitation team. Decreasing length of hospital stay after the acute event or intervention has made the traditional program of multiple rehabilitation steps obsolete, as many uncomplicated patients are seen for only 3 to 4 days before discharge. Activities during the first 48 hours after MI or cardiac surgery should be restricted to self-care activities, arm and leg range of motion, and postural change (4). Simple exposure to orthostatic or gravitational stress, such as intermittent sitting or standing during hospital convalescence, reduces much of the deterioration in exercise performance that generally follows an acute cardiac event (16,17). Patients may progress from self-care activities, to walking short to moderate distances of 50 to 500 feet (15–152 m) with minimal or no assistance 3–4 times $\cdot$ d^{-1}, to independent ambulation on the hospital unit. The optimal dosage of exercise for inpatients depends in part on their medical history, clinical status, and symptoms. The rating of perceived exertion (RPE) provides a useful and complementary guide to heart rate (HR) to gauge exercise intensity (Chapter 7). In general, the criteria for terminating an inpatient exercise session are similar to or slightly more conservative than those for terminating a low-level exercise test (Box 9.3) (2).

Recommendations for inpatient exercise programming include the Frequency, Intensity, Time, and Type of Exercise (FITT) framework as well as progression. Activity goals should be built into the overall plan of care (5). The exercise

BOX 9.2	Clinical Indications and Contraindications for Inpatient and Outpatient Cardiac Rehabilitation

INDICATIONS
- Medically stable post–myocardial infarction (MI)
- Stable angina
- Coronary artery bypass graft surgery (CABG)
- Percutaneous transluminal coronary angioplasty (PTCA) or other transcatheter procedure
- Compensated congestive heart failure (CHF)
- Cardiomyopathy
- Heart or other organ transplantation
- Other cardiac surgery, including valvular and pacemaker insertion (including implantable cardioverter defibrillator [ICD])
- Peripheral arterial disease (PAD)
- High-risk cardiovascular disease (CVD) ineligible for surgical intervention
- Sudden cardiac death syndrome
- End-stage renal disease
- At risk for coronary artery disease (CAD) with diagnoses of diabetes mellitus, dyslipidemia, hypertension, obesity, or other diseases and conditions
- Other patients who may benefit from structured exercise and/or patient education based on physician referral and consensus of the rehabilitation team

CONTRAINDICATIONS
- Unstable angina
- Resting systolic BP (SBP) >200 mm Hg or resting diastolic BP (DBP) >110 mm Hg that should be evaluated on a case-by-case basis
- Orthostatic BP drop of >20 mm Hg with symptoms
- Critical aortic stenosis (i.e., peak SBP gradient of >50 mm Hg with an aortic valve orifice area of <0.75 cm^2 in an average-size adult)
- Acute systemic illness or fever
- Uncontrolled atrial or ventricular dysrhythmias
- Uncontrolled sinus tachycardia (>120 beats · min^{-1})
- Uncompensated CHF
- Third-degree atrioventricular (AV) block without pacemaker
- Active pericarditis or myocarditis
- Recent embolism
- Thrombophlebitis
- Resting ST-segment depression or elevation (>2 mm)
- Uncontrolled diabetes mellitus (See Chapter 10 for additional information on exercise prescription recommendations for individuals with diabetes mellitus.)
- Severe orthopedic conditions that would prohibit exercise
- Other metabolic conditions, such as acute thyroiditis, hypokalemia, hyperkalemia, or hypovolemia.

BOX 9.3	Adverse Responses to Inpatient Exercise Leading to Exercise Discontinuation

- Diastolic blood pressure (DBP) ≥110 mm Hg
- Decrease in systolic blood pressure (SBP) >10 mm Hg during exercise
- Significant ventricular or atrial dysrhythmias with or without associated signs/symptoms
- Second- or third-degree heart block
- Signs/symptoms of exercise intolerance, including angina, marked dyspnea, and electrocardiogram (ECG) changes suggestive of ischemia

Used with permission from American Association of Cardiovascular and Pulmonary Rehabilitation. *Guidelines for Cardiac Rehabilitation and Secondary Prevention Programs.* 4th ed. Champaign (IL): Human Kinetics. 2004. p. 36 and 119.

program components for patients with CVD are essentially the same as for people who are apparently healthy (Chapter 7) or are in the low-risk category (see Table 2.1).

FREQUENCY

- Early mobilization: 2–4 times $\cdot$ d^{-1} for the first 3 days of the hospital stay
- Later mobilization: 2 times $\cdot$ d^{-1} beginning on day 4 of the hospital stay with exercise bouts of increased duration

INTENSITY

The intensity recommendations that follow reflect the advised upper intensity limits (18).

- To tolerance if asymptomatic
- RPE ≤13 on a scale of 6–20
- Post-MI/congestive heart failure (CHF): HR ≤120 beats $\cdot$ min^{-1} or HR$_{rest}$ + 20 beats $\cdot$ min^{-1} as the arbitrary upper limit
- Postsurgery: HR$_{rest}$ + 30 beats $\cdot$ min^{-1} as the arbitrary upper limit

TIME (DURATION)

- Begin with intermittent bouts lasting 3 to 5 minutes as tolerated.
- Rest period may be a slower walk (or complete rest, at the patient's discretion) that is shorter than the duration of the exercise bout. Attempt to achieve a 2:1 exercise/rest ratio.

PROGRESSION

- When continuous exercise duration reaches 10 to 15 minutes, increase intensity as tolerated.

By hospital discharge, the patient should demonstrate an understanding of physical activities that may be inappropriate or excessive. Moreover, a safe, progressive plan of exercise should be formulated before leaving the hospital. Until evaluated with a submaximal or maximal exercise test or entry into a clinically supervised outpatient cardiac rehabilitation program, the upper limit of exercise should not exceed levels observed during the inpatient program while closely monitoring for signs and symptoms of exercise intolerance. All patients also should be educated and encouraged to investigate outpatient exercise program options and be provided with information regarding the use of home exercise equipment. All patients, especially moderate- to high-risk patients (see Table 2.1), should be strongly encouraged to participate in a clinically supervised outpatient rehabilitation program. Patients should be counseled to identify abnormal signs and symptoms suggesting exercise intolerance and the need for medical evaluation. Although not all patients may be suitable candidates for inpatient exercise, virtually all benefit from some level of inpatient intervention, including risk-factor assessment, activity counseling, and patient and family education.

OUTPATIENT EXERCISE PROGRAMS

Outpatient cardiac rehabilitation programs may begin as soon as hospital dismissal (i.e., discharge). Most patients are capable of beginning a supervised exercise program within 1 to 2 weeks of leaving the hospital (6). The goals for the outpatient rehabilitation are listed in Box 9.4. At program entry, the following assessments should be performed:

- Medical and surgical history, including the most recent cardiovascular event, comorbidities, and other pertinent medical history
- Physical examination, with an emphasis on the cardiopulmonary and musculoskeletal systems

---

BOX 9.4   Goals for Outpatient Cardiac Rehabilitation

- Develop and assist the patient to implement a safe and effective formal exercise and lifestyle physical activity program.
- Provide appropriate supervision and monitoring to detect deterioration in clinical status and provide ongoing surveillance data to the patients' healthcare providers to enhance medical management.
- Return the patient to vocational and recreational activities or modify these activities contingent on the patient's clinical status.
- Provide patient and family education to maximize secondary prevention (e.g., risk-factor modification) through aggressive lifestyle management and judicious use of cardioprotective medications.

- Review of recent cardiovascular tests and procedures, including 12-lead electrocardiogram (ECG), coronary angiogram, echocardiogram, stress test (exercise or imaging studies), revascularization, and pacemaker/implantable defibrillator implantation
- Current medications, including dose, route of administration, and frequency
- CVD risk factors

Although exercise training is safe and effective for cardiac patients, all patients should be stratified for risk of occurrence of cardiac events during exercise training (Chapter 2) (7). Routine pre-exercise assessment of risk for exercise should be performed at each rehabilitation session and include:

- Consideration of ECG surveillance that may consist of telemetry or hardwire monitoring, "quick-look" monitoring using defibrillator paddles, or periodic rhythm strips
- Blood pressure (BP)
- Body weight
- Heart rate (HR)
- Symptoms or evidence of change in clinical status not necessarily related to activity (e.g., dyspnea at rest, lightheadedness/dizziness, palpitations or irregular pulse, and chest discomfort)
- Symptoms and evidence of exercise intolerance
- Medication compliance

EXERCISE PRESCRIPTION

Prescriptive techniques for determining exercise dosage or FITT framework for the general apparently healthy population are detailed in Chapter 7. The techniques used for the apparently healthy adult population or for those classified as low risk for occurrence of cardiac events during exercise training (see Table 2.1) may be applied to many low- and moderate-risk patients with cardiac disease. This chapter provides specific considerations and modifications of the exercise prescription for patients with known CVD.

Key variables to be considered in the development of an exercise prescription for cardiac patients include (8):

- Safety factors, including clinical status, risk-stratification category, exercise capacity, ischemic/anginal threshold, and cognitive/psychological impairment that might result in nonadherence to exercise guidelines
- Associated factors, including vocational and avocational requirements, musculoskeletal limitations, premorbid activity level, and personal health/fitness goals

Frequency

Exercise frequency should include participation in sessions most days of the week, i.e., $4–7 \, d \cdot wk^{-1}$. For patients with very limited exercise capacities, multiple short (1–10 min) daily sessions may be prescribed. Patients should be encouraged to perform some of the exercise sessions independently (i.e., without direct supervision).

Intensity

Exercise intensity may be prescribed using one or more of the following methods (9,23):

- RPE of 11 to 16 on a scale of 6 to 20.
- 40% to 80% of exercise capacity using the HR reserve (HRR) or Karvonen method, percent oxygen uptake reserve ($\dot{V}O_2R$) or %$\dot{V}O_{2peak}$) techniques if maximal exercise test data are available. Please review Table 9.1 when exercise test data are not available.
- Exercise intensity should be prescribed at a HR below the ischemic threshold if such a threshold has been determined for the patient. The presence of classic angina pectoris that is induced with exercise and relieved with rest or nitroglycerin is sufficient evidence for the presence of myocardial ischemia.

For the purposes of the exercise prescription, it is preferable for patients to take their prescribed medications at the recommended time. However, dependent on the purposes of the exercise test (e.g., diagnosis in a changing clinical condition), medications may be withheld before testing with physician approval. Nonetheless, individuals on β-blockers may have an attenuated HR response to exercise and an increased or decreased maximal exercise capacity. For patients whose β-blocker dose was altered after an exercise test or during the course of rehabilitation, a new graded exercise test would be beneficial. However, another exercise test may not be medically necessary or may even be impractical. When these patients are exercising without a new exercise test, signs and symptoms should be monitored and RPE and HR responses recorded at previously performed workloads. These new HRs may serve as patients' new exercise target HR range (THR). In addition, individuals on diuretic therapy may become volume depleted or suffer from hypokalemia or orthostatic hypotension. For these patients, the BP response to exercise, potential symptoms of dizziness or lightheadedness, and dysrhythmias should be monitored while providing education regarding proper hydration (11). Please see Appendix A (Common Medications) for other medications that may influence the exercise and postexercise response.

Time (Duration)

Warm-up and cool-down activities of 5 to 10 minutes—including static stretching, range of motion, and low-intensity (<40%$\dot{V}O_2R$) aerobic activities—should be a component of each exercise session and precede and follow the conditioning phase, respectively. The goal for the duration of the aerobic conditioning phase is generally 20 to 60 minutes per session. After a cardiac event, many patients begin with 5- to 10-minute sessions with a gradual progression in aerobic exercise time of 1 to 5 minutes per session or an increase in time per session of 10% to 20% per week. However, there is no set format for the rate of progression in exercise session duration. Thus, progression should be individualized to patient tolerance. Factors to consider in this regard include initial physical fitness level, patient motivation and goals, symptoms, and musculoskeletal limitations. Exercise sessions may include continuous or intermittent exercise,

TABLE 9.1. RECOMMENDED *FREQUENCY, INTENSITY, TIME* AND *TYPE* OF EXERCISE (FITT) FRAMEWORK FOR CARDIAC PATIENTS WITHOUT AN ENTRY EXERCISE TEST (21,22)

	TRAINING HR	INITIAL MET LEVEL	MONITORING	RPE	MET PROGRESSION INCREMENTS
No exercise or pharmacologic test available	Upper limit of HR_{rest} + 20 beats · min^{-1} (15). Gradually titrate to higher levels according to RPE, signs and symptoms, normal physiologic responses.	2–4	ECG, BP, RPE, and signs or symptoms of ischemia	11–14	1–2
Pharmacologic test available (negative for ischemia)	If good HR increase: 70%–85% HR_{max}. If HR does not increase: HR_{rest} + 20 beats · min^{-1} with progression as described for no exercise or pharmacologic test available.	2–4	ECG, BP, RPE, and signs or symptoms of ischemia	11–14	1–2
Pharmacologic test available (positive for ischemia)	10 beats · min^{-1} below ischemic threshold (if determined). If ischemic threshold not determined, use procedure for no exercise or pharmacologic test available.	2–4	ECG, BP, RPE, and signs or symptoms of ischemia	11–14	1–2

HR, heart rate; MET, metabolic equivalent; RPE, rating of perceived exertion; HRmax, maximal heart rate; HRrest, resting heart rate; ECG, electrocardiogram; BP, blood pressure.

Initial workload of 2–4 METs is equivalent to treadmill: 1.7 mph/0–7.5% grade; 2.0 mph/0–5.0% grade; 2.5 mph/0–2.5% grade; leg cycle ergometry: ≤0 W; and arm ergometry: ≤25 W (1,2). Progression of 1–2 METs is equivalent to treadmill: 1–1.5 mph or 1%–2% grade; leg cycle ergometry: 25–50 W; and arm ergometry: ≤25 W.

See Table 7.3 for additional information regarding the FITT framework, including caloric expenditure, time (duration), frequency, and steps per day.

TABLE 9.2. EXAMPLE OF EXERCISE PROGRESSION USING INTERMITTENT EXERCISE (15)

			FUNCTIONAL CAPACITY ≥4 METs		
WEEK	**% FC**	**TOTAL MIN AT % FC**	**EXERCISE BOUT (min)**	**REST BOUT (min)**	**REPETITIONS**
1–2	50–60	15–20	3–10	2–5	3–4
3–4	60–70	20–40	10–20	Optional	2

			FUNCTIONAL CAPACITY <4 METs		
WEEK	**% FC**	**TOTAL MIN AT % FC**	**EXERCISE BOUT (min)**	**REST BOUT (min)**	**REPETITIONS**
1–2	40–50	10–20	3–7	3–5	3–4
3–4	50–60	15–30	7–15	2–5	2–3
5	60–70	25–40	12–20	2	2

Continue with two repetitions of continuous exercise, with one rest period or progress to a single continuous bout.
MET, metabolic equivalent; FC, functional capacity.

depending on the capability of the patient (10,17). Table 9.2 provides a recommended progression using intermittent exercise (15).

Type

The aerobic exercise portion of the session should include rhythmic, large-muscle-group activities with an emphasis on increased caloric expenditure for maintenance of a healthy body weight (Chapters 7 and 10). To promote whole-body physical fitness conditioning that includes the upper and lower extremities, multiple forms of aerobic activities and exercise equipment should be incorporated into the exercise program for patients with cardiac disease. The different types of exercise equipment may include:

- Arm ergometer
- Combination upper/lower extremity ergometer
- Upright and recumbent cycle ergometer
- Elliptical
- Rower
- Stair climber
- Treadmill for walking

Lifestyle Physical Activity

In addition to formal exercise sessions, patients should be encouraged to gradually return to general activities of daily living such as household chores, yard work, shopping, hobbies, and sports as evaluated and appropriately modified by the rehabilitation staff. Relatively inexpensive pedometers may enhance compliance with walking programs. Walking for 30 $min \cdot d^{-1}$ equates to 3,000 to 4,000 steps, whereas a 1 mile (1.6 km) walk equates to ~1,500 to 2,000 steps. For overall health/fitness benefits, a minimum of 10,000 $steps \cdot d^{-1}$ is recommended (Chapter 7).

TYPES OF OUTPATIENT EXERCISE PROGRAMS

Ideally, most patients with cardiac disease should participate in a medically supervised exercise program for at least a few weeks to facilitate exercise and lifestyle changes and a return to work. However, patients who experience an acute coronary syndrome and receive percutaneous coronary intervention for revascularization often return to work within 1 week of hospital discharge and may not be able to exercise during the operating hours of a supervised exercise program. Additionally, although all patients with CVD should be encouraged to attend a formal and supervised exercise rehabilitation program, some patients live in regions without a local program or do not wish to attend a program for a variety of reasons. In these cases, an independent program with follow-up by the patient's healthcare providers may be the only option. Some programs provide programmatic options for these patients, such as regular telephone, Internet, or mail contact, and should be investigated as alternatives to direct supervision.

Most patients will transition from a medically supervised program to an independent one (i.e., nonmonitored, unsupervised home exercise program). The optimal number of weeks of attendance at a supervised program before entering an independent program is not known and is likely patient specific. Unfortunately, insurance reimbursement often determines the length of time of participation in a supervised program. The patient and rehabilitation team should investigate thoroughly the limits of reimbursement and the ability of the patient to continue the program to develop the proper progression of exercise to ready the patient for eventual transfer into an independent program. Some programs offer long-term supervision. Suggestions for criteria to determine when a patient is appropriate for an independent exercise program are as follows:

- Cardiac symptoms stable or absent
- Appropriate ECG, BP, and HR responses to exercise
- Demonstrated knowledge of proper exercise principles and awareness of abnormal symptoms
- Motivation to continue to exercise regularly without close supervision

SPECIAL CONSIDERATIONS

Patients with a Sternotomy

For 5 to 8 weeks after cardiothoracic surgery, lifting with the upper extremities should be restricted to 5 to 8 pounds (2.27–3.63 kg). Range of motion (ROM) exercises and lifting 1 to 3 pounds (0.45–1.36 kg) with the arms is permissible if there is no evidence of sternal instability, as detected by movement in the sternum, pain, cracking, or popping. Patients should be advised to limit ROM within the onset of feelings of pulling on the incision or mild pain.

Continuous Electrocardiographic Monitoring

ECG monitoring during supervised exercise sessions is routinely performed during the first several weeks. Insurance reimbursement sometimes requires ECG monitoring. The following recommendations for ECG monitoring are related to patient-associated risks of exercise training (see Table 2.1) (5):

- Low-risk cardiac patients may begin with continuous ECG monitoring and decrease to intermittent ECG monitoring after 6 to 12 sessions as deemed appropriate by the rehabilitation staff.
- Moderate-risk patients may begin with continuous ECG monitoring and decrease to intermittent ECG monitoring after 12 to 18 sessions as deemed appropriate by the rehabilitation staff.
- High-risk patients may begin with continuous ECG monitoring and decrease to intermittent ECG monitoring after 18, 24, or 30 sessions as deemed appropriate by the rehabilitation staff.

Recent Pacemaker/Implantable Cardioverter Defibrillator Implantation

Implantable cardioverter defibrillators (ICDs) are small, battery-powered devices implanted into the body to monitor the electrical impulses in the heart. ICDs deliver electrical stimuli to make the heart beat or contract in a more normal rhythm when necessary. Cardiac pacemakers are used to restore more optimal cardiac function when there is a loss of normal sequence of atrial and ventricular filling and contraction that results in deterioration of cardiovascular function and the onset of signs and symptoms. Specific indications for pacemakers include sick sinus syndrome with symptomatic bradycardia, acquired atrioventricular (AV) block, and persistent advanced AV block after MI. There are different types of pacemakers that fulfill specific functions as detailed below:

- Rate-responsive pacemakers are programmed to increase or decrease HR to match the level of physical activity (i.e., sitting rest or walking).
- Single-chambered pacemakers have only one lead placed into the right atrium or the right ventricle.
- Dual-chambered pacemakers have two leads; one placed in the right atrium and one in the right ventricle.
- Cardiac resynchronization therapy pacemakers have three leads; one in right atrium, one in right ventricle, and one in left ventricle.

The type of pacemaker is identified by a four-letter code as indicated below:

- The first letter of the code describes the chamber paced, e.g, atria (A), ventricle (V), or dual (A and V).
- The second letter of the code describes the chamber sensed.
- The third letter of the code describes the pacemaker's response to a sensed event.
- The fourth letter of the code describes the rate-response capabilities of the pacemaker, e.g., inhibited (I) or rate responsive (R).

For example, a VVIR code pacemaker means that (a) the ventricle is paced and sensed; (b) when the pacemaker senses a normal ventricular contraction, it is inhibited; and (c) the pulse generator is rate responsive.

ICDs are devices that monitor heart rhythms and deliver shocks if dangerous rhythms are detected. ICDs are used for high-rate ventricular tachycardia or fibrillation in patients who are at risk for these conditions as a result of previous cardiac arrest, heart failure, or ineffective drug therapy for abnormal heart rhythms. When ICDs detect a too-rapid or irregular heartbeat, they deliver a shock that resets the heart to a more normal HR and electrical pattern (i.e., cardioversion). Thus, ICDs protect against sudden cardiac death from ventricular tachycardia and ventricular fibrillation.

Exercise prescription considerations for those with pacemakers are as follows:

- Pacemakers may improve functional capacity as a result of an improved HR response to exercise.
- The upper HR limit of dual-sensor rate responsive and VVIR pacemakers should be set 10% below the ischemic threshold (i.e., the 10% safety margin).
- When an ICD is present, exercise training intensity should be maintained at least 10 beats $\cdot$ min^{-1} below the programmed HR threshold for defibrillation.
- To minimize the risk of lead dislocation, for 3 weeks after implantation, all pacemaker patients should avoid activities that require raising the hands above the level of the shoulders.

Patients after Cardiac Transplantation

The purpose of medical management for the cardiac transplant patient is to control immune system rejection while avoiding possible adverse side effects of immunosuppressive therapy, such as infections, dyslipidemia, hypertension, obesity, osteoporosis, renal dysfunction, and diabetes mellitus.

For the first several months after surgery, the transplanted heart does not respond normally to sympathetic nervous stimulation (19). The clinician and cardiac rehabilitation professional should be aware of the following hemodynamic alterations during this time: (a) resting HR (HR$_{rest}$) is elevated; and (b) the HR response to exercise is abnormal, such that the increase in HR during exercise is delayed, and the peak HR (HR$_{peak}$) is below normal. Exercise prescription for these patients does not include use of a THR. For these patients, the clinician and cardiac rehabilitation professional should consider (a) an extended warm-up and cool-down if limited by muscular deconditioning; (b) using RPE to monitor exercise intensity; and (c) incorporation of stretching and ROM exercises (Chapter 7). However, at 1 year after surgery, approximately one third of patients exhibit a partially normalized HR response to exercise and may be given a THR based on results from a graded exercise test (GXT) (25).

EXERCISE PRESCRIPTION WITHOUT A PRELIMINARY EXERCISE TEST

With shorter hospital stays, more aggressive interventions, and greater sophistication of diagnostic procedures, it is not unusual for patients to begin cardiac rehabilitation before having a GXT. Reasons for not having a GXT are presented

BOX 9.5	**Reasons for No Available Preliminary Exercise Test (21,22)**

- Pharmacologic stress test without sufficient data to formulate an exercise prescription
- Extreme deconditioning
- Orthopedic limitations
- Left ventricular dysfunction limited by shortness of breath
- Known coronary anatomy; therefore, exercise test felt clinically nonessential
- Recent successful percutaneous intervention or revascularization surgery
- Uncomplicated or stable myocardial infarction (MI)

in Box 9.5. For those without exercise tests, exercise prescription procedures are based on what was accomplished during the inpatient phase, home exercise activities, and close surveilance for signs and symptoms of exercise intolerance, such as excessive fatigue, dizziness or lightheadness, inotropic or chronotropic incompetence, and signs or symptoms of ischemia (Box 9.1). Suggestions for developing an exercise prescription in the event of no available GXT are presented in Table 9.1.

RESISTANCE TRAINING FOR CARDIAC PATIENTS

The development of muscular strength and endurance is essential for resumption of work and efficient performance of activities of daily living. Most patients with cardiac disease should be encouraged to participate in resistance training. The specific reasons that patients with CVD should participate in resistance training are listed in Box 9.6. Patient criteria for participation in resistance training are located in Box 9.7 with guidelines for resistance training in Box 9.8.

BOX 9.6	**Purposes of Resistance Training for Patients with Cardiac Disease (14,20)**

- Improve muscular strength and endurance
- Improve self-confidence
- Increase ability to perform activities of daily living
- Maintain independence
- Decrease cardiac demands of muscular work (i.e., reduced rate pressure product [RPP]) during daily activities
- Prevent and attenuate the development of other diseases and conditions, such as osteoporosis, type 2 diabetes mellitus, and obesity
- Slow age- and disease-related declines in muscle strength and mass

(*text continues on page 222*)

BOX 9.7	Patient Criteria for a Resistance Training Program[a] (10)

- Low- to moderate-risk patients and possibly higher-risk patients with supervision (see Table 2.1)
- Those who require strength for work or recreational activities, particularly in their upper extremities
- Initiate a minimum of 5 weeks after date of myocardial infarction (MI) or cardiac surgery, *including* 4 weeks of consistent participation in a supervised cardiac rehabilitation endurance training program[b] (Range of motion [ROM] and very light resistance exercise of 1–3 lb [0.45–1.36 kg] may be started earlier if tolerated.)
- Initiate a minimum of 2 to 3 weeks following transcatheter procedure (i.e., PTCA or other), *including* 2 weeks of consistent participation in a supervised cardiac rehabilitation endurance training program[b] (ROM and very light resistance exercise of 1–3 lb [0.45–1.36 kg] may be started earlier if tolerated.)
- No evidence of congestive heart failure (CHF), uncontrolled dysrhythmias, severe valvular disease, uncontrolled hypertension, and unstable symptoms

[a]In this box, a resistance-training program is defined as one in which patients lift weights ≥50% one repetition maximum (1-RM). The use of elastic bands, 1- to 3-lb (0.45–1.36-kg) hand weights, and light free weights may be initiated in a progressive fashion at outpatient program entry provided no other contraindications exist. See Chapter 7 for further information on the FITT framework for resistance training.

[b]Entry should be a rehabilitation staff decision with approval of the medical director and surgeon as appropriate.

BOX 9.8	Resistance Training Guidelines[a]

- Equipment (*Type*)
  - Elastic bands
  - Light (1–5 lb; 0.45–2.27 kg) cuff and hand weights
  - Light free weights (1–5 lb; 0.45–2.27 kg)
  - Wall pulleys
  - Machines (dependent on weight of lever arms and range of motion)
- Proper technique
  - Raise and lower weights with slow, controlled movements to full extension.
  - Maintain regular breathing pattern. >

> Box 9.8. continued

- Avoid straining.
- Avoid sustained, tight gripping, which may evoke an excessive blood pressure (BP) response.
- A rating of perceived exertion (RPE) of 11 to 13 ("light" to "somewhat hard") on a scale of 6 to 20 may be used as a subjective guide to effort.
- Terminate exercise if warning signs or symptoms occur, including dizziness, dysrhythmias, unusual shortness of breath, or anginal discomfort.
- Initial load should allow 12 to 15 repetitions that can be lifted comfortably (~30%–40% one repetition maximum [1-RM] for the upper body; ~50%–60% for the lower body).
  - Increase loads by 5% increments when the patient can comfortably lift 12 to 15 repetitions.
  - Low-risk patients may progress to 8 to 12 repetitions with a resistance of ~60% to 80% 1-RM.
  - Because of the potential for an elevated BP response, the rate pressure product (RPP) should not exceed that during prescribed endurance exercise as determined from the graded exercise test (GXT).
  - RPE is 11 to 13 ("light" to "somewhat hard") on a scale of 6 to 20.
- Each major muscle group (i.e., chest, shoulders, arms, abdomen, back, hips, and legs) should be trained with two to four sets.
  - Sets may be of the same exercise or from different exercises affecting the same muscle group.
  - Gains in muscular strength and endurance are obtained with one set, particularly in novices.
  - Perform eight to 10 exercises of the major muscle groups.
  - Exercise large muscle groups before small muscle groups.
  - Include multijoint exercises or "compound" exercises that affect more than one muscle group.
- Frequency: 2–3 d · wk^{-1} with at least 48 hours separating training sessions for the same muscle group. All muscle groups to be trained may be done in the same session, i.e., whole body, or each session may "split" the body into selected muscle groups so that only a few are trained in any one session.
- Progression: Increase slowly as the patient adapts to the program (~2–5 lb · wk^{-1} [0.91–2.27 kg] for arms and 5–10 lb · wk^{-1} for legs [0.91–4.5 kg]).

^{a}For additional information on resistance training, see Chapter 7.

BOX 9.9   Exercise Prescription and Return to Work

- Assess patient's work environment
  - Nature of work
  - Muscle groups used at work
  - Work demands that primarily involve muscular strength and endurance
  - Primary movements performed doing work
  - Periods of high metabolic demands versus periods of low metabolic demands
  - Environmental factors
  - Average metabolic demands for 8 hours of work should not exceed 50% of maximal functional capacity
- Exercise prescription
  - Use exercise modalities that use muscle groups involved in work tasks.
  - Prescribe intensity versus duration in intermittent fashion as is similar to that of work tasks.
  - If possible, use exercises that mimic movement patterns used during work tasks.
  - Balance resistance versus aerobic training relative to work tasks.
  - If environmental stress occurs at work, educate the patient about appropriate precautions; expose them to similar environmental conditions while performing activities similar to work tasks (see the ACSM positions stands (11–13,24) and Chapter 8 for additional information on environmental precautions).
  - Monitor the physiologic responses to a simulated work environment.

EXERCISE TRAINING FOR RETURN TO WORK

For those returning to work, exercise training must be specific to the muscle groups and energy systems used for occupational tasks, particularly for those whose employment involves manual labor. Exercise results in better appreciation of the ability to perform physical work, improved safety, enhanced self-efficacy, greater willingness to resume work, greater willingness to remain employed long term following a cardiac event, and appropriate perception of job demands (20,24). Box 9.9 discusses the exercise prescription regarding preparation for returning to work.

REFERENCES

1. American Association of Cardiovascular and Pulmonary Rehabilitation. *Guidelines for Cardiac Rehabilitation and Secondary Prevention Programs*. 4th ed. Champaign (IL): Human Kinetics; 2004. p. 32.

2. American Association of Cardiovascular and Pulmonary Rehabilitation. *Guidelines for Cardiac Rehabilitation and Secondary Prevention Programs.* 4th ed. Champaign (IL): Human Kinetics; 2004. p. 36.

3. American Association of Cardiovascular and Pulmonary Rehabilitation. *Guidelines for Cardiac Rehabilitation and Secondary Prevention Programs.* 4th ed. Champaign (IL): Human Kinetics; 2004. p. 63.

4. American Association of Cardiovascular and Pulmonary Rehabilitation. *Guidelines for Cardiac Rehabilitation and Secondary Prevention Programs.* 4th ed. Champaign (IL): Human Kinetics; 2004. p. 37.

5. American Association of Cardiovascular and Pulmonary Rehabilitation. *Guidelines for Cardiac Rehabilitation and Secondary Prevention Programs.* 4th ed. Champaign (IL): Human Kinetics; 2004. p. 44.

6. American Association of Cardiovascular and Pulmonary Rehabilitation. *Guidelines for Cardiac Rehabilitation and Secondary Prevention Programs.* 4th ed. Champaign (IL): Human Kinetics; 2004. p. 65.

7. American Association of Cardiovascular and Pulmonary Rehabilitation. *Guidelines for Cardiac Rehabilitation and Secondary Prevention Programs.* 4th ed. Champaign (IL): Human Kinetics; 2004. p. 62.

8. American Association of Cardiovascular and Pulmonary Rehabilitation. *Guidelines for Cardiac Rehabilitation and Secondary Prevention Programs.* 4th ed. Champaign (IL): Human Kinetics; 2004. p. 115.

9. American Association of Cardiovascular and Pulmonary Rehabilitation. *Guidelines for Cardiac Rehabilitation and Secondary Prevention Programs.* 4th ed. Champaign (IL): Human Kinetics; 2004. p. 116.

10. American Association of Cardiovascular and Pulmonary Rehabilitation. *Guidelines for Cardiac Rehabilitation and Secondary Prevention Programs.* 4th ed. Champaign (IL): Human Kinetics; 2004. p. 36 and 119.

11. American College of Sports Medicine. Position Stand. Exercise and fluid replacement. *Med Sci Sports Exerc.* 2007;39(2):377–90.

12. American College of Sports Medicine. Position Stand. Exertional heat illness during training and competition. *Med Sci Sports Exerc.* 2007;39(3):556–72.

13. American College of Sports Medicine. Position Stand. Prevention of cold injuries during exercise. *Med Sci Sports Exerc.* 2006;38:2012–29.

14. American College of Sports Medicine. Position Stand. The recommended quantity and quality of exercise for developing and maintaining cardiorespiratory and muscular fitness, and flexibility in healthy adults. *Med Sci Sports Exerc.* 1998;30:975–91.

15. American College of Sports Medicine's *Guidelines for Exercise Testing and Prescription.* 7th ed. Philadelphia (PA): Lippincott Williams & Wilkins, 2005.

16. Convertino VA. Effect of orthostatic stress on exercise performance after bed rest: relation to in-hospital rehabilitation. *J Cardiac Rehab.* 1983;3:660–3.

17. Franklin BA. Myocardial infarction. In: Durstine JL, Moore GE, editors. *ACSM's Exercise Management for Persons with Chronic Diseases and Disabilities.* 2nd ed. Champaign (IL): Human Kinetics; 2003. p. 24–31.

18. Joo KC, Brubaker PH, MacDougall AS, Saikin AM, Ross JH, Whaley MH. Exercise prescription using heart rate plus 20 or perceived exertion in cardiac rehabilitation. *J Cardiopulm Rehabil.* 2004;24:178–86.

19. Keteyian SJ, Brawner C. Cardiac transplant. In: Durstine JL, Moore GE, editors. *ACSM's Exercise Management for Persons with Chronic Diseases and Disabilities.* 2nd ed. Champaign (IL): Human Kinetics; 2003. p. 70–5.

20. Leon AS, Franklin BA, Costa F, et al. Cardiac rehabilitation and secondary prevention of coronary heart disease: an American Heart Association Scientific Statement from the Council on Clinical Cardiology (Subcommittee on Exercise, Cardiac Rehabilitation, and Prevention and the Council on Nutrition, Physical Activity, and Metabolism [Subcommittee on Physical Activity]), in Collaboration with the American Association of Cardiovascular and Pulmonary Rehabilitation. *Circulation.* 2005;111:369–76.

21. McConnell TR. Exercise prescription when the guidelines do not work. *J Cardiopulm Rehabil.* 1996;16:34–7.

22. McConnell TR, Klinger TA, Gardner JK, Laubach CA, Herman CE, Hauck CA. Cardiac rehabilitation without exercise tests for post-myocardial infarction and post-bypass surgery patients. *J Cardiopulm Rehabil.* 1998;18:458–63.

23. Schairer JR, Keteyian SJ. Exercise training in patients with cardiovascular disease. In: American College of Sports Medicine. In *ACSM's Resource Manual for Guidelines for Exercise Testing and Prescription*. 5th ed. Philadelphia (PA): Lippincott Williams & Wilkins; 2006. p. 439–51.
24. Sheldahl LM, Wilke NA, Tristani FE. Evaluation and training for resumption of occupational and leisure-time physical activities in patients after a major cardiac event. *Med Exerc Nutr Health*. 1995;4:273–89.
25. Squires RW, Leung TC, Cyr NS, et al. Partial normalization of the heart rate response to exercise after cardiac transplantation: frequency and relationship to exercise capacity. *Mayo Clin Proc*. 2002;77:1295–300.

Exercise Prescription for Other Clinical Populations

ARTHRITIS

Arthritis and rheumatic diseases are leading causes of pain and disability. These diseases currently affect more than 40 million individuals in the United States and are expected to affect about 60 million by the year 2020 (27,28,49). There are more than 100 rheumatic diseases, the two most common being osteoarthritis and rheumatoid arthritis. Osteoarthritis is a local degenerative joint disease affecting one or multiple joints (most commonly the hands, hips, spine, and knees). Rheumatoid arthritis is a chronic, systemic inflammatory disease in which there is pathologic activity of the immune system against joint tissues (58). Other common rheumatic diseases include fibromyalgia, systemic lupus erythematosus, gout, and bursitis.

Medications are a core component in the treatment of arthritis, including analgesics, nonsteroidal anti-inflammatory drugs, and disease-modifying antirheumatic drugs for rheumatoid arthritis. However, optimal treatment of arthritis involves a multidisciplinary approach, including patient education in self-management and weight loss, physical therapy, and occupational therapy. In the later stages of disease, when pain is refractory to conservative management, total joint replacement and other surgeries provide substantial relief (58). Although pain and functional limitations present challenges to physical activity among individuals with arthritis, regular exercise is essential for managing these conditions (16). Specifically, exercise reduces pain, maintains muscle strength around affected joints, reduces joint stiffness, prevents functional decline, and improves mental health and quality of life.

EXERCISE TESTING

Most individuals with arthritis tolerate symptom-limited exercise testing. Special considerations for people with arthritis are indicated below.

- Vigorous-intensity exercise is contraindicated when there is acute inflammation (i.e., until hot, swollen, and flare has subsided).
- Although some people with arthritis tolerate treadmill walking, use of a cycle ergometer alone or combined with arm ergometry may be less painful and

Category-Ration Scale

0	Nothing at all	"No pain"
0.3		
0.5	Extremely weak	Just noticable
0.7		
1	Very weak	
1.5		
2	Weak	Light
2.5		
3	Moderate	
4		
5	Strong	Heavy
6		
7	Very strong	
8		
9	Extremely strong	"Maximum pain"
10		
11		
?		
•	Absolute maximum	Highest possible

FIGURE 10.1. The Borg CR 10 Customized for Pain Measurement Scale (Copyright Gunnar Borg. Reproduced with permission. For correct use of the Borg scales, it is necessary to follow the administration and instructions given in Borg G. *Borg's Perceived Exertion and Pain Scales*. Champaign (IL): Human Kinetics; 1998).

allow better assessment of cardiovascular function. The mode of exercise used should be the least painful for the person being tested.
- Allow ample time for individuals to warm up at a low intensity level before beginning the graded exercise test.
- Monitor pain levels during testing using a scale such as the Borg CR10 Customized for Pain Measurement Scale (23) (Fig. 10.1).
- Isotonic, isokinetic, or isometric muscle strength may be measured (37). A one-repetition maximum test (1-RM) is tolerated by many individuals with arthritis, though pain may limit maximum muscle contraction in affected joints.

EXERCISE PRESCRIPTION

In general, recommendations for Frequency, Intensity, Time, and Type of exercise (or the FITT framework) are consistent with those for apparently healthy adults (Chapter 7). However, there are several considerations for people with arthritis that are noted below.

Frequency: Aerobic exercise 3–5 d · wk^{-1}; resistance exercise 2–3 d · wk^{-1}; flexibility/range of motion exercises should be emphasized and performed at least daily.

Intensity: General recommendations for exercise intensity apply for aerobic exercise, however, the intensity level may be limited by pain. For resistance exercise, start with a relatively low amount of weight, about 10% of the individual's maximum, and progress at a maximal rate of a 10% increase per week as tolerated to the point of pain tolerance and/or low to moderate intensity (i.e., 40%–60% 1-RM) for 10 to 15 repetitions per exercise (37).

Time: Aerobic exercise: start with short bouts of 5 to 10 minutes to accumulate 20–30 min · d^{-1} as tolerated, with a goal of progressing to total 150 minutes per week of moderate-intensity activity. Resistance exercise: perform one or more sets involving 10 to 15 repetitions per exercise (37).

Type: Aerobic exercise: participate in activities having low joint stress, such as walking, cycling, or swimming. Resistance exercise: individuals with significant joint pain or muscle weakness may benefit from beginning with maximum voluntary isometric contractions around the affected joint, then progressing to dynamic training (37). A strength-training program should include all major muscle groups as recommended for healthy adults (10) (Chapter 7). Flexibility exercise: perform stretching or range of motion (ROM) exercises of all major muscle groups.

Special Considerations

Additional considerations when prescribing exercise for people with arthritis are indicated below.

- Avoid strenuous exercises during acute flares and periods of inflammation. However, it is appropriate to gently move joints through their full range of motion during these periods.
- Progression in duration of activity should be emphasized over increased intensity (67).
- Adequate warm-up and cool-down periods of 5 to 10 minutes are critical for minimizing pain. Warm-up and cool-down activity may involve slow movement of joints through their range of motion.
- Inform individuals with arthritis that some discomfort during or immediately after exercise can be expected, and this discomfort does not necessarily mean joints are being further damaged. However, if joint pain persists for 2 hours after exercise and exceeds pain severity before exercise, the duration and/or intensity of exercise should be reduced in future sessions.
- Encourage individuals with arthritis to exercise during the time of day when pain is typically least severe and/or in conjunction with peak activity of pain medications.
- Appropriate shoes that provide shock absorption and stability are particularly important for people with arthritis. Shoe specialists may provide recommendations for appropriate shoes to meet individuals' biomechanical profiles.

- Because many patients with osteoarthritis of the lower extremities are overweight and obese, healthy weight loss maintenance should be encouraged. See Chapter 10 on overweight and obesity for additional information.
- Incorporate functional exercises such as the sit-to-stand and step-ups as tolerated to improve neuromuscular control, balance, and maintenance of activities of daily living.
- For water exercise, the temperature should be 83°F to 88°F (28°C–31°C), as warm water helps to relax muscles and reduce pain.
- A majority of older persons will have arthritis. Older people experience similar training adaptations as younger people. See Chapter 8, Nelson et al. (73), and the American College of Sports Medicine (ACSM) Position Stand (8) on Exercise Prescription for the Older Adult for additional information.

CANCER

Cancer is a group of diseases characterized by the uncontrolled growth and spread of abnormal cells resulting from damage to deoxyribonucleic acid (DNA) by internal factors (e.g., inherited mutations) and environmental exposures (e.g., tobacco smoke). Most cancers are classified according to the cell type from which they originate. Carcinomas develop from the epithelial cells of organs and compose at least 80% of all cancers. Other cancers arise from the cells of the blood (leukemias), immune system (lymphomas), and connective tissues (sarcomas). The lifetime prevalence of cancer is one in two for men, and one in three for women (3). Cancer affects all ages but is most common in older adults. About 76% of all cancers are diagnosed in persons aged 55 years and older (3), hence, there is a strong likelihood of cancer comorbidities, such as cardiopulmonary disease, diabetes mellitus, osteoporosis, and arthritis.

Treatment for cancer may involve surgery, radiation, chemotherapy, hormones, and immunotherapy. In the process of destroying cancer cells, some treatments also damage healthy tissue. Patients may experience side effects that may limit their ability to exercise during treatment and afterward. Furthermore, overall physical function is generally diminished because of losses of aerobic capacity, muscle tissue, and range of motion. Even among cancer survivors who are 5 years or more posttreatment, more than half report physical performance limitations, including crouching/kneeling, standing for 2 hours, lifting/carrying 10 pounds (4.5 kg), and walking quarter of a mile (0.4 km) (74).

EXERCISE TESTING

There is an absence of expert consensus or position statements on the safety of exercise testing and training in people with cancer. Nonetheless, a set of guidelines relating to safety considerations for this population that are based on existing evidence and clinical experience have been published and can be found in Table 10.1 (65). These guidelines are deliberately conservative. They will not necessarily apply to every person with cancer because of the diversity of this patient population; however, they provide a fundamental framework for the

TABLE 10.1. CONTRAINDICATIONS AND PRECAUTIONS TO EXERCISE TESTING AND TRAINING FOR PATIENTS WITH CANCER

	CONTRAINDICATIONS TO EXERCISE TESTING AND TRAINING	PRECAUTIONS REQUIRING MODIFICATION AND/OR PHYSICIAN APPROVAL
Factors related to cancer treatment	• No exercise on days of intravenous chemotherapy or within 24 h of treatment • No exercise before blood draw • Severe tissue reaction to radiation therapy	• Caution if on treatments that affect the lungs and/or heart: recommend medically supervised exercise testing and training • Mouth sores/ulcerations: avoid mouthpieces for maximal testing; use face masks
Hematologic	• Platelets <50,000 • White blood cells <3,000 • Hemoglobin <10 g · dL^{-1}	• Platelets >50,000–150,000: avoid tests that increase risk of bleeding • White blood cells >3,000–4,000: ensure proper sterilization of equipment • Hemoglobin >10 g · dL^{-1}–11.5/13.5 g · dL^{-1}: caution with maximal tests
Musculoskeletal	• Bone, back, or neck pain of recent origin • Unusual muscular weakness • Severe cachexia • Unusual/extreme fatigue • Poor functional status: avoid exercise testing if Karnofsky performance status score ≤60%	• Any pain or cramping: investigate • Osteopenia: avoid high-impact exercise if risk of fracture • Steroid-induced myopathy • Cachexia: multidisciplinary approach to exercise • Mild to moderate fatigue: closely monitor response to exercise
Systemic	• Acute infections • Febrile illness: fever >100°F (38°C) • General malaise	• Recent systemic illness or infection: avoid exercise until asymptomatic for >48 h
Gastrointestinal	• Severe nausea • Vomiting or diarrhea within 24–36 h • Dehydration • Poor nutrition: inadequate fluid and/or intake	• Compromised fluid and/or food intake: recommend multidisciplinary approach/ consultation with nutritionist

(continued)

TABLE 10.1. CONTRAINDICATIONS AND PRECAUTIONS TO EXERCISE TESTING AND TRAINING FOR PATIENTS WITH CANCER (*Continued*)

	CONTRAINDICATIONS TO EXERCISE TESTING AND TRAINING	PRECAUTIONS REQUIRING MODIFICATION AND/OR PHYSICIAN APPROVAL
Cardiovascular	• Chest pain • Resting HR >100 beats · min^{-1} or <50 beats · min^{-1} • Resting SBP >145 mm Hg and/or DBP >95 mm Hg • Resting SBP <85 mm Hg • Irregular HR • Swelling of ankles	• Caution if at risk of cardiac disease: recommend medically supervised exercise testing and training • If on antihypertensive medications that affect HR, THR may not be attainable; avoid overexertion • Lymphedema: wear compression garment on limb when exercising
Pulmonary	• Severe dyspnea • Cough, wheezing • Chest pain increased by deep breath	• Mild to moderate dyspnea: avoid maximal tests
Neurologic	• Significant decline in cognitive status • Dizziness/lightheadedness • Disorientation • Blurred vision • Ataxia (i.e., inability to co-ordinate voluntary movement)	• Mild cognitive changes: ensure that patient is able to understand and follow instructions • Poor balance/peripheral sensory neuropathy: use well-supported positions for exercise

HR, heart rate; SBP, systolic blood pressure; DBP, diastolic blood pressure; THR, target heart rate.

Reprinted with permission from McNeely ML, Peddle C, Parliament M, Courneya KS. Cancer rehabilitation: recommendations for integrating exercise programming in the clinical practice setting. *Curr Cancer Ther Rev.* 2006; 2:351–60.

health/fitness professional to consider for exercise testing and prescription. Standard exercise testing methods are generally appropriate for cancer patients who have been cleared for exercise testing (Chapter 5). The presence of comorbidities, specific disease-related symptoms, or treatment-related side effects may require modifications to testing procedures as indicated below.

• Cancer and cancer therapy have the potential to affect the health-related components of physical fitness (i.e., cardiovascular fitness, muscular strength and endurance, body composition, flexibility, and gait and balance). Ideally, cancer patients should receive a comprehensive fitness assessment involving all components of health-related fitness.
• A thorough screening for cancer comorbidities and exercise contraindications should take place before exercise testing, including a medical history, physical examination, and laboratory tests, such as a complete blood count, lipid profile, and pulmonary function test.

- Medical supervision of symptom-limited or maximal exercise testing is strongly recommended.
- Decisions regarding testing protocols may be influenced by the specific disease or treatment-related limitations of the individual. For example, submaximal tests may be most appropriate for older patients or those with advanced cancer for whom increasing or maintaining daily activity is the primary goal. However, the submaximal exercise test should stress the individual to at least the anticipated intensity level of the daily activity to be performed.
- Decisions regarding testing modes may be influenced by the specific disease or treatment-related limitations of the individual. For example, a treadmill rather than cycle ergometer may be the more appropriate modality for patients who have undergone rectal or prostate surgery or radiation.

EXERCISE PRESCRIPTION

Insufficient evidence exists for the precise recommendations regarding the optimal components of exercise prescription for each cancer type. The currently recommended components of an exercise program for cancer patients (65) are consistent with the ACSM general principles of exercise prescription for aerobic, resistance, and flexibility exercise (Chapter 7). They are also compatible with the American Cancer Society's recommendation of 30 to 60 minutes of moderate- to vigorous-intensity physical activity at least 5 $d \cdot wk^{-1}$ for cancer survivors (35).

Safety considerations for exercise training for cancer patients are presented in Table 10.1 (65). Medical clearance should be obtained before vigorous-intensity exercise. Blood pressure (BP), heart rate (HR), and other relevant vital signs should be monitored before, during, and after the exercise sessions. Exercise should be stopped if unusual symptoms are experienced (e.g. dizziness, nausea, or chest pain).

Frequency: Aerobic exercise 3–5 $d \cdot wk^{-1}$; resistance exercise 2–3 $d \cdot wk^{-1}$ with at least 48 hours of recovery between sessions; and flexibility exercise 2–7 $d \cdot wk^{-1}$.

Intensity: Aerobic exercise: 40% to <60% oxygen uptake reserve ($\dot{V}O_2R$) or heart rate reserve (HRR). Resistance exercise: 40% to 60% 1-RM; and flexibility exercise, slow static stretching to the point of tension.

Time: Aerobic exercise: 20–60 $min \cdot d^{-1}$ with accumulated shorter bouts if necessary. Resistance exercise: 1 to 3 sets of 8 to 12 repetitions per exercise, with an upper limit of 15 repetitions appropriate for deconditioned, fatigued, or frail individuals. Flexibility exercise: 4 repetitions of 10 to 30 seconds per stretch for flexibility.

Type: Aerobic exercise: prolonged, rhythmic activities using large muscle groups (e.g., walking, cycling, and swimming). Resistance exercise: weights, resistance machines, or weight-bearing functional tasks (e.g., sit to stand) targeting all major muscle groups. Flexibility exercise: stretching or ROM exercises of all major muscle groups also addressing specific areas of joint or muscle restriction that may have resulted from treatment with steroids, radiation, or surgery.

Special Considerations

- Cancer-related fatigue is prevalent in patients receiving chemotherapy and radiation and may prevent or restrict the ability to exercise. In some cases, fatigue may persist for months or years after treatment completion.
- Bone is a common site of metastases in many cancers, particularly breast, prostate, and lung cancer. Lesions are reported to occur most frequently in the vertebra, pelvis, femur, and skull. High-impact activities and contact sports should be avoided to minimize fracture risk.
- Cachexia or muscle wasting is prevalent in individuals with incurable cancer and is likely to limit the exercise, depending on the extent of muscle wasting.
- Patients who have received bone-marrow transplants and those with low white blood cell counts should avoid exercising in public places that have high risk of microbial contamination.
- Swimming should not be prescribed for patients with indwelling catheters or central lines and feeding tubes, or for those who are receiving radiation.
- Patients receiving chemotherapy may experience fluctuating periods of sickness and fatigue during treatment cycles that require frequent modifications to exercise prescription, such as reducing the intensity and/or duration of the exercise session.

DIABETES MELLITUS

Diabetes mellitus is a group of metabolic diseases characterized by an elevated fasting blood glucose level (i.e., hyperglycemia) as a result of either defects in insulin secretion or an inability to use insulin. Sustained elevated blood glucose levels place patients at risk for micro- and macrovascular diseases as well as neuropathies (peripheral and autonomic). Currently, 7% of the United States population has diabetes mellitus, with 1.5 million new cases diagnosed each year (26). Four types of diabetes are recognized based on etiologic origin: type 1, type 2, gestational (i.e., diagnosed during pregnancy), and other specific origins (i.e., genetic defects and drug induced); however, most patients have type 2 (90% of all cases) followed by type 1 (5%–10% of all cases) (14).

Type 1 diabetes mellitus is most often caused by the autoimmune destruction of the insulin producing β cells of the pancreas, although some cases are idiopathic in origin. The primary characteristics of patients with type 1 diabetic mellitus are absolute insulin deficiency and a high propensity for ketoacidosis. Type 2 diabetes mellitus is caused by insulin resistance with an insulin secretory defect. Type 2 diabetes mellitus is associated with excess body fat. A common feature of type 2 diabetes is an upper-body fat distribution regardless of the amount of total body fat (9). In contrast to type 1 diabetes mellitus, type 2 is often associated with elevated insulin concentrations.

The fundamental goal for the management of diabetes mellitus is glycemic control using diet, exercise, and, in many cases, medications such as insulin or oral hypoglycemic agents (Appendix A, Common Medications). Intensive treatment to control blood glucose reduces the risk of progression of diabetic complications in adults with type 1 and type 2 diabetes mellitus (14). The criteria for

TABLE 10.2. DIAGNOSTIC CRITERIA FOR DIABETES MELLITUS

NORMAL	PREDIABETES	DIABETES MELLITUS
Fasting plasma glucose <100 mg · dL^{-1} (5.55 mmol · L^{-1})	IFG = Fasting plasma glucose 100 mg · dL^{-1} (5.55 mmol · L^{-1})– 125 mg · dL^{-1} (6.94 mmol · L^{-1}) IGT = 2-h plasma glucose 140 mg · dL^{-1} (7.77 mmol · L^{-1})– 199 mg/dL (11.04 mmol·L^{-1}) during an OGTT	Symptomatic with casual glucose ≥200 mg · dL^{-1} (11.10 mmol · L^{-1}) Fasting plasma glucose ≥126 mg · dL^{-1} (6.99 mmol·L^{-1}) 2-h plasma glucose ≥200 mg · dL^{-1} (11.10 mmol·L^{-1}) during an OGTT

IFG, impaired fasting glucose (at least 8 h); IGT, impaired glucose tolerance; OGTT, oral glucose tolerance test.

Adapted from American Diabetes Association. Standards of medical care in diabetes—2007. *Diabetes Care.* 2007;30:S4–41.

diagnosis of diabetes mellitus (14) are presented in Table 10.2. Prediabetes is a risk factor for future diabetes mellitus and atherosclerotic cardiovascular disease (CVD). Glycosylated hemoglobin (HbA$_{1C}$) reflects mean blood glucose control over the past 2 to 3 months with a general patient goal of <7%. HbA$_{1C}$ may be used as an additional blood chemistry test for patients with diabetis mellitus to provide information on long-term glycemic control (9). However, it is not recommended at the present time as a screening tool for diabetes mellitus.

EXERCISE TESTING

The special considerations for exercise testing people with diabetes mellitus are listed below.

- Before beginning an exercise program, patients with diabetes mellitus should undergo an extensive medical evaluation, particularly of the cardiovascular, nervous, renal, and visual systems to identify related diabetic complications.
- When beginning an exercise program of low to moderate intensity (i.e., physical activities that increase HR and breathing), exercise testing may not be necessary for individuals with diabetes mellitus who are asymptomatic for CVD and low risk (<10% risk of cardiac event over a 10-year period) (106) (Tables 2.2 and 2.4).
- People with diabetes mellitus with ≥10% risk of a cardiac event over a 10-year period and who want to begin a vigorous-intensity exercise program (i.e., ≥60% $\dot{V}O_2R$ that substantially increases HR and breathing) should undergo a medically supervised graded exercise test (GXT) with electrographic (ECG) monitoring (14).
- Patients with an abnormal exercise ECG and those unable to perform a GXT for various reasons—such as deconditioning, peripheral artery disease (PAD), orthopedic disabilities, and neurologic diseases—may require a radionuclide stress test or stress echocardiography (14).
- Autonomic neuropathy in people with diabetes mellitus increases the likelihood of CVD. Patients with this complication wanting to engage in any activity at an intensity greater than they are accustomed to should undergo a thorough cardiac screening, including thallium scintigraphy (95).

- Current guidelines to detect CVD in patients with diabetes mellitus often fail to detect silent ischemia (113). Consequently, annual CVD risk-factor identification should be conducted by a healthcare provider (14).

EXERCISE PRESCRIPTION

The benefits of regular exercise in patients with type 2 diabetes mellitus include improved glucose tolerance, increased insulin sensitivity, decreased HbA_{1C}, and decreased insulin requirements. Additional exercise benefits for people with type 1 and type 2 diabetes mellitus include improvement in CVD risk factors (i.e., lipid profiles, BP, body weight, and functional capacity) and well being (9,14). Regular exercise participation may also prevent type 2 diabetes mellitus in those considered at high risk (i.e., prediabetic) for developing the disease (59) (Table 10.2).

The general recommendations for exercise prescription apply to people with diabetes mellitus (Chapter 7). However, the reasons for participating in an exercise program may differ among those with type 1 and type 2 diabetes mellitus. For example, a primary purpose for a person with type 1 diabetes mellitus to undertake an exercise program is often cardiovascular health/fitness related; whereas for a person with type 2 diabetes mellitus, the primary purposes are often healthy weight loss maintenance and improved glucose disposal. See the other sections of Chapter 10 for more specific information on how the exercise prescription should be adapted for these various diseases and conditions should they be present. The aerobic exercise training exercise prescription recommendations for those with diabetes mellitus follow.

Frequency: 3–7 d · wk^{-1}

Intensity: 50%–80% $\dot{V}O_2R$ or HRR corresponding to a rating of perceived exertion (RPE) of 12 to 16 on a 6 to 20 scale (23)

Time: 20–60 min · d^{-1} continuous or accumulated in bouts of at least 10 minutes to total 150 minutes per week of moderate physical activity with additional benefits of increasing to 300 minutes or more of moderate-intensity physical activity.

Type: Emphasize activities that use large muscle groups in a rhythmic and continuous fashion. Personal interest and desired goals of the exercise program should be considered.

Resistance training should be encouraged for people with diabetes mellitus in the absence of contraindications (Chapters 2 and 3), retinopathy, and recent laser treatments. The recommendations for healthy persons generally apply to persons with diabetes mellitus (10) (Chapter 7). An optimal resistance-training program should include the following components (14).

Frequency: 2–3 d · wk^{-1} with at least 48 hours separating the exercise sessions

Intensity: 2 to 3 sets of 8 to 12 repetitions at 60% to 80% 1-RM

Time: 8 to 10 multijoint exercises of all major muscle groups in the same session (whole body) or sessions split into selected muscle groups

Type: Given that many patients may present with comorbidities, it may be necessary to tailor the resistance-exercise prescription accordingly. Emphasize proper technique, including minimizing sustained gripping, static work, and the Valsalva manuever to prevent an exacerbated BP response.

Those without contraindications for exercise (Chapters 2 and 3) should strive to accumulate a minimum of 1,000 kcal $\cdot$ wk^{-1} either through 150 min $\cdot$ wk^{-1} of moderate-intensity (40%–60% $\dot{V}O_2R$ or 55%–70% age-predicted maximum heart rate [HR$_{max}$]) or 90 min $\cdot$ wk^{-1} of vigorous-intensity ($\geq$60% $\dot{V}O_2R$ or $\geq$70% HR$_{max}$) exercise, or some combination of moderate- and vigorous-intensity physical activity for health/fitness benefits (14). Moreover, no more than two consecutive days of physical inactivity per week should be allowed. A greater emphasis should eventually be placed on vigorous-intensity exercise if cardiovascular fitness is a primary goal. On the other hand, greater amounts of moderate-intensity exercise that result in a caloric energy expenditure of $\geq$2,000 kcal $\cdot$ wk^{-1}, including daily exercise, may be required if weight loss maintanence is the goal, as is the case for most people with type 2 diabetes mellitus (5). See Chapter 10 and the ACSM position stand (5) on overweight and obesity and the metabolic syndrome, and the American Diabetes Association (ADA) standards of care (14) for additional information.

Special Considerations

- Hypoglycemia is the most common problem for people with diabetes mellitus who exercise and is usually only a concern in individuals taking insulin or oral hypoglycemic agents (14) (Appendix A). Hypoglycemia, defined as blood glucose level <70 mg $\cdot$ dL^{-1} (<3.89 mmol $\cdot$ L^{-1}), is relative (14). Rapid drops in blood glucose may occur with exercise and render patients symptomatic even in elevated glycemic states. Common symptoms associated with hypoglycemia include shakiness, weakness, abnormal sweating, nervousness, anxiety, tingling of the mouth and fingers, and hunger. Neuroglycopenic symptoms may include headache, visual disturbances, mental dullness, confusion, amnesia, seizures, and coma (2).
- Blood glucose monitoring before and following exercise, especially when beginning or modifying the exercise program, is prudent.
- The timing of exercise should be considered in individuals taking insulin or hypoglycemic agents. Exercise is not recommended during peak insulin action because hypoglycemia may result. Moreover, given the risk of a delayed postexercise hypoglycemia, exercise before bed is not recommended. However, if exercising late in the evening is necessary, an increased consumption of carbohydrates may be required to minimize the risk of nocturnal hypoglycemia. When possible, scheduling similar timing of exercise into the daily routine may be beneficial to minimize potential hypoglycemic events.
- Adjust carbohydrate intake and/or medications before and after exercise based on blood glucose levels and exercise intensity to prevent hypoglycemia associated with exercise (95). If pre- or postexercise blood glucose is <100 mg $\cdot$ dL^{-1} (<5.55 mmol $\cdot$ L^{-1}), 20 to 30 g of additional carbohydrates should be ingested.
- Avoid injecting insulin into exercising limbs. Use an abdominal injection site instead to lower the risk of hypoglycemia associated with exercise.

- Exercise with a partner or under supervision to reduce the risk of problems associated with hypoglycemic events.
- Hyperglycemia with or without ketosis is a concern for people with type 1 diabetes mellitus who are not in glycemic control. Common symptoms associated with hyperglycemia include polyuria, fatigue, weakness, increased thirst, and acetone breath (2). Patients who present with hyperglycemia, provided they feel well and have *no* ketone bodies present in either the blood or urine, may exercise, but they should refrain from vigorous-intensity exercise (14,95).
- Dehydration resulting from polyuria, a common occurrence of hyperglycemia, may contribute to a compromised thermoregulatory response (110). Thus, a patient with hyperglycemia should be treated as having an elevated risk for heat illness requiring more frequent monitoring of signs and symptoms. Please see Chapter 8 and the ACSM positions stands (6,11) for additional information on exercising in the heat and fluid replacement.
- Patients with diabetes mellitus and retinopathy are at risk for retinal detachment and vitreous hemorrhage associated with vigorous-intensity exercise. However, risk may be minimized by avoiding activities that dramatically elevate BP. Thus, for those with severe nonproliferative and proliferative diabetic retinopathy, vigorous-intensity aerobic and resistance exercise should be avoided (14,95).
- During exercise, autonomic neuropathy may cause chronotropic incompetence, a blunted systolic blood pressure (SBP) response, attenuated $\dot{V}O_2$ kinetics, and anhydrosis (14,110). In this situation, the following should be considered:
  - Monitor the signs and symptoms of hypoglycemia because of the inability of the patient to recognize them. Also, monitor the signs and symptoms of silent ischemia because of the inability to perceive angina.
  - Monitor BP following exercise to manage hypotension and hypertension associated with vigorous-intensity exercise (110). See this chapter's exercise prescription recommendations for those with hypertension for additional information.
  - The HR and BP responses to exercise may be blunted. RPE should also be used to assess exercise intensity (110).
- Given the likelihood that thermoregulation in hot and cold environments is impaired (14), additional precautions for heat and cold illness are warranted. See Chapter 8 and the ACSM positions stands (6,11,13) on environmental considerations for additional information.
- For the patient with peripheral neuropathy, take proper care of the feet to prevent foot ulcers (14). Special precautions should be taken to prevent blisters on the feet. Feet should be kept dry and the use of silica gel or air midsoles as well as polyester or blend socks should be used. Consider non–weight-bearing activities such as cycling because they may be better tolerated and aid healing.
- For the patient with nephropathy (14), although protein excretion acutely increases postexercise, there is no evidence that vigorous-intensity exercise accelerates the rate of progression of kidney disease. Although there are no current exercise intensity restrictions for patients with diabetic nephropathy, it is prudent to encourage sustainable exercise programming, which more likely includes tolerable moderate intensities.

- Because a majority of people with diabetes mellitus will be overweight, see this chapter and the ACSM position stand (5) on overweight and obesity and the metabolic syndrome for additional information.
- Because a majority of people with diabetes mellitus will develop or have CVD, see Chapter 9 on exercise prescription for those with cardiac disease for additional information.

DISABILITIES

CEREBRAL PALSY

Cerebral palsy (CP) is a nonprogressive lesion of the brain occurring before, at, or soon after birth that interferes with normal brain development. CP is caused by damage to areas of the brain that control and coordinate muscle tone, reflexes, posture, and movement. The resulting impact on muscle tone and reflexes depend on the location and extent of the injury within the brain. Consequently, type and severity of dysfunction varies considerably between individuals with CP. In developed countries the incidence of CP is reported to be between 1.5 and 5 live births per 1,000.

Despite its diverse manifestations, CP predominantly exists in two forms: spastic (70% of those with CP) (63) and athetoid (102). Spastic CP is characterized by an increased muscle tone typically involving the flexor muscle groups of the upper extremity (e.g., biceps brachialis and pronator teres) and extensor muscle groups of the lower extremities (e.g., quadriceps femoris and triceps surae). The antagonistic muscles of the hypertonic muscles are usually weak. Spasticity is a dynamic condition decreasing with slow stretching, warm external temperature, and good positioning. However, quick movements, cold external temperature, fatigue, and emotional stress increase hypertonicity. Athetoid CP is characterized by involuntary and/or uncontrolled movement that occurs primarily in the extremities. These extraneous movements may increase with effort and emotional stress.

CP can further be categorized topographically (e.g., quadriplegia, diplegia, and hemiplegia); however, in the context of exercise prescription, a functional classification as developed by the Cerebral Palsy International Sport and Recreation Association (CP-ISRA) is more relevant (29). CP-ISRA has developed an eight-part comprehensive classification scheme for sports participation based on the degree of neuromotor function. Athletes are classified in eight classes, with class CP1 representing an athlete with severe spasticity and/or athetosis resulting in poor functional ROM and poor functional strength in all extremities and the trunk. The athlete will be dependent on a power wheelchair or assistance for mobility. An athlete in class CP8 will demonstrate minimal neuromuscular involvement and may appear to have near-normal function. See the CP-ISRA manual for a detailed description of classes of CP (29).

The variability in motor control pattern in CP is large and becomes even more complex because of the persistence of primitive reflexes. In normal motor development, reflexes appear, mature, and disappear, whereas other reflexes become controlled or mediated at a higher level (i.e., the cortex). In CP, primitive reflexes (e.g., the palmar and tonic labyrinthine reflexes) may persist, and higher-level reflex activity (i.e., postural reflexes) may be delayed or absent. Severely involved individuals with CP may primarily move in reflex patterns, whereas those with mild involvement may be only hindered by reflexes during extreme effort or emotional stress (63).

Exercise Testing

The hallmark of CP is disordered motor control; however, CP is often associated with other sensory (e.g., vision or hearing impairment) or cognitive (e.g., intellectual disability or perceptual motor disorder) disabilities that may limit participation as much as or perhaps more than the motor limitations (31). Convulsive seizures (i.e., epilepsy) is an associated condition that may interfere significantly with exercise testing and programming in people with CP, occurring in about 25% of the CP population.

People with CP have decreased physical fitness levels compared with their able-bodied peers. The limited investigation in this area has focused almost entirely on children and adolescents and tends to involve only persons with minimal or moderate involvement (i.e., those who are ambulatory) (32,33,85,102). When exercise testing individuals with CP, consider the following issues.

- Initially, a functional assessment should be taken of the trunk and upper- and lower-extremity involvement that includes measures of ROM, flexibility, and balance. This assessment will facilitate the choice of exercise testing equipment, protocols, and adaptations. Medical clearance should be sought before any physical fitness testing.
- All testing should be conducted using adaptive equipment, such as straps and holding gloves, and guarantee safety and optimal testing conditions for mechanical efficiency.
- The testing mode used to assess cardiovascular physical fitness is dependent on the functional capacity of the person and—if an athlete with CP—the desired sport. In general:
  - Arm cranking and cycling ergometry are preferred for people with athetoid CP because of the benefit of moving in a closed chain.
  - In CP1 individuals, minimal efforts result in work levels that are above the anaerobic threshold and in some instances may be maximal efforts so that aerobic conditioning will not be possible.
  - In CP3 and CP4 individuals with good functional strength and minimal coordination problems in the upper extremities and trunk, wheelchair ergometry is recommended.
  - In CP5 to CP8 individuals who are ambulatory, treadmill ergometry may be recommended, but care should be taken at the final stages of the protocol when fatigue occurs and the athlete's walking or running skill may deteriorate.
- Because of the heterogeneity of the CP population, a maximal exercise test protocol can not be generalized. It is recommended to test the new participant at two or three submaximal levels, starting with a minimal power output, before determining the maximal exercise protocol.

- Maximal cardiovascular physical fitness testing should involve submaximal steady-state workloads at levels comparable with sporting conditions. Movement during these submaximal workloads should be controlled to optimize economy of movement (i.e., mechanical efficiency). For example, with cycle ergometry, the choice of resistance or gearing is extremely important in people with CP. Whereas some individuals will benefit from a combination of low resistance and high segmental velocity, others will have optimal economy of movement with a high resistance, low segmental velocity combination.
- In people with moderate and severe CP, motion is considered a series of discrete bursts of activity. Hence, the assessment of anaerobic power derived from the Wingate anaerobic test gives a good indication of the performance potential of the individual.
- In people with athetoid CP, strength tests should be performed through movement in a closed chain (e.g., exercise machines that control the path of the movement). Always check the impact of primitive reflexes on performance (i.e., position of head, trunk, and proximal joints of the extremities) and whether there is enough control to exercise with free weights.
- Results from any exercise test in the same person with CP may vary considerably from day to day because of fluctuations in muscle tone.

Exercise Prescription

In principle, for the person with CP, the exercise prescription guidelines for the general population should be applied (10,47) (Chapter 7). However, because of the impact of CP on the neuromotor function, the following considerations should be noted.

- The Frequency, Intensity, Time (duration), and Type of exercise (or FITT framework) for health/fitness benefits in persons with CP are unknown. Even though the design of exercise training programs to enhance health/fitness benefits should be based on the same principles as the general population, modifications to the training protocol may have to be made based on the person's functional mobility level, number and type of associated conditions, and degree of involvement of each limb (88).
- Because of lack of movement control, energy expenditure is high even at low power-output levels. In people with severe involvement (CP1 and CP2), aerobic exercise programs should start with frequent but short bouts of moderate intensity (i.e., 40%–50% $\dot{V}O_2R$). Recovery periods should begin each time the moderate-intensity level is exceeded. Progressively, exercise bouts should be extended to reach an intensity of 50% to 85% $\dot{V}O_2R$ for a duration of 20 minutes. Because of poor economy of movement, some CP1 individuals will not be able to work at submaximal levels over these longer periods of time, so that shorter durations that can be accumulated should be considered.
- In CP3 to CP8 individuals, aerobic exercise training should follow the guidelines for the general population (10,47) (Chapter 7). Cycling with a tricycle to facilitate balance for the lower extremities and hand cycling for the upper extremities are recommended because (a) they allow for a wide range of

power output, (b) movements occur in a closed chain, (c) muscle contraction velocity can be changed without changing the power output through the use of resistance or gears, and (d) there is minimal risk for injuries caused by lack of movement or balance control.

- Persons with CP fatigue easily because of poor economy of movement. Fatigue has a disastrous effect on hypertonic muscles and will further deteriorate the voluntary movement patterns. Training sessions will be more effective, particularly for athletes with high muscle tone, if (a) several short training sessions are conducted rather than one longer session, (b) relaxation and stretching routines are included throughout the session, and (c) new skills are introduced early in the session.

- Resistance training increases strength in people with CP without an adverse effect on muscle tone (33,84). Emphasize the role of flexibility training in conjunction with any resistance-training program designed for people with CP.

- Resistive exercises designed to target weak muscle groups that oppose hypertonic muscle groups improve the strength of the weak muscle group and normalize the tone in the opposing hypertonic muscle group through reciprocal inhibition. For example, slow concentric elbow extensor activity will normalize the tone in a hypertonic elbow flexor. Other techniques, such as neuromuscular electrical stimulation (84) and whole-body vibration (1), increase muscle strength without negative effects on spasticity.

- Dynamic strengthening exercises over the full ROM that are executed at slow contraction speed to avoid stretch reflex activity in the opposing muscles are recommended.

- Hypertonic muscles should be stretched slowly to their limits throughout the workout program to maintain length. Ballistic stretching should be avoided.

Special Considerations

- In young participants, activities that are in conflict with rehabilitation programs should be avoided. Generally the focus with young people is on inhibiting abnormal reflex activity, normalizing muscle tone, and developing reactions to increase equilibrium. The focus with adolescents and adults is more likely to be on functional outcomes and performance. Experienced athletes will learn to use hyperactive stretch reflexes and primitive reflexes to better execute sport-specific tasks.

- During growth, hypertonicity in the muscles—and consequently, muscle balance around the joints—may change significantly because of inadequate adaptations in muscle length. Training programs should be adapted continuously to accommodate these changing conditions (84). Medical interventions, such as Botox injections, a medication which decreases spasticity, may drastically change the functional potential of the individual.

- Good positioning of the head, trunk, and proximal joints of extremities to control persistent primitive reflexes is preferred to strapping. Inexpensive modifications that enable good position, such as Velcro gloves to attach the hands to the equipment, should be used whenever needed.

- Persons with CP are more susceptible to overuse injuries because of their higher incidence of inactivity and associated conditions (i.e., hypertonicity, contractures, and joint pain) (1).

SPINAL CORD INJURIES

Spinal cord injury results in an incomplete to complete loss of somatic, sensory, and autonomic functions below the lesion level. Lesions in the cervical (C) region typically result in quadriplegia, whereas lesions in the thoracic (T) and lumbar (L) regions lead to paraplegia. Approximately 50% of those with spinal cord injury have quadriplegia, and 80% are male (97). Spinal cord injury of traumatic origin is often incurred at an early age. People with spinal cord injury have a high risk for the development of secondary complications (e.g., urinary tract infections, pressure ulcers, CVD, obesity, and type 2 diabetes mellitus). Exercise and sports participation reduces the prevalence of secondary complications and improves the quality of life among individuals with spinal cord injury.

The spinal cord injury level has a direct impact on physical function and the cardiopulmonary and metabolic response to exercise. When exercise testing and prescribing exercise for those with spinal cord injury, it is crucial to take into account the spinal cord injury lesion level. Those with spinal cord lesions from:

- L2–sacral (S) 2 lack voluntary control of the bladder, bowels, and sexual function; however, the trunk has maximal range of motion.
- T6–L2 have respiratory and motor control that depends on the functional capacity of the abdominal muscles (i.e., minimal control at T6 to maximal control at L2).
- T1–T6 experience autonomic dysreflexia (i.e., an uncoordinated, spinally mediated reflex response called the "mass reflex"), poor thermoregulation, and orthostatic hypotension. In instances in which there is no sympathetic innervation to the heart, HR_{max} is limited to ~115 to 130 beats $\cdot$ min^{-1}. Breathing capacity is further diminished because of intercostal muscle paralysis; however, arm function is normal.
- C5–8 are quadriplegic. Those with C8 lesions have voluntary control of the shoulder, elbow, and wrist, but minimized hand function; whereas those with C5 lesions rely on the biceps brachialis and shoulder muscles for manual wheelchair propulsion.
- C4 require artificial support for breathing.

Exercise Testing

When exercise testing individuals with spinal cord injury, consider the following issues.

- Initially, a functional assessment should be taken, including trunk ROM, wheelchair mobility, transfer ability, and upper- and lower-extremity involvement. This assessment will facilitate the choice of exercise testing equipment, protocols, and adaptations.

- Body mass index (BMI) is prone to measurement error, does not adequately discriminate between those with obesity and those who are normal weight, and is not as accurately correlated with percent fat mass and CVD risk factors as in able-bodied populations (24). Skinfold prediction equations systematically underestimate percent body fat in individuals with spinal cord injury. Therefore, skinfold measurements should be made separately and include sublesion regions.
- Consider the purposes of the exercise test, the level of spinal cord injury lesion, and the physical fitness level of the participant to optimize equipment and protocol selection.
- Voluntary arm cranking ergometry is the easiest to perform and norm referenced for the assessment of cardiovascular physical fitness (45). This form of exercise testing, however, is not wheelchair-propulsion-sport specific, and the equipment is not accurate in the lower work rate ranges needed for quadriplegics (i.e., 0–50 W).
- Stationary wheelchair roller systems and motor-driven treadmills should be used with the participant's proper wheelchair. Motor-driven treadmill protocols allow for realistic simulation of external conditions, such as slope and speed alterations (109).
- Incremental exercise tests for the assessment of cardiovascular physical fitness in the laboratory should begin at 0 W with increment increases of 5 to 10 W per stage among quadriplegics; among paraplegics, begin at 30 to 40 W with increment increases of 10 to 15 W per stage.
- For sport-specific indoor cardiovascular physical fitness assessments in the field, an incremental test adapted from the Léger and Boucher shuttle run test around a predetermined rectangular court is recommended. Floor surface characteristics and wheelchair user interface should be standardized (109).
- There are no special considerations for the assessment of muscular strength regarding the exercise testing mode beyond those for the general population with the exception of the lesion level and mode of locomotion. See Chapter 7 on exercise prescription recommendations for resistance training for additional information.
- Individuals with spinal cord injury requiring a wheelchair for locomotion may develop contractures because of their position in the wheelchair (i.e., hip flexors/adductors and knee flexors) and excessive wheelchair pushing (i.e., the anterior shoulder). Therefore, intensive sport-specific training should be complemented with a stretching (e.g., the prime movers) and strengthening (e.g., the antagonists) program to promote muscular balance around the joints.

Exercise Prescription/Special Considerations

In principle, the exercise prescription guidelines for the general population should be applied (10,47) (Chapter 7). For this reason and because of the impact of spinal cord injury on neuromotor, cardiopulmonary, and metabolic function, exercise prescription recommendations and special considerations are combined in this section and are listed below.

- Participants should empty their urinary bag before exercising because autonomic dysreflexia can be triggered by a full bladder or bowel distension.
- Pressure sores should be avoided at all times and potential risk areas should be checked on a regular basis.
- Decreased cardiovascular performance may be found in individuals with complete spinal cord lesions above T6, particularly among individuals with complete quadriplegia who have no sympathetic innervation to the heart with HR_{max} limited to ~115 to 130 beats·min^{-1}. Individuals with high spinal lesions may reach their maximum HR, cardiac output ($\dot{Q}$), and oxygen uptake ($\dot{V}O_2$) at lower exercise levels than paraplegics with injuries below T5–6 (53).
- During exercise, autonomic dysreflexia results in an increased release of catecholamines that increases exercise capacity, HR, $\dot{V}O_2$, and BP (94). In some instances, BP may be elevated to levels high enough to produce a stroke (i.e., SBP 250–300 mm Hg and/or diastolic blood pressure [DBP] 200–220 mm Hg). In these situations, immediate response is needed (i.e., stopping exercise, sitting straight to decrease BP, and identifying and removing the irritating stimulus such as a catheter, leg bag, tight clothing, or braces). If the symptoms (i.e., headaches, piloerection, sweating above the lesion level, stuffy nose, and bradycardia) persist, medical attention should be sought. In international competition, athletes with a resting SBP $\geq$180 mm Hg should not be allowed to start the event.
- Novice and unfit participants will suffer from peripheral fatigue before any central training effect is achieved. Initially, the exercise sessions should consist of short bouts of 5 to 10 minutes of moderate intensity (i.e., 40%–50% $\dot{V}O_2R$) alternated with active recovery periods of 5 minutes.
- Quadriplegics have a minimal amount of active musculature and will experience peripheral fatigue before central fatigue occurs. Aerobic exercise programs should progress over time from short bouts of 5 to 10 minutes of moderate intensity (i.e., 40%–50% $\dot{V}O_2R$) alternated with active recovery periods of 5 minutes of vigorous intensity (i.e., 85%–90% $\dot{V}O_2R$) performed for 10 to 20 minutes.
- Beneficial hemodynamic effects (i.e., lower HR and higher stroke volume [SV]) of lower-body positive pressure on the legs by applying stockings and an abdominal binder during arm work compensate for blood pooling below the lesion. This benefit seems to be related to the level of spinal cord injury, with quadriplegics responding best to lower-body positive pressure. Also, functional neuromuscular stimulation of the paralyzed lower limbs (87) increases venous return. However, this response only occurs in individuals classified as responders (i.e., those for whom stimulation intensities can be set high enough to induce static or dynamic contractions). No such effects were found in more pain-sensitive nonresponders or in able-bodied individuals.
- Muscle strength-training sessions from a seated position in the wheelchair should be complemented with nonwheelchair exercise bouts to involve all trunk-stabilizing muscles. However, transfers (e.g., from wheelchair to the exercise apparatus) should be limited as they result in a significant hemodynamic load and increase the glenohumeral contact forces and the risk of repetitive-strain injuries, especially in quadriplegics (108). Special attention

should be given to muscle imbalance and the prevention of repetitive-strain injuries. The prime movers of wheelchair propulsion should be lengthened (i.e., muscles of the anterior shoulder), and antagonists should be strengthened (i.e., muscles of the upper back and posterior shoulder).

- Tenodesis allows quadriplegics who do not have use of the hand muscles to functionally grasp (i.e., to passively pull the fingers into flexion by extending the wrist). These individuals must never stretch the finger flexor muscles to keep the tenodesis effect intact (i.e., maximal and simultaneous extension of wrist and fingers should be avoided).

- Persons with spinal cord injuries tend to endure higher core temperatures during endurance exercise than their able-bodied counterparts. Despite this enhanced thermoregulatory drive, they generally have lower sweat rates. The following factors reduce heat tolerance and should be avoided: lack of acclimatization, dehydration, glycogen depletion, sleep loss, alcohol, and infectious disease. During training and competition, the use of light clothing, ice vests, protective sun cream, and mist spray is recommended (6,11).

DYSLIPIDEMIA

When genetic, environmental or pathologic conditions abnormally alter blood lipid and lipoprotein concentrations, the condition is known as *dyslipidemia* (i.e., abnormal blood lipid and lipoprotein levels). See Table 3.2 for the National Cholesterol Education Program (NCEP) blood lipid and lipoprotein classification scheme. Although severe forms of dyslipidemia are linked to genetic defects in cholesterol metabolism, less severe cases may result in response to other diseases (e.g., diabetes mellitus) or as a result of combining a specific genetic pattern with various environmental exposures (e.g., diet, exercise, and smoking). Dyslipidemia is a major modifiable cause of CVD (68).

Improvements in cholesterol awareness and more effective treatments are responsible for the decline in the prevalence of elevated blood cholesterol levels in recent years. These improvements have contributed to a 30% decline in CVD (100). Recent clinical trials indicate the added value of cholesterol-lowering therapy in high-risk individuals (Chapters 2 and 3), people with diabetes mellitus, and older persons with a treatment goal to lower baseline low-density lipoprotein cholesterol (LDL-C) concentrations by 30% to 40% (44). Current detection, evaluation, and treatment guidelines for dyslipidemia are available in the updated NCEP Adult Treatment Panel (ATP) III report (44) (Chapter 3). The NCEP ATP III report recognizes the importance of lifestyle modification in the treatment of dyslipidemia (68). These recommendations include increased physical activity and weight reduction if warranted.

Although exercise has been shown to improve lipid profiles in many individuals, these changes are not universal, particularly among patients with dyslipidemia. Nevertheless, exercise is valued for controlling other CVD risk factors and should be a primary component to leading a healthy lifestyle. The ACSM makes the following recommendations regarding exercise testing and training of persons with dyslipidemia.

EXERCISE TESTING

- Individuals with dyslipidemia should be screened and risk stratified before exercise testing (Chapters 2 and 3).
- Use caution when testing patients with dyslipidemia because underlying CVD may be present.
- Standard exercise testing methods and protocols are appropriate for use with patients with dyslipidemia cleared for exercise testing. Special consideration should be given to the presence of other conditions (e.g., the metabolic syndrome, obesity, and hypertension) that may require modifications to standard exercise testing protocols and modalities. See other sections of Chapter 10 for additional information on exercise testing individuals with these diseases and conditions.
- Alternative testing modes may be required if the individual has xanthomas (i.e., a macrophage containing lipid material) that cause biomechanical problems.

EXERCISE PRESCRIPTION

The exercise prescription for individuals with dyslipidemia without comorbities is very similar to an exercise prescription for healthy adults (10,47) (Chapter 7). A major difference in the exercise prescription for patients with dyslipidemia as compared with healthy adults is that healthy weight maintenance should be emphasized. Accordingly, aerobic exercise becomes the foundation of the exercise prescription. Resistance and flexibility exercises are adjunct to an aerobic training program designed for the treatment of dyslipidemia primarily because these modes of exercise do not substantially contribute to the overall caloric expenditure goals that appear to be beneficial for improvements in blood lipid and lipoprotein concentrations. Additionally, the evidence is limited suggesting that resistance exercise improves lipid profiles (38). The FITT framework recommended for people with dylipidemia are listed below.

Frequency: ≥ 5 d $\cdot$ wk^{-1} to maximize caloric expenditure

Intensity: 40% to 75% $\dot{V}O_2R$ or HRR

Time: 30–60 min $\cdot$ d^{-1}. However, to promote or maintain weight loss, 50–60 min $\cdot$ d^{-1} or more of daily exercise is recommended (5). Performance of intermittent exercise of at least 10 minutes in duration to accumulate these duration recommendations is an effective alternative to continuous exercise.

Type: The primary mode should be aerobic physical activities that involve the large muscle groups. As part of a balanced exercise program, resistance-training exercise should be incorporated. People with dyslipidemia without comorbidities may follow the resistance-training guidelines for healthy adults (Chapter 7).

These FITT recommendations for people with dyslipidemia are consistent with the recommendations for healthy weight loss maintenance of 200–300 min $\cdot$ wk^{-1} that results in an energy expenditure of $\geq 2,000$ kcal $\cdot$ wk^{-1} (5). See this chapter on exercise prescription recommendations for people with the metabolic syndrome and overweight and obesity for additional information.

Special Considerations

- The exercise prescription may need to be modified should the patient present with other conditions, such as the metabolic syndrome, obesity, and hypertension. See this chapter for additional information on exercise testing individuals with these diseases and conditions.
- Individuals taking lipid-lowering medications that have the potential to cause muscle damage (i.e., HMG CoA reductase inhibitors or statins and fibric acid) may experience muscle weakness and soreness termed *myalgia* (Appendix A). Physicians should be consulted if the patient experiences unusual muscle soreness when exercising while taking these medications.
- Improvement in blood lipids and lipoproteins with aerobic exercise training may take several weeks to months depending on a variety of factors, including initial blood lipid and lipoprotein levels, weekly caloric expenditure, and the blood lipid parameter that is being targeted with exercise training (38).

HUMAN IMMUNODEFICIENCY VIRUS

Human Immunodeficiency virus (HIV) is a cytopathic retrovirus that may lead to acquired immunodeficiency syndrome (AIDS). Prevalence rates of HIV infection among adults differ widely, from near 0% in Norway to 0.3% in the United States to greater than 25% in some African countries. The severity of HIV/AIDS may be assessed using a measure of immune function (i.e., a low immune cell count [CD4] <200 cells $\cdot$ mL^{-1} indicates active AIDS). Complex treatment regimes (i.e., highly active antiretroviral therapy [HAART]) have greatly reduced HIV-associated mortality; however, patients now frequently present with chronic health impairments and disabilities (76,77). HAART improves immune status, reduces muscle wasting, and increases survival but results in lipodystrophy (i.e., abnormal distributions of body fat and elevated blood lipid levels) and may increase the risk of cardiovascular dysfunction and CVD (112,116). Hypertension, osteopenia, opportunistic infections, and insulin resistance may remain or become elevated in the presence of HAART (112,116). Persistent weight loss is still observed in some patients despite HAART. Additional treatment options include dietary interventions, anabolic steroids, growth hormone, and growth factors (116).

Aerobic and resistance exercise provide important health benefits for patients with HIV/AIDS. Improved psychological status (i.e., enhanced body image and quality of life) and reduced lipodystrophy results from aerobic training and improved body composition from resistance training (76,77). Regular participation in moderate-intensity exercise does not adversely affect immune function (77,93).

EXERCISE TESTING

The increased prevalence of cardiovascular pathology, metabolic disorders, and the complex medication routines of patients with HIV/AIDS require physician consultation before exercise testing. The following list of issues should be considered.

- Exercise testing should be postponed in patients with acute infections.
- When conducting cardiopulmonary exercise tests, infection control measures should be employed (57). Transmission of the virus through saliva has

not been observed. Increased prevalence of infectious agents, including respiratory pathogens, makes use of measures such as disposable equipment advisable.

- The increased prevalence of cardiovascular impairments requires monitoring of BP and ECG.
- Maximal muscle strength testing or alternatively testing to determine the maximum weight lifted over four to eight repetitions may be used to establish a resistance-training regime.

EXERCISE PRESCRIPTION

The impairments and activity limitations experienced by patients with HIV/AIDS may be improved with habitual exercise participation. The varied presentation of patients requires a flexible approach. However, a combined program of aerobic and resistive exercise as outlined below is recommended (76,77,93).

Frequency: Aerobic exercise 3–4 $d \cdot wk^{-1}$; resistance exercise 2–3 $d \cdot wk^{-1}$

Intensity: Aerobic exercise: 40% to <60% $\dot{V}O_2R$ or HRR to avoid possible immune suppression with more intense exercise. Resistance exercise: select a weight that can be lifted 8 to 10 repetitions before failure for resistance training. Severe HIV/AIDS and presence of comorbidities will require further restriction of the intensity range.

Time: Aerobic and resistance exercise combined to total 30–60 $min \cdot d^{-1}$ that may be accumulated in shorter duration bouts if better tolerated. Resistance exercise should involve 10 to 12 muscle groups with 8 to 10 repetitions in 2 to 3 sets.

Type: Modality will vary with the health status and interests of the patient. Presence of osteopenia will require weight-bearing activities. Contact sports and high-risk sports are not recommended because of risk of bleeding.

Special Considerations

- There are no currently established guidelines regarding contraindications for exercise for patients with HIV/AIDS so that the guidelines in Chapters 2 and 3 should generally apply.
- Supervised exercise whether in the community or at home is recommended because of HIV/AIDS comorbidities.
- Asymptomatic patients with HIV may participate in more vigorous-intensity exercise than patients with lower cell counts and pronounced health impairments.
- Day-to-day variations in health may affect participation. General fatigue should not preclude participation, but dizziness, swollen joints, or vomiting should.
- Monitoring of progress of the health-related components of physical fitness and CVD risk factors is critical for clinical management and continued exercise participation.

HYPERTENSION

Approximately 65 million Americans have hypertension, which is defined as having a resting SBP ≥140 mm Hg and/or DBP ≥90 mm Hg, taking antihypertensive medication, or being told by a physician or other health professional on at least two occasions that a person has high BP (see Chapter 3, Table 3.1, for the BP classification scheme) (5). Hypertension leads to an increased risk of CVD, stroke, heart failure, PAD, and chronic kidney disease (7,15). BP readings as low as 115/75 mm Hg are associated with a higher-than-normal risk of ischemic heart disease and stroke. The risk of CVD doubles for each increment increase in SBP of 20 mm Hg or DBP of 10 mm Hg (69). The underlying cause of hypertension is not known in 90% of the cases (i.e., essential hypertension). In the other 5% to 10% of cases, hypertension is secondary to a variety of known diseases, including chronic kidney disease, coarctation of the aorta, Cushing syndrome, and pheochromocytoma (69).

Recommended lifestyle changes include the adoption of the Dietary Approaches to Stop Hypertension diet and participation in habitual physical activity that leads to reductions in body weight (69). There are a variety of medications that are effective in the treatment of hypertension (Appendix A). Most patients may need to be on at least two medications to achieve targeted BP levels (7).

EXERCISE TESTING

Individuals with hypertension are stratified into one of three risk groups (A, B, or C) depending upon their BP level and presence of other CVD risk factors, target organ damage, or clinical CVD (7) (see Chapter 3, Table 3.1, for BP classification scheme and the management of BP). Recommendations regarding exercise testing vary depending on the risk group to which the individual belongs.

- Individuals with hypertension should have a medical evaluation before exercise testing. The extent of the evaluation will vary depending on the exercise intensity to be performed and the clinical status of the individual being tested.
- Individuals with hypertension who plan to perform vigorous-intensity exercise (i.e., ≥60% $\dot{V}O_2R$) should have a medically supervised symptom-limited exercise test.
- For persons in asymptomatic risk group A or B (BP <180/110 mm Hg) who want to engage in light- or very-light- (i.e., <40% $\dot{V}O_2R$) to moderate-intensity activity (i.e., 40% to <60% $\dot{V}O_2R$), a symptom-limited GXT may not be necessary beyond the routine medical evaluation.
- Individuals in risk group C should have an exercise test before engaging in moderate-intensity exercise, but testing is not necessary before engaging in light- or very-light-intensity activity.
- Although formal evaluation is taking place, the majority of patients with hypertension may begin moderate-intensity aerobic exercise training.
- Resting SBP >200 mm Hg and/or DBP >110 mm Hg are contraindications to exercise testing (see Chapter 3 for contraindications to exercise testing).
- If the exercise test is for nondiagnostic purposes, individuals may take their prescribed medications at the recommended time. When testing is for

diagnostic purposes, BP medication may be withheld before testing with physician approval.
- Individuals on β blockers will have an attenuated HR response to exercise and reduced maximal exercise capacity. Individuals on diuretic therapy may experience hypokalemia, cardiac dysrhythmias, or potentially a false-positive exercise test.
- The exercise test should generally be stopped with SBP >250 mm Hg and/or DBP >115 mm Hg.

EXERCISE PRESCRIPTION

Aerobic exercise training leads to reductions in resting BP of 5 to 7 mm Hg in individuals with hypertension (7). Exercise training also lowers BP at fixed submaximal exercise workloads. Emphasis should be placed on aerobic activities; however, these may be supplemented with moderate-intensity resistance training. Flexibility exercise should be performed after a thorough warm-up and during the cool-down period. In persons with hypertension, the following exercise prescription is recommended.

Frequency: Aerobic exercise on most, preferably all days of the week; resistance exercise 2–3 d · wk^{-1}

Intensity: Moderate-intensity aerobic exercise (i.e., 40% to <60% $\dot{V}O_2R$) supplemented by resistance training at 60% to 80% 1-RM

Time: 30–60 min · d^{-1} of continuous or intermittent aerobic exercise. If intermittent, use a minimum of 10-minute bouts accumulated to total 30–60 min · d^{-1} of exercise. Resistance training should consist of at least one set of 8 to 12 repetitions.

Type: Emphasis should be placed on aerobic activities such as walking, jogging, cycling, and swimming. Resistance training using either machine weights or free weights may supplement aerobic training. Such training programs should consist of 8 to 10 different exercises targeting the major muscle groups. See Chapter 7 for additional information on resistance training.

Special Considerations

- Patients with severe or uncontrolled BP should add exercise training to their treatment plan only after first being evaluated by their physician and being prescribed antihypertensive medication.
- For patients with documented CVD, such as ischemic heart disease, heart failure, or stroke, vigorous-intensity exercise training is best initiated in rehabilitation centers under medical supervision. See Chapter 9 on exercise prescription recommendations for patients with cardiac disease for additional information.
- If resting SBP >200 mm Hg and/or DBP >110 mm Hg, do not exercise. When exercising, it appears prudent to maintain SBP ≤220 mm Hg and/or DBP ≤105 mm Hg).

- β-blockers and diuretics may adversely affect thermoregulatory function and cause hypoglycemia in some individuals. In these situations, educate patients about the signs and symptoms of heat intolerance (6,11) and hypoglycemia, and the precautions that should be taken to avoid these situations. See this chapter on exercise prescription recommendations for those with diabetes mellitus for additional information.
- β-blockers, particularly the nonselective types, may reduce submaximal and maximal exercise capacity primarily in patients without myocardial ischemia. Consider using perceived exertion to monitor exercise intensity in these individuals.
- Antihypertensive medications such as α-blockers, calcium channel blockers, and vasodilators may lead to sudden reductions in postexercise BP. Extend and monitor the cool-down period carefully in these situations.
- Many individuals with hypertension are overweight or obese. Exercise prescriptions for these individuals should focus on increasing caloric expenditure coupled with reducing caloric intake to facilitate weight reduction. See this chapter and the ACSM position stand (5) on exercise prescriptions recommendations for promoting and sustaining weight loss for additional information.
- A majority of older persons will have hypertension. Older people experience similar exercise-induced BP reductions as younger people. See Chapter 8, Nelson et al. (73), and the ACSM position stand (8) on exercise prescription recommendations for the older adults for additional information.
- The BP-lowering effects of aerobic exercise are immediate, a physiologic response referred to as *postexercise hypotension*. To enhance patient adherence, educate patients about the acute or immediate BP-lowering effects of exercise, although investigation is limited that education about acute BP effects of exercise will improve adherence.
- For individual with documented episodes of ischemia during exercise, the exercise intensity should be set ($\geq$10 beats $\cdot$ min^{-1}) below the ischemic threshold.
- Avoid the Valsalva maneuver during resistance training.

METABOLIC SYNDROME

The metabolic syndrome is characterized by a constellation of CVD risk factors (Chapters 2 and 3). Based on the NCEP ATP III Guidelines (68), the diagnosis of metabolic syndrome is made when at least three of the CVD risk factors shown in Table 10.3 are present. The cut-off thresholds for the CVD risk factors that meet the definition of the metabolic syndrome are typically less than those of the ACSM risk stratification shown in Table 2.2. The reason for lower CVD risk-factor thresholds used to categorize those with the metabolic syndrome is that they occur in aggregate and thus confer greater risk than when they occur alone. However, these criteria are based on expert opinion. At this time, it is underdetermined whether the metabolic syndrome represents a distinct pathophysiologic condition or disease (41). Nonetheless, the metabolic syndrome is often encountered in clinical practice and health/fitness settings.

Age-adjusted prevalence data from the National Health and Nutrition Examination Survey (NHANES 1999–2000) indicates that 27% of adults in the United

TABLE 10.3. CLINICAL CRITERIA FOR THE METABOLIC SYNDROME

CARDIOVASCULAR DISEASE RISK FACTOR	NCEP (68) CRITERIA[a]	IDF (55) CRITERIA[b]
Abdominal obesity		
Men	>102 cm (>40 in)	Country/ethnic-specific
Women	>88 cm (>35 in)	Country/ethnic-specific
Triglycerides	$\geq$150 mg $\cdot$ dL^{-1} (1.69 mmol $\cdot$ L^{-1})	$\geq$150 mg $\cdot$ dL^{-1} (1.69 mmol $\cdot$ L^{-1}) or specific treatment of this abnormality
High-density lipoprotein cholesterol		
Men	<40 mg $\cdot$ dL^{-1} (1.04 mmol $\cdot$ L^{-1})	<40 mg $\cdot$ dL^{-1} (1.04 mmol $\cdot$ L^{-1}) or specific treatment of this abnormality
Women	<50 mg $\cdot$ dL^{-1} (1.30 mmol $\cdot$ L^{-1})	<50 mg $\cdot$ dL^{-1} (1.30 mmol $\cdot$ L^{-1}) or specific treatment of this abnormality
Blood pressure (systolic/ diastolic)	$\geq$130 and/or $\geq$85 mm Hg	$\geq$130 and/or $\geq$85 mm Hg or treatment of previously diagnosed hypertension
Fasting glucose	$\geq$110 mg $\cdot$ dL^{-1} (6.11 mmol $\cdot$ L^{-1})	>100 mg $\cdot$ dL^{-1} (5.55 mmol $\cdot$ L^{-1})

[a]National Cholesterol Education Program (NCEP) metabolic syndrome diagnosis is established when three of the criteria are present (59).

[b]International Diabetes Federation (IDF) metabolic syndrome diagnosis is established when abdominal obesity and two additional criteria are present (55).

States meet the criteria for metabolic syndrome, an increase compared with the prevalence of 24% in NHANES III (40). The International Diabetes Federation (IDF) proposed a new definition for metabolic syndrome in 2005 (55) that was based on the presence of abdominal adiposity and two additional CVD risk factors shown in Table 10.3. When the metabolic syndrome classifications are compared, the NCEP and IDF definitions gave the same classification in 93% of individuals (39), indicating their compatibility.

The treatment guidelines for metabolic syndrome recommended by NCEP focus on three interventions, including (a) weight control, (b) physical activity, and (c) treatment of the associated CVD risk factors that may include pharmacotherapy (68). The IDF guidelines for primary intervention include (55) (a) moderate restriction in energy intake to achieve a 5% to 10% weight loss within 1 year, (b) moderate increases in physical activity consistent with the consensus public health recommendations of 30 minutes of moderate-intensity physical activity on most days of the week (47,104), and (c) change in dietary intake composition that may require changes in macronutrient composition consistent with modifying specified CVD risk factors. The IDF secondary intervention includes pharmacotherapy for associated CVD risk factors (55).

EXERCISE TESTING

- The appropriate risk stratification to be established for individuals with metabolic syndrome should be based on the presence of dyslipidemia, hypertension, and hyperglycemia. This risk stratification may result in the need for additional medical screening before exercise testing and/or appropriate medical supervision during exercise testing (Chapters 2 and 3).
- Special consideration should be given to associated CVD risk factors as outlined in previous sections on exercise testing (Chapters 2 and 3) and in this chapter for individuals with dyslipidemia, hypertension, and hyperglycemia.
- Because many individuals with the metabolic syndrome are either overweight or obese, exercise testing considerations specific to those individuals should be followed. See this chapter and the ACSM position stand (5) on exercise prescription recommendations for those who are overweight or obese for additional information.
- The potential for low exercise capacity in people who are overweight or obese may necessitate a low initial workload (i.e., 2–3 metabolic equivalents [METs]) and small increments per testing stage (0.5–1.0 MET).
- Because of the potential presence of elevated BP, strict adherence to protocols for assessing BP before and during exercise testing should be followed (7).

EXERCISE PRESCRIPTION/SPECIAL CONSIDERATIONS

The minimal FITT framework is consistent with the recommendations for healthy adults regarding aerobic, resistance, and flexibility exercise (Chapter 7). Similarly, the minimal dose of physical activity to improve health/fitness outcomes is consistent with the consensus public health recommendations of 150 $min \cdot wk^{-1}$ or 30 minutes of physical activity on most days of the week (47,104). For these reasons and because of the impact of the clustering of diseases and conditions that accompany the metabolic syndrome, exercise prescription recommendations and special considerations are combined in this section and listed below.

- Individuals with the metabolic syndrome will likely present with multiple CVD risk factors (i.e., dyslipidemia, hypertension, obesity, and hyperglycemia). Special consideration should be given to the exercise prescription based on the presence of these associated CVD risk factors and the goals of the participant and/or healthcare provider. See other sections of this chapter on the exercise prescription recommendations for these other conditions and diseases for additional information.
- Initial exercise training should be performed at a moderate intensity (i.e., 40%–60% $\dot{V}O_2R$ or HRR) and, when appropriate, progress to more vigorous intensity (i.e., 50%–75% $\dot{V}O_{2max}$ or HRR) to allow for optimal health/fitness improvements.
- Because of the high likelihood of overweight and obesity, most individuals with the metabolic syndrome may benefit by gradually increasing their physical activity levels to approximately 300 $min \cdot wk^{-1}$ or 50 to 60 minutes on 5 $d \cdot wk^{-1}$ when appropriate (5,91,105). This amount of physical activity may be accumulated in multiple daily bouts of at least 10 minutes in duration or through increases in other forms of moderate-intensity lifestyle activities. For

some individuals to promote or maintain weight loss, progression to 60–90 min · d^{-1} may be necessary. See the next section in this chapter and the ACSM position stand (5) on exercise prescription recommendations for those with overweight and obesity for additional information.

OVERWEIGHT AND OBESITY

Overweight and obesity are characterized by excess body weight with BMI commonly used as the criterion to define these conditions. Recent estimates indicate that more than 66% of adults are classified as overweight (BMI ≥25 kg · m^{-2}), 32% as obese (BMI ≥30 kg · m^{-2}), and 5% extremely obese (BMI ≥40 kg · m^{-2}) (78). Obesity is also an increasing concern in youth, with ~14% to 18% of children and adolescents classified as overweight, defined as ≥95th percentile of BMI for age and sex (78). Overweight and obesity are linked to numerous chronic diseases, including CVD, diabetes mellitus, many forms of cancer, and numerous musculoskeletal problems (70). It is estimated that obesity-related conditions account for ~7% of total healthcare costs in the United States, and the direct and indirect costs of obesity are in excess of $117 billion annually (98).

The management of body weight is dependent on energy balance, which is affected by energy intake and energy expenditure. For a person who is overweight or obese to reduce body weight, energy expenditure must exceed energy intake. A weight loss of 5% to 10% provides significant health benefits (70), and these benefits are more likely to be sustained through the maintenance of weight loss and/or participation in habitual physical activity. Weight loss maintenance is challenging, with weight regain averaging approximately 33% to 50% of initial weight loss within 1 year of terminating treatment (114).

Lifestyle interventions for weight loss that combine reductions in energy intake with increases in energy expenditure through exercise and other forms of physical activity typically result in an initial 9% to 10% reduction in body weight (114). However, physical activity appears to have little impact on the magnitude of weight loss observed across the initial 6-month intervention compared with reductions in energy intake (70). Thus, the combination of modest reductions in energy intake with adequate levels of physical activity is necessary to maximize weight loss in people with overweight and obesity (5,70). Despite the minimal impact of physical activity for initial weight loss periods of ≤6 months in duration, physical activity appears to be important for sustaining significant weight loss and to prevent weight regain (5,70,91,105).

Based on the scientific evidence and practical clinical guidelines, the ACSM makes the following recommendations regarding exercise testing and training for overweight and obese individuals.

EXERCISE TESTING

- The presence of other comorbidities (e.g., dyslipidemia, hypertension, hyperinsulinemia, hyperglycemia, etc.) may increase the risk stratification for overweight and obese individuals, resulting in the need for additional medical screening before exercise testing and/or appropriate medical supervision during exercise testing (Chapters 2 and 3).

- The timing of medications to treat comorbidities relative to exercise testing should be considered (Appendix A).
- The presence of musculoskeletal and/or orthopedic conditions may require modifications to the exercise testing procedure that may require the need for leg or arm ergometry.
- The potential for low exercise capacity in overweight and obese individuals may necessitate a low initial workload (i.e., 2–3 METs) and small increments per testing stage of 0.5 to 1.0 MET.
- Because of ease of test administration for the healthcare provider/exercise specialist and the patient, consider a cycle ergometer (with an oversized seat) versus a treadmill.
- Overweight and obese adults may have difficulty achieving traditional physiologic criteria indicative of maximal exercise testing so that standard termination criteria may not apply to these individuals (Chapters 5 and 6).
- Appropriate cuff size should be used to measure BP in people who are overweight and obese to minimize the potential for inaccurate measurement.

EXERCISE PRESCRIPTION

The minimal FITT framework of exercise is consistent with the recommendations for healthy adults for aerobic, resistance, and flexibility exercise (10,47) (Chapter 7). Similarly, the minimal dose of physical activity to improve health/fitness outcomes is consistent with the consensus public health recommendations of 150 min · wk^{-1} or 30 minutes of physical activity on most days of the week (47,104). The following is the recommended minimal FITT framework for people who are overweight and obese.

Frequency: $\geq$5 d · wk^{-1} to maximize caloric expenditure

Intensity: Moderate- to vigorous-intensity physical activity should be encouraged. Initial exercise training intensity should be moderate (i.e., 40%–60% $\dot{V}O_2R$ or HRR). Eventual progression to more vigorous-exercise intensity (i.e., 50%–75% $\dot{V}O_2R$ or HRR) may result in further health/fitness benefits.

Time: 30–60 min · d^{-1} to total 150 minutes per week, progressing to 300 minutes per week, of moderate physical activity; 150 minutes of vigorous physical activity; or an equivalant combination of moderate and vigorous physical activity. Performance of intermittent exercise of at least 10 minutes in duration; accumulating these duration recommendations is an effective alternative to continuous exercise.

Type: The primary mode should be aerobic physical activities that involve the large muscle groups. As part of a balanced exercise program, resistance-training exercise should be incorporated. See Chapter 7 on exercise prescription recommendations for resistance training for additional information.

Special Considerations

The amount of physical activity that may be required to sustain weight loss and prevent weight regain may be more than the consensus public health recommendation for physical activity of 150 min · wk^{-1} or 30 minutes of physical activity on most days of the week (47,104). For these reasons, the following considerations should be noted.

- Overweight and obese adults may benefit from *progression* to approximately 250–300 min · wk^{-1} or 50 to 60 min on 5 d · wk^{-1} as this magnitude of physical activity appears to enhance long-term weight-loss maintenance (5,91,105). For some individuals to promote or maintain weight loss, progression to 60–90 min · d^{-1} of daily exercise may be necessary.
- Adequate amounts of physical activity should be performed on 5–7 d · wk^{-1}.
- The duration of moderate- to vigorous-intensity physical activity should initially progress to at least 30 min · d^{-1} (47,104) and when appropriate progress to 50–60 min · d^{-1} or more to enhance long-term weight control. Adults with overweight and obesity may accumulate this amount of physical activity in multiple daily bouts of at least 10 minutes in duration or through increases in other forms of moderate-intensity lifestyle activities. In addition, these strategies may enhance the adoption and maintenance of physical activity (47).
- The addition of resistance exercise to energy restriction does not appear to prevent the loss of fat-free mass or the observed reduction in resting energy expenditure (34). However, resistance exercise may enhance muscular strength and physical function in people with overweight and obesity. Moreover, there may be additional health benefits of participating in resistance exercise in this population. See Chapter 7 on the exercise prescription recommendations for resistance training for additional information.

BEHAVIORAL WEIGHT LOSS PROGRAM RECOMMENDATIONS

An effective behavioral weight loss program should include reductions in energy intake and increases in energy expenditure through physical activity. Thus, ACSM makes the following recommendations for weight-loss programs (5).

- Target adults with a BMI ≥25 kg · m^{-2} and children exceeding the 95th percentile of BMI based on age and sex.
- Target a minimal reduction in body weight of at least 5% to 10% of initial body weight over a 3- to 6-month period.
- Incorporate opportunities to enhance communication between healthcare professionals, dietitians, and exercise professionals and people with overweight and obesity following the initial weight loss period.
- Target changing eating and exercise behaviors, as sustained changes in both behaviors result in significant long-term weight loss.
- Target reducing current energy intake by 500 to 1,000 kcal · d^{-1} to achieve weight loss. This reduced energy intake should be combined with a reduction in dietary fat to <30% of total energy intake.
- Target progressively increasing to a minimum of 150 min · wk^{-1} of moderate-intensity physical activity to optimize health/fitness benefits for overweight and obese adults.
- Progress to higher amounts of exercise (i.e., 200–300 min · wk^{-1} or ≥2,000 kcals · wk^{-1}) of physical activity to promote long-term weight control.

- Consider resistance exercise as a supplement to the combination of aerobic exercise and modest reductions in energy intake to lose weight.
- Incorporate behavioral modification strategies to facilitate the adoption and maintenance of the desired changes in behavior.

OSTEOPOROSIS

Osteoporosis is a skeletal disease that is characterized by low bone mineral density (BMD) and changes in the microarchitecture of bone that increase susceptibility to fracture. The burden of osteoporosis on society and the individual patient is significant (103). More than 10 million Americans 50 years of age and older have osteoporosis, and another 34 million are at risk. Hip fractures, in particular, are associated with increased risk of disability and death. The 2005 position stand of the International Society of Clinical Densitometry, which has been endorsed by the American Society for Bone and Mineral Research, the International Osteoporosis Foundation, and the American Association of Clinical Endocrinologists, defines osteoporosis in postmenopausal women and men ≥50 years as a BMD T-score of the lumbar spine, total hip, or femoral neck of ≤−2.5 (22,46). However, it is important to recognize that osteoporotic fractures may occur at BMD levels above this threshold, particularly in the elderly.

Physical activity is essential to bone health (12,89,103). Physical activity may reduce the risk for osteoporotic fractures by enhancing the peak bone mass achieved during growth and development, by slowing the rate of bone loss with aging, and/or by reducing the risk of falls via benefits on muscle strength and balance (20,89). Accordingly, physical activity plays a prominent role in primary (at risk for) and secondary (treatment) prevention of osteoporosis (103).

EXERCISE TESTING

There are no special considerations for exercise testing of individuals at risk for osteoporosis, regarding when a test is clinically indicated, beyond those for the general population. However, when exercise tests are performed in individuals with osteoporosis, the following issues should be considered.

- Use of cycle ergometry as an alternative to treadmill exercise testing to assess cardiovascular function may be indicated in patients with severe vertebral osteoporosis for whom walking is painful.
- Vertebral compression fractures leading to a loss of height and spinal deformation can compromise ventilatory capacity and result in a forward shift in the center of gravity. The latter may affect balance during treadmill walking.
- Maximal muscle strength testing may be contraindicated in patients with severe osteoporosis, although there are no established guidelines for contraindications for maximal muscle strength testing.

EXERCISE PRESCRIPTION

The exercise prescription recommendations for osteoporosis are categorized into two types of populations: (a) individuals at risk for osteoporosis defined as having

≥1 risk factor for osteoporosis (e.g., current low bone mass, age, and being female) (103), and (b) those with osteoporosis.

- In individuals *at risk* for osteoporosis, the following FITT framework is recommended to help *preserve bone health.*

Frequency: Weight-bearing aerobic activities 3–5 d · wk^{-1} and resistance exercise 2–3 d · wk^{-1}

Intensity: Moderate (e.g., 60%–80% 1-RM, 8 to 12 repetitions for resistance exercise) to high (e.g., 80%–90%, 5 to 6 repetitions for resistance exercise) intensity in terms of bone-loading forces

Time: 30–60 min · d^{-1} of a combination of weight-bearing aerobic and resistance activities

Type: Weight-bearing aerobic activities (e.g., tennis, stair climbing/descending, and walking with intermittent jogging), activities that involve jumping (e.g., volleyball and basketball), and resistance exercise (e.g., weight lifting)

- In individuals *with osteoporosis,* the following FITT framework is recommended to help *prevent disease progression.*

Frequency: Weight-bearing aerobic activities 3–5 d · wk^{-1} and resistance exercise 2–3 d · wk^{-1}

Intensity: Moderate intensity (i.e., 40% to <60% $\dot{V}O_2R$ or HRR) for weight-bearing aerobic activities and moderate intensity (e.g., 60%–80% 1-RM, 8 to 12 repetitions for resistance exercise) in terms of bone-loading forces, although some individuals may be able to tolerate more intense exercise

Time: 30–60 min · d^{-1} of a combination of weight-bearing aerobic and resistance activities

Type: Weight-bearing aerobic activities (e.g., stair climbing/descending, walking, and other activities as tolerated) and resistance exercise (e.g., weight lifting)

Special Considerations

- It is difficult to quantify exercise intensity in terms of bone-loading forces. However, the magnitude of bone-loading force generally increases in parallel with exercise intensity quantified by conventional methods (e.g., %HR$_{max}$ or %1-RM). See Chapter 7 on exercise prescription recommendation for resistance training for additional information.
- There are currently no established guidelines regarding contraindications for exercise for people with osteoporosis. The general recommendation is to prescribe moderate intensity exercise that does not cause or exacerbate pain. Exercises that involve explosive movements or high-impact loading should be avoided. Exercises that cause twisting, bending, or compression of the spine should also be avoided.
- BMD of the spine may appear *normal* or *increased* after osteoporotic compression fractures have occurred or in people with osteoarthritis of the

spine. Hip BMD is a more reliable indicator of risk for osteoporosis than spine BMD (62).

- For older women and men at increased risk for falls, the exercise prescription should also include activities that improve balance. See Chapter 8, Nelson et al. (73), and the ACSM position stand (8) on exercise prescription recommendations for the older adult for additional information.

- In light of the rapid and profound effects of immobilization and bed rest on bone loss, and the poor prognosis for recovery of mineral after remobilization, even the frailest elderly should remain as physically active as their health permits to preserve skeletal integrity.

PERIPHERAL ARTERY DISEASE

PAD affects 5 to 10 million adults in the United States, is more common in men than women, and increases in prevalence with advancing age (99). Major risk factors for PAD include diabetes mellitus, hypertension, and smoking (69). Patients with PAD have a 6.6 times greater risk of dying from CVD compared with individuals without PAD (99). Intermittent claudication, the major symptom of PAD, is characterized by a reproducible aching or cramping sensation in one or both legs that typically is triggered by weight-bearing exercise (96). Intermittent claudication is reported in 5% of the U.S. population older than the age of 55 years and in 15% to 40% of individuals with PAD (42,52). As the symptoms worsen, they may become severe enough to limit the individual from performing activities of daily living (42).

PAD is caused by the development of atherosclerotic plaque in systemic arteries that leads to significant stenosis, resulting in the reduction of blood flow to regions distal to the area of occlusion. This reduction in blood flow creates a mismatch between oxygen supply and demand, causing ischemia to develop in the affected areas, typically the calf, thigh, or buttocks (50). When the stenosis in the lower extremity results in necrosis in the dependent tissues, leg amputation may be indicated (50,99). PAD is staged based on the presence of symptoms as described in Table 10.4 and by the ABI (ankle-brachial index), with values ranging

TABLE 10.4. FONTAINE CLASSIFICATION OF PERIPHERAL ARTERY DISEASE

STAGE	SYMPTOMS
1	Asymptomatic
2	Intermittent claudication
2a	Distance to pain onset >200 m
2b	Distance to pain onset <200 m
3	Pain at rest
4	Gangrene, tissue loss

Updated from Squires RW. Pathophysiology and clinical features of cardiovascular diseases. In: Kaminsky LA, editor. *ACSM's Resource Manual for Guidelines for Exercise Testing and Prescription.* 5th ed. Philadelphia (PA): Lippincott Williams & Wilkins; 2006. p. 411–38.

TABLE 10.5. ANKLE-BRACHIAL INDEX SCALE FOR PERIPHERAL ARTERIAL DISEASE

	SUPINE RESTING ANKLE BRACHIAL INDEX	POSTEXERCISE ANKLE BRACHIAL INDEX
Normal	>1.0	No change or increase
Mild disease	0.8–0.9	>0.5
Moderate disease	0.5–0.8	>0.2
Severe disease	<0.5	<0.2

Reprinted with permission from Squires RW. Pathophysiology and clinical features of cardiovascular diseases. In: Kaminsky LA, editor. *ACSM's Resource Manual for Guidelines for Exercise Testing and Prescription*. 5th ed. Philadelphia (PA): Lippincott Williams & Wilkins; 2006. p. 411 38. Reprinted with permission from Squires RW.

from >1 to <0.5 (Table 10.5) (96). The recommended treatments for PAD include medications (e.g., cilostazol), revascularization, and exercise (50).

EXERCISE TESTING

Exercise testing is performed in patients with PAD to determine the time of onset of claudication pain pre- and posttherapeutic intervention, measure the postexercise ABI, and diagnose the presence of CVD (115).

- Patients with PAD are classified as high risk; therefore, exercise testing under medical supervision is indicated.
- Medication intake should be noted and repeated in an identical manner in subsequent exercise tests.
- Ankle and brachial artery SBP should be measured bilaterally after 15 minutes of rest in the supine position. The ABI should be calculated by dividing the higher ankle SBP reading by the higher brachial artery SBP reading.
- A treadmill protocol beginning with a slow speed with gradual increments in grade is recommended (115).
- Claudication pain perception may be monitored using the following scale: 0 = no pain, 1 = onset of pain, 2 = moderate pain, 3 = intense pain, and 4 = maximal pain (115), or the Borg CR10 Customized for Pain Measurement Scale (23) (Fig. 10.1). The time and distance for the onset of pain, and the time and distance to achieve maximal pain, should be recorded.
- Following the completion of the exercise test intended for research purposes, patients should recover in the supine position for 5 minutes, and ABI should be calculated during this time. The time taken for the pain to resolve after exercise should also be recorded (115).
- In addition to the GXT, the 6-minute walking test may be used to assess function in patients with PAD (115).

EXERCISE PRESCRIPTION

Exercise training is effective in the treatment of individuals with PAD because chronic training using an interval-training approach leads to increases in the initial and absolute distance that can be walked without pain (42). The exercise program should also be designed to target the CVD risk factors that are often associated with PAD (115). The following exercise prescription is recommended for people with PAD.

Frequency: Weight-bearing aerobic exercise 3–5 $d \cdot wk^{-1}$; resistance exercise at least 2 $d \cdot wk^{-1}$

Intensity: Moderate intensity (i.e., 40% to <60% $\dot{V}O_2R$) that allows the patient to walk until he/she reaches a pain score of 3 (i.e., intense pain) on the 4-point pain scale (115). Between bouts of activity, individuals should be given time to allow ischemic pain to subside before resuming exercise (51,115).

Time: 30–60 min $\cdot d^{-1}$, but initially some patients may need to start with 10-minute bouts and exercise intermittently to accumulate a total of 30–60 min $\cdot d^{-1}$

Type: Weight-bearing aerobic exercise, such as walking, and non–weight-bearing activity, such as arm ergometry. Cycling may be used as a warm-up, but should not be the primary type of activity. Resistance training is recommended to enhance and maintain muscular strength and endurance. See Chapter 7 on exercise prescription recommendations for resistance training for additional information.

Special Considerations

- The optimal work-to-rest ratio has not been determined for individuals with PAD. The work-to-rest ratio may need to be adjusted for each patient.
- A cold environment may aggravate the symptoms of intermittent claudication; therefore, a longer warm-up may be necessary (13).
- Encourage patients to stop smoking if they are current smokers.
- For optimal benefit, patients should participate in a supervised exercise program for a minimum of 5 to 6 months. Following exercise training programs of this length, improvements in pain-free walking of 106% to 177%, and 64% to 85% in absolute walking ability, may occur (25).

PULMONARY DISEASES

Pulmonary diseases typically result in dyspnea or shortness of breath with exertion. As a result of dyspnea, patients with pulmonary disease limit physical activity, and deconditioning results. Consequently, patients with pulmonary disease experience dyspnea even at low levels of physical exertion. This adverse cycle can lead to eventual functional impairment and disability. Exercise is an effective intervention that lessens the development of functional impairment and disability in patients with pulmonary disease (4,72,86). The beneficial effects of exercise occur mainly through adaptations in the musculoskeletal and cardiovascular systems, which in turn reduce stress on the pulmonary system during exercise (19,86).

The focus of this section is on pulmonary function abnormalities resulting from chronic bronchitis, emphysema, asthma, and cystic fibrosis. Chronic bronchitis, emphysema, and cystic fibrosis are classified as chronic obstructive

BOX 10.1	Classification of Pulmonary Diseases

- Chronic obstructive lung disease (COPD)—a permanent reduction in airflow
  - Bronchitis—mucus hyperexcretion and chronic cough
  - Emphysema—destruction of alveolar walls
  - Cystic fibrosis—a genetic disease of the exocrine glands resulting in excessive thick mucus that obstructs the gastrointestinal system and lungs
- Asthma—a reversible component to airway obstruction consisting of bronchospasm and inflammation

pulmonary diseases (COPD), resulting in a permanent diminution of airflow; whereas asthma has a reversible component to airway obstruction (see Box 10.1 for pulmonary disease classification). Detailed guidelines for exercise testing and prescription exist elsewhere for persons with these pulmonary diseases (19,72). Individuals with mild COPD and well-controlled asthma may exercise following the general principles of exercise prescription guidelines presented in Chapter 7. However, persons with asthma, particularly those with exercise-induced asthma (EIA), should avoid environmental triggers, such as cold, dry, dusty air, and inhaled pollutants. Individuals suffering from acute exacerbations of their pulmonary disease should limit exercise until symptoms have subsided.

EXERCISE TESTING

- Assessment of physiologic function should include cardiopulmonary capacity, pulmonary function, and determination of arterial blood gases or arterial oxygen saturation (S_aO_2) via direct or indirect methods.
- Modifications of traditional protocols (e.g., extended stages, smaller increments, and slower progression) may be warranted depending on functional limitations and the early onset of dyspnea. For example, in patients with severe COPD, the Naughton protocol may be modified such that only the speed but not the grade increases every 2 minutes instead of 3 minutes.
- As indicated in Chapter 5, submaximal exercise testing may be used depending on the reason for the test and the clinical status of the patient. However, it should be noted that persons with pulmonary disease may have ventilatory limitations to exercise; thus, prediction of peak $\dot{V}O_2$ based on age-predicted HR_{max} may not be appropriate. In recent years, the 6-minute walk test has become popular for assessing functional exercise capacity in persons with more severe pulmonary disease and in settings that lack exercise testing equipment (17).
- In addition to standard termination criteria, exercise testing may be terminated because of severe arterial oxygen desaturation (i.e., $S_aO_2 \leq 80\%$) (18).

- The exercise testing mode is typically walking or stationary cycling. Walking protocols may be more suitable for persons with severe disease who may lack the muscle strength to overcome the increasing resistance of cycle ergometers. Furthermore, if arm ergometry is used, upper-extremity aerobic exercise may result in increased dyspnea that may limit the intensity and duration of the activity.

EXERCISE PRESCRIPTION

The recommended FITT framework for pulmonary disease is generally consistent with the general principles of exercise prescription in Chapter 7 (10,47). The exercise prescription for those with pulmonary disease is categorized into two types of populations: (a) individuals with well-controlled asthma or mild COPD and (b) individuals with moderate to severe COPD.

- For individuals with *well-controlled asthma or mild COPD*, the following exercise prescription for cardiovascular fitness is recommended.

Frequency: At least 3–5 d·wk^{-1}

Intensity: Presently there is no consensus as to the "optimal" exercise intensity for patients with pulmonary disease. The exercise-intensity recommendations for older, healthy adults found in Chapter 8 and Nelson et al. (73) may be used for persons with COPD. The recommendations for children and adolescents in Chapter 8 may be used for younger persons with asthma or cystic fibrosis.

Time: 20–60 min·d^{-1} of continuous or intermittent physical activity

Type: Walking is strongly recommended because it is involved in most activities of daily living. Stationary cycling may be used as an alternate type of training. Additionally, resistance training and flexibility exercises should be incorporated into the exercise prescription using the guidelines presented in Chapter 7.

- For individuals with *moderate to severe COPD*, the following exercise prescription for cardiovascular fitness is recommended.

Frequency: At least 3–5 d·wk^{-1}

Intensity: For those patients with severe COPD whose exercise tolerance may be ventilatory limited, exercise intensities as high as 60% to 80% of peak work rates are suggested (72,101). Intensity may also be based on dyspnea ratings determined from the GXT with ratings between 3 (moderate shortness of breath) to 5 (strong or hard breathing) on a scale of 0 to 10 corresponding to the desired exercise intensity that can be tolerated (23).

Time: Persons with moderate or severe COPD may be able to exercise only at a specified intensity for a few minutes at the start of the training program. Intermittent exercise may also be used for the initial training sessions until the patient tolerates exercise at sustained higher intensities and durations of activity.

Type: Walking and or cycling. Additionally, resistance training and flexibility exercises should be incorporated into the exercise prescription using the guidelines presented in Chapter 7.

Special Considerations

- Pulmonary diseases and their treatments not only affect the lungs but skeletal muscles as well (19). Resistance training of skeletal muscle should be an integral part of exercise prescription for pulmonary patients. The exercise prescription for resistance training with pulmonary patients who have controlled asthma or mild COPD should follow the same principles for healthy adults presented in Chapter 7, whereas the prescription for those with moderate to severe COPD should follow the principles for older adults in Nelson et al. (73) and Chapter 8 (72,101).
- Because pulmonary disease patients may experience greater dyspnea while performing activities of daily living involving the upper extremities, it may be beneficial for these patients to focus on the muscles of the shoulder girdle when performing resistance exercises.
- Inspiratory muscle weakness is a contributor to exercise intolerance and dyspnea in patients with COPD. Training of these muscles increases respiratory muscle strength and endurance, and ultimately reduces dyspnea and improves exercise tolerance, particularly in patients presenting with inspiratory muscle weakness (36,64,92).

The guidelines for *inspiratory muscle training* are included below.

Frequency: A minimum of 4–5 $d \cdot wk^{-1}$

Intensity: 30% of maximal inspiratory pressure measured at functional residual capacity

Time: 30 $min \cdot d^{-1}$ or two 15-minute $sessions \cdot d^{-1}$

- Regardless of the prescribed exercise intensity, the exercise or health/fitness professional should closely monitor initial exercise sessions and adjust intensity and duration according to patient responses and tolerance. In many cases, the presence of symptoms, particularly dyspnea/breathlessness, supersedes objective methods of exercise prescription.
- The traditional method for monitoring the exercise intensity is HR, as discussed in Chapter 7. As previously mentioned, an alternative approach to HR is using the dyspnea rating obtained from a GXT as a "target" intensity for exercise training (54). Most patients with COPD accurately and reliably produce a dyspnea rating obtained from an incremental exercise test as a target to regulate/monitor the exercise intensity. A dyspnea rating between 3 (moderate shortness of breath) to 5 (strong or hard breathing) on a scale of 0 to 10 is the recommended exercise intensity for patients with moderate to severe COPD (23).
- Unlike most healthy individuals and persons with heart disease, patients with moderate to severe COPD may exhibit oxyhemoglobin desaturation with exercise. Therefore, a measure of blood oxygenation, either the partial pressure of arterial oxygen (P_aO_2) or $\%S_aO_2$, should be made during the initial GXT. In addition, oximetry is recommended for the initial exercise training sessions to evaluate possible exercise-induced oxyhemoglobin desaturation.
- Based on the recommendations of the Nocturnal Oxygen Therapy Trial (75), supplemental O_2 is indicated for patients with a $P_aO_2 \leq 55$ mm Hg or an $\%S_aO_2 \leq 88\%$ while breathing room air. These same guidelines apply when considering supplemental oxygen during exercise.

- To reduce the risk of exercise-induced bronchoconstriction, persons with asthma should use inhaled bronchodilator therapy (i.e., 2 to 4 puffs) 15 minutes before the start of exercise and should warm up gradually by engaging in low-intensity exercise for several minutes before increasing exercise intensity (72).
- For persons with cystic fibrosis, rigorous precautions, including frequent hand and equipment washing, should be used in exercise testing and training facilities to minimize exposure to multiresistant pathogens (30,43).

RENAL DISEASE

Individuals are diagnosed with chronic kidney disease if they have kidney damage evidenced by microalbuminuria or a glomerular filtration rate <60 mL $\cdot$ min^{-1} $\cdot$ 1.73 m$^{2-1}$ for $\geq$3 months (71). Based on National Kidney Foundation Kidney Disease Outcomes Quality Initiative (K/DOQI) guidelines, chronic kidney disease is divided into five stages, primarily depending on the glomerular filtration rate (see Table 10.6 for chronic kidney disease staging criteria) (71). Approximately 20 million Americans have chronic kidney disease (107). When individuals progress to stage 5 of the disease (i.e., glomerular filtration rate <15 mL $\cdot$ min^{-1} $\cdot$ 1.73 m$^{2-1}$), their treatment options include renal replacement therapy (hemo or peritoneal dialysis) or kidney transplantation.

Diabetes mellitus and hypertension are the major causes of end-stage renal disease, accounting for 45% and 27.2% of the cases, respectively (107). The incident rate of individuals progressing to the end-stage renal disease has decreased, with the rate of 343 people per million in 2003 to 339 people per million in 2004 (107). However, the prevalence of the disease is still high, reaching 1,542 people per million in 2004, which is 5.4 times greater than the corresponding number in 1980. End-stage renal disease is about 1.5 times more prevalent in men than women and 4.2 times greater in blacks than whites.

EXERCISE TESTING

Individuals with chronic kidney disease tend to have low functional capacity that is approximately 50% of that recorded in healthy age- and sex-matched

---

TABLE 10.6. STAGES OF CHRONIC KIDNEY DISEASE

STAGE	DESCRIPTION	GLOMERULAR FILTRATION RATE (mL $\cdot$ min^{-1} $\cdot$ 1.73 m$^{2-1}$)
1	Kidney damage with normal or ↑ glomerular filtration rate	$\geq$90
2	Kidney damage with mild ↓ glomerular filtration rate	60–89
3	Moderate ↓ glomerular filtration rate	30–59
4	Severe ↓ glomerular filtration rate	15–29
5	Kidney failure	<15 (or dialysis)

Reprinted from the National Kidney Foundation. K/DOQI clinical practice guidelines for chronic kidney disease: evaluation, classification, and stratification. *Am J Kidney Dis.* 2002;39(2 suppl 1):S1–266, with permission from Elsevier.

controls (60,61). This reduced functional capacity is thought to be related to several factors, including a sedentary lifestyle, cardiac dysfunction, anemia, and musculoskeletal dysfunction. Exercise testing of individuals with chronic kidney disease should be supervised by trained medical personnel with the use of standard test termination criteria and test interpretation methods (Chapters 5 and 6). The following exercise testing considerations should be noted.

- Medical clearance should be sought from the patient's nephrologist.
- Patients are likely to be on multiple medications, including those that are commonly used in the treatment of hypertension and diabetes mellitus (Appendix A).
- When performing a GXT on individuals with chronic kidney disease (stages 1–4), standard testing procedures should be followed.
- Treadmill and cycle ergometer protocols may be used to test patients with kidney disease, with the treadmill being more popular.
- Because of the low functional capacity among this patient population, treadmill protocols such as the modified Bruce, Balke, Naughton, or branching protocols are appropriate (80).
- If the cycle ergometer is used, recommended initial warm-up work rates are 20 to 25 W. The work rate should be increased by 10 to 30 W increments every 1 to 3 minutes (111).
- In patients receiving maintenance hemodialysis, exercise testing should be scheduled on nondialysis days and BP should be monitored in the arm that does not contain the arteriovenous fistula (81). In addition, peak HR (HR_{peak}) is ~75% of the age-predicted HR_{max} (82).
- Patients receiving continuous ambulatory peritoneal dialysis should be tested without dialysate fluid in their abdomens (81).
- Because HR may not always be a reliable indicator of exercise intensity in individuals with chronic kidney disease, perceived exertion should always be monitored.
- Standard procedures are used to exercise test transplant recipients.
- Dynamic strength testing should be done using a 3-RM or higher load (e.g., 10–12-RM), as 1-RM testing is generally thought to be contraindicated in persons with chronic kidney disease because of the fear of spontaneous avulsion fractures (21,56,81,90).
- Muscular strength and endurance may be safely assessed using isokinetic dynamometry with angular velocities in the 60°–180° · s $^{-1}$ range (48,80).
- A variety of physical performance tests may be used to test individuals with kidney disease. Tests to assess cardiovascular fitness (e.g., 6-minute walk test), muscular strength (e.g., sit-to-stand-to-sit test), and balance (e.g., functional reach test) are appropriate (79,83).

EXERCISE PRESCRIPTION

The ideal exercise prescription for individuals with chronic kidney disease has not been fully developed (56). The recommendations for the general population should be modified by using low (i.e., <40% $\dot{V}O_2R$) to moderate (i.e., 40% to <60% $\dot{V}O_2R$) initial exercise intensities and gradually progressing over time based on patient tolerance (Chapter 7). Medically cleared transplant recipients may initiate exercise training as early as 8 days following the transplant operation (66). Resistance exercise is important for the overall well-being of persons with stable chronic kidney disease. The following are exercise recommendations for patients with chronic kidney disease.

Frequency: Aerobic exercise 3–5 d·wk^{-1}; resistance exercise 2–3 d·wk^{-1}

Intensity: Moderate-intensity (i.e., 40% to <60% $\dot{V}O_2R$, RPE 11–13 on a scale of 6–20) aerobic and resistance exercise 60% to 75% 1-RM

Time: Aerobic exercise: 20–60 min·d^{-1} of continuous aerobic activity; however, if this duration cannot be tolerated, 10-minute bouts of intermittent exercise to accumulate 20–60 min·d^{-1}. Resistance training: 1 set of 10 to 15 repetitions. Multiple sets may be done depending on patient tolerance and time (10).

Type: Aerobic exercise, such as walking and cycling. Use machines or free weights for resistance exercise. Choose 8 to 10 different exercises to work the major muscle groups. See Chapter 7 on exercise prescription recommendations on resistance training for additional information.

Special Considerations

Hemodialysis Patients

* Training should not be done immediately postdialysis but may be performed on nondialysis days. If training is done during dialysis, exercise should be attempted during the first half of the treatment to avoid hypotensive episodes.
* Because HR may be an unreliable indicator of exercise intensity, use RPE.
* Exercise the arm with the arteriovenous access so long as the patient does not directly rest weight on this area of the arm (56).

Peritoneal Patients

* Patients on continuous ambulatory peritoneal dialysis may try exercising with fluid in their abdomens; however, if this produces discomfort, they should be encouraged to drain the fluid (56).

Transplant Patients

* During periods of rejection, the intensity and time of exercise should be reduced, but exercise may still be performed (79,83).

REFERENCES

1. Ahlborg L, Andersson C, Julin P. Whole-body vibration training compared with resistance training: effect on spasticity, muscle strength and motor performance in adults with cerebral palsy. *J Rehabil Med.* 2006;38:302–8.
2. Albright A. Diabetes. In: Ehrman JK, Gordon PM, Visich PS, Keteyian SJ, editors. *Clinical Exercise Physiology.* Champaign (IL): Human Kinetics; 2003. 133 p.
3. American Cancer Society. *Cancer Facts and Figures 2006.* Atlanta (GA): American Cancer Society; 2006.

4. American College of Chest Physicians/American Association of Cardiovascular and Pulmonary Rehabilitation Pulmonary Rehabilitation Guidelines Panel. Pulmonary rehabilitation: joint ACCP/AACVPR evidence-based guidelines. Chest. 1997;112;1363–96.

5. American College of Sports Medicine. Position Stand. Appropriate intervention strategies for weight loss and prevention of weight regain for adults. Med Sci Sports Exerc. 2001;33:2145–56.

6. American College of Sports Medicine. Position Stand. Exercise and fluid replacement. Med Sci Sports Exerc. 2007;39(2):377–90.

7. American College of Sports Medicine. Position Stand. Exercise and hypertension. Med Sci Sports Exerc. 2004;36:533–53.

8. American College of Sports Medicine. Position Stand. Exercise and physical activity for older adults. Med Sci Sports Exerc. 1998;30(6):992–1008.

9. American College of Sports Medicine. Position Stand. Exercise and type 2 diabetes. Med Sci Sports Exerc. 2000;32:1345–62.

10. American College of Sports Medicine. Position Stand. The recommended quantity and quality of exercise for developing and maintaining cardiorespiratory and muscular fitness and flexibility in adults. Med Sci Sports Exerc. 1998;30:975–91.

11. American College of Sports Medicine. Position Stand. Exertional heat illness during training and competition. Med Sci Sports Exerc. 2007;39(3):556–72.

12. American College of Sports Medicine. Position Stand. Physical activity and bone health. Med Sci Sports Exerc. 2004;36:1985–96.

13. American College of Sports Medicine. Position Stand. Prevention of cold injuries during exercise. Med Sci Sports Exerc. 2006;38:2012–29.

14. American Diabetes Association. Standards of medical care in diabetes—2007. Diabetes Care. 2007;30:S4–41.

15. American Heart Association. Heart Disease and Stroke Statistics—2006 Update: A report from the American Heart Association Statistics Committee and Stroke Statistics Subcommittee. Circulation. 2006;113:e85–151.

16. American Geriatrics Society Panel on Exercise and Osteoarthritis. Exercise prescription for older adults with osteoarthritis pain: consensus practice recommendations. J Am Geriatr Soc. 2001; 48:808–23.

17. American Thoracic Society. ATS statement: guidelines for the six-minute walk test. Am. J Respir Crit Care Med. 2002;166:111–7.

18. American Thoracic Society and American College of Chest Physicians. ATS/ACCP statement on cardiopulmonary exercise testing. Am J Respir Crit Care Med. 2003;167:211–77.

19. American Thoracic Society and European Respiratory Society. Skeletal muscle dysfunction in chronic obstructive pulmonary disease. Am J Respir Crit Care Med. 1999;159:S1–40.

20. Beck BR, Snow CM. Bone health across the lifespan—exercising our options. Exerc Sport Sci Rev. 2003;31:117–22.

21. Bhole RJ, Flynn JC, Marbury TC. Quadriceps tendon ruptures in uremia. Clin Orthop Relat Res. 1985;195:200–6.

22. Binkley N, Bilezikian JP, Kendler DL, Leib ES, Lewiecki EM, Petak SM. Official positions of the International Society for Clinical Densitometry and Executive Summary of the 2005 Position Development Conference. J Clin Densitom. 2006;9:4–14.

23. Borg G. Scaling pain and related subjective somatic symptoms. In: Borg's Perceived Exertion and Pain Scales. Champaign (IL): Human Kinetics; 1998;63–5.

24. Buchholz AC, Bugaresti JM. A review of body mass index and waist circumference as markers of obesity and coronary heart disease risk in persons with chronic spinal cord injury. Spinal Cord. 2005;43:513–8.

25. Bulmer AC, Coombes JS. Optimizing exercise training in peripheral arterial disease. Sports Med. 2004;34:983–92.

26. Centers for Disease Control and Prevention. National diabetes fact sheet: general information and national estimates on diabetes in the United States, 2005.

27. Centers for Disease Control and Prevention. Prevalence of disabilities and associated health conditions among adults—United States, 1999. MMWR Morb Mortal Wkly Rep 2001;50:120–5.

28. Centers for Disease Control and Prevention. Prevalence of doctor-diagnosed arthritis and arthritis-related activity limitation—United States, 2003–2005. MMWR Morb Mortal Wkly Rep 2006;55:1089–92.

29. Cerebral Palsy—International Sport and Recreation Association. *Classification and Sports Rules Manual.* 9ᵗʰ ed. Nottingham, England: CP-ISRA, 2006.

30. Cystic Fibrosis Foundation. 2006 *Burkholderia cepacia* and the CF Foundation's Participation Policy [Internet]. 2006 [cited 2007 December 1]. Available from http://www.cff.org/LivingWithCF/ StayingHealthy/Germs/Bcepacia/

31. Damiano DL Activity, activity, activity: rethinking our physical therapy approach to cerebral palsy. *Phys Ther.* 2006;86:1–7.

32. Darrah J, Wessel J, Nerainagburg P, O'Connor M. Evaluation of a community fitness program for adolescents with cerebral palsy. *Ped Phys Ther.* 1999;11:18–23.

33. Dodd KJ, Taylor NF, Damiano DL. A systematic review of the effectiveness of strength training programs for people with cerebral palsy. *Arch Phys Med Rehabil.* 2002;83:1157–64.

34. Donnelly JE, Jakicic JM, Pronk NP, Smith BK, Kirk EP, Jacobsen DJ, Washburn R. Is resistance exercise effective for weight management? *Evidenced Based Preventive Medicine.* 2004;1:21–9.

35. Doyle C, Kushi LH, Byers T, et al. 2006 Nutrition, Physical Activity and Cancer Survivorship Advisory Committee. Nutrition and physical activity during and after cancer treatment: an American Cancer Society guide for informed choices. *CA Cancer J Clin.* 2006;56:323–53.

36. Enright SK, Chatham AA, Ionescu V, Unnithan B, Shale DJ. Inspiratory muscle training improves lung function and exercise capacity in adults with cystic fibrosis. *Chest.* 2004;126:405–11.

37. Fisher NM. Osteoarthritis, rheumatoid arthritis, and fibromyalgia. In: Myers JN, Herbert WG, Humphrey R, editors. *ACSM's Resources for Clinical Exercise Physiology: Musculoskeletal, Neuromuscular, Neoplastic, Immunologic, and Hematologic Conditions.* Philadelphia (PA): Lippincott Williams & Wilkins; 2002. p. 111–24.

38. Fletcher B, Berra K, Ades P, et al. AHA Scientific Statement: Managing blood lipids a collaborative approach. *Circulation.* 2005;112:3184–209.

39. Ford ES. Prevalence of the metabolic syndrome defined by the international diabetes federation among adults in the US. *Diabetes Care.* 2005;28:2745–9.

40. Ford ES, Giles WH, Mokdad AH. Increasing prevalence of the metabolic syndrome among US adults. *Diabetes Care.* 2004;27:2444–9.

41. Franks PW, Olsson T. Metabolic syndrome and early death getting to the heart of the problem. *Hypertension* 2007;49:10–2.

42. Gardner AW, Montgomery PS, Flinn WR, Katzel LI. The effect of exercise intensity on the response to exercise rehabilitation in patients with intermittent claudication. *J Vasc Surg.* 2005;42:702–9.

43. Geddes DM. Of isolates and isolation: pseudomonas aeruginosa in adults with cystic fibrosis. *Lancet* 2001;358:522–3.

44. Grundy S, Cleeman JI, Merz NB, et al. Implications of recent clinical trials for the National Cholesterol Education Program Adult Treatment Panel III Guidelines. *Circulation.* 2004;110:227–39.

45. Haisma JA, Van der Woude LHV, Stam HJ, Bergen MP, Sluis TAR, Bussmann JBJ. Physical capacity in wheelchair dependent persons with a spinal cord injury: a critical review of the literature. *Spinal Cord.* 2006;44:1–11.

46. Hans D, Downs RW, Duboeuf F, Greenspan S, Jankowski LG, Kiebzak GM, Petak SM. Skeletal sites for osteoporosis diagnosis: the 2005 ISCD Official Positions. *J Clin Densitom.* 2006;9:15–21.

47. Haskell WL, Lee IM, Pate RR, et al. Physical activity and public health updated recommendations from the American College of Sports Medicine and the American Heart Association. *Med Sci Sports Exerc.* 2007;39(8):1423–34.

48. Headley S, Germain M, Mailloux P, et al. Resistance training improves strength and functional measures in patients with end-stage renal disease. *Am J Kidney Dis.* 2002;40:355–64.

49. Helmick CG, Lawrence RC, Pollard RA, Lloyd E, Heyse SP. Arthritis and other rheumatic conditions: who is affected now, who will be affected later? *Arthritis Care Res.* 1995;8:203–11.

50. Hiatt WR, Cox L, Greenwalt M, Griffin A, Schechter C. Quality of assessment of primary and secondary endpoints in claudication and critical leg ischemia trials. *Vasc Med.* 2005;10:207–13.

51. Hiatt WR, Wolfel EE, Meier RH, Regensteiner JG. Superiority of treadmill walking exercise versus strength training for patients with peripheral arterial disease. *Circulation.* 1994;90:1866–74.

52. Hirsch AT, Criqui MH, Treat-Johnson D, et al. Peripheral arterial disease detection, awareness, and treatment in primary care. *JAMA.* 2001;286:1317–24.

53. Hopman MT, Oeseburg B, Binkhorst RA. Cardiovascular responses in persons with paraplegia to prolonged arm exercise and thermal stress. *Med Sci Sports Exerc.* 1993;25:577–83.

54. Horowitz MB, Littenberg B, Mahler DA. Dyspnea ratings for prescribing exercise intensity in patients with COPD. *Chest.* 1996;109:1169–75.

55. International Diabetes Federation. The IDF consensus world-wide definition of the metabolic syndrome [Internet]. 2007. Available from: http://www.idf.org/webdata/docs/MetSyndrome_FINAL.pdf

56. Johansen KL. Exercise and chronic kidney disease: current recommendations. *Sports Med.* 2005;35:485–99.

57. Kendrick AH, Johns DP, Leeming JP. Infection control of lung function equipment: a practical approach. *Respir Med.* 2003;97:1163–79.

58. Klippel JH, editor. *Primer on the Rheumatic Diseases.* Atlanta (GA): Arthritis Foundation, 2001.

59. Knowler WC, Barrett-Connor E, Fowler SE, Hamman RF, Lachin JM, Walker EA, Nathan DM. Reduction in the incidence of type 2 diabetes with lifestyle intervention or metformin. *N Engl J Med.* 2002;346:393–403.

60. Kouidi EJ. Central and peripheral adaptations to physical training in patients with end-stage renal disease. *Sports Med.* 2001;31:651–65.

61. Lin K, Stewart D, Cooper S, Davis CL. Pre-transplant cardiac testing for kidney-pancreas transplant candidates and association with cardiac outcomes. *Clin Transplant.* 2001;15:269–75.

62. Liu G, Peacock M, Eilam O, Dorulla G, Braunstein E, Johnston CC. Effect of osteoarthritis in the lumbar spine and hip on bone mineral density and diagnosis of osteoporosis in elderly men and women. *Osteoporos Int.* 1997;7:564–9.

63. Lockette K, Keys A. *Conditioning with Physical Disabilities.* Champaign (IL): Human Kinetics; 1995. p. 65–90.

64. Lotters F, van Tol B, Kwakkel G, Gosselink R. Effects of controlled inspiratory muscle training in patients with COPD: a meta-analysis. *Eur Respir J.* 2002;20:570–6.

65. McNeely MI, Peddle C, Parliament M, Courneya KS. Cancer rehabilitation: recommendations for integrating exercise programming in the clinical practice setting. *Curr Cancer Ther Rev.* 2006;2(4):351–60.

66. Miller TD, Squires RW, Gau GT, Ilstrup DM, Frohnert PP, Sterioff S. Graded exercise testing and training after renal transplantation: a preliminary study. *Mayo Clin Proc.* 1987;62:773–7.

67. Minor MA, Kay DR. Arthritis. In: Durstine J.L. Moore GE, editors. *ACSM's Exercise Management for Persons with Chronic Diseases and Disabilities.* 2nd ed. Champagne (IL): Human Kinetics; 2003. p. 210–6.

68. National Cholesterol Education Program. Third Report of the National Cholesterol Education Program (NCEP) Expert Panel on the Detection, Evaluation, and Treatment of High Blood Cholesterol in Adults (Adult Treatment Panel III). 2002. Bethesda, MD, NIH Publication No. 02-5215.

69. National Heart Lung and Blood Institute. Seventh Report of the Joint National Committee on Prevention, Detection, Evaluation and Treatment of High Blood Pressure—JNC VII. Bethesda (MD): U.S. Department of Health and Human Services. 2004. 04-52302003.

70. National Institutes of Health and National Heart, Lung, and Blood Institute. Clinical guidelines on the identification, evaluation, and treatment of overweight and obesity in adults—the evidence report. *Obes Res.* 1998;6(suppl.2), p. 515–2095.

71. National Kidney Foundation. K/DOQI clinical practice guidelines for chronic kidney disease: evaluation, classification, and stratification. *Am J Kidney Dis.* 2002;39(2 suppl 1):S1–266.

72. Nici L, Donner C, Wouters E, et al. American Thoracic Society/European Respiratory Society statement on pulmonary rehabilitation. *Am J Respir Crit Care Med.* 2006;173:1390–413.

73. Nelson ME, Rejeski WJ, Blair SN, et al. Physical activity and public health in older adults: recommendation from the American College of Sports Medicine and the American Heart Association. *Med Sci Sports Exer.* 2007;39(8):1435–45.

74. Ness KK, Wall MM, Oakes JM, Robison LL, Gurney JG. Physical performance limitations and participation restrictions among cancer survivors: a population-based study. *Ann Epidemiol.* 2006;16:197–205.

75. Nocturnal Oxygen Therapy Trial Group. Continuous or nocturnal oxygen therapy in hypoxemic chronic obstructive lung disease: a clinical trial. *Ann Intern Med.* 1980;93:391–8.

76. O'Brien K, Nixon S, Glazier RH, Tynan AM. Progressive resistive exercise interventions for adults living with HIV/AIDS. *Cochrane Database Syst Rev.* 2004;CD004248.

77. O'Brien K, Nixon S, Tynan AM, Glazier RH. Effectiveness of aerobic exercise in adults living with HIV/AIDS: systematic review. *Med Sci Sports Exerc.* 2004;36:1659–66.

78. Ogden CL, Carroll MD, Curtin LR, McDowell MA, Tabak CJ, Flegal KM. Prevalence of overweight and obesity in the United States, 1999–2004. *JAMA.* 2006;295:1549–55.

79. Painter PL. Exercise after renal transplantation. *Adv Ren Replace Ther.* 1999;6:159–64.

80. Painter PL, Hector L, Ray K, et al. Randomized trial of exercise training after renal transplantation. *Transplantation.* 2002;74:42–8.

81. Painter PL, Krasnoff JB. End-stage metabolic disease: renal failure and liver failure. In: J.L. Durstine, editor. *ACSM's Exercise Management for Persons with Chronic Diseases and Disabilities.* 2nd ed. Champaign (IL): Human Kinetics; 2003. p. 126–32.

82. Painter P, Moore GE. The impact of recombinant human erythropoietin on exercise capacity in hemodialysis patients. *Adv Ren Replace Ther.* 1994;1:55–65.

83. Painter PL, Stewart AL, Carey S. Physical functioning: definitions, measurement, and expectations. *Adv Ren Replace Ther.* 1999;6:110–23.

84. Palisano RJ, Snider LM, Orlin MN. Recent advances in physical and occupational therapy for children with cerebral palsy. *Semin Pediatr Neurol.* 2004;11:66–77.

85. Pitetti K, Fernandez J, Lanciault M. Feasibility of an exercise program for adults with cerebral palsy: a pilot study. *Adapted Physical Activity Quarterly.* 1991;8:833–41.

86. Ram FS, Robinson SM, Black PN, Picot J. Physical training for asthma. *Cochrane Database Syst Rev.* 2005;CD001116.

87. Raymond J, Davis GM, Clarke J, Bryant G. Cardiovascular responses during arm exercise and orthostatic challenge in individuals with paraplegia. *Eur J Appl Physiol.* 2001;85:89–95.

88. Rimmer JH. Physical fitness levels of persons with cerebral palsy. *Develop Med Child Neurol.* 2001;43:208–12.

89. Robertson MC, Campbell AJ, Gardner MM, Devlin N. Preventing injuries in older people by preventing falls: a meta-analysis of individual-level data. *J Am Geriatr Soc.* 2002;50:905–11.

90. Ryuzaki M, Konishi K, Kasuga A, et al. Spontaneous rupture of the quadriceps tendon in patients on maintenance hemodialysis—report of three cases with clinicopathological observations. *Clin Nephrol.* 1989;32:144–8.

91. Saris WHM, Blair SN, van Baak MA, et al. How much physical activity is enough to prevent unhealthy weight gain? Outcome of the IASO 1st Stock Conference and consensus statement. *Obes Rev.* 2003;4:101–14.

92. Sawyer EH, Clanton TL. Improved pulmonary function and exercise tolerance with inspiratory muscle conditioning in children with cystic fibrosis. *Chest.* 1993;104:1490–7.

93. Scevola D, Di Matteo A, Lanzarini P, et al. Effect of exercise and strength training on cardiovascular status in HIV-infected patients receiving highly active antiretroviral therapy. *AIDS* 2003;17(Suppl 1):S123–9.

94. Schmid A, Schmidt-Trucksass A, Huonker M, et al. Catecholamines response of high performance wheelchair athletes at rest and during exercise with autonomic dysreflexia. *Int J Sports Med.* 2001;22:2–7.

95. Sigal RJ, Kenny GP, Wasserman DH, Castaneda-Sceppa C, White RD. Physical activity/exercise and type 2 diabetes: a consensus statement from the American Diabetes Association. *Diabetes Care.* 2006;29:1433–8.

96. Squires RW. Pathophysiology and clinical features of cardiovascular diseases. In: Kaminsky LA, editor. *ACSM's Resource Manual for Guidelines for Exercise Testing and Prescription.* 5th ed. Philadelphia (PA): Lippincott Williams & Wilkins; 2006. p. 411–38.

97. Steadward R. Musculoskeletal and neurological disabilities: implications for fitness appraisal, programming and counseling. *Can J Appl Physiol.* 1998;23:131–65.

98. Stein CJ, Colditz GA. The epidemic of obesity. *J Clin Endocrinol Metab.* 2004;89:2522–5.

99. Stein R, Hriljac I, Halperin JL, et al. Limitation of the resting ankle-brachial index in symptomatic patients with peripheral arterial disease. *Vasc Med.* 2006;11:29–33.

100. Thom T, Haase N, Rosamond W, et al. Heart disease and stroke statistics—2006 update: a report from the American Heart Association Statistics Committee and Stroke Statistics Subcommittee. *Circulation.* 2006;113:85–151.

101. Troosters T, Casaburi R, Gosselink R, DeCramer M. Pulmonary rehabilitation in chronic obstructive pulmonary disease. *Am J Respir Crit Care Med.* 2005;172:19–38.

102. Unnithan VB, Clifford C, Bar-Or O. Evaluation by exercise testing of the child with cerebral palsy. *Sports Med.* 1998;26:239–51.

103. U.S. Department of Health and Human Services. *Bone Health and Osteoporosis: A Report of the Surgeon General*. Rockville (MD): U.S. Department of Health and Human Services, Office of the Surgeon General; 2004.

104. U.S. Department of Health and Human Services. *Physical Activity and Health: A Report of the Surgeon General*. Atlanta (GA): U.S. Department of Health and Human Services, Centers for Disease Control and Prevention, and National Center for Chronic Disease Prevention and Health Promotion; 1996.

105. U.S. Department of Health and Human Services and U.S. Department of Agriculture. *Dietary Guidelines for Americans* [Internet]. 2005 [cited 2007 June 15]. Available from: www.healthierus.gov/dietaryguidelines

106. U.S. Preventive Task Force. Screening for coronary artery disease: recommendations statement. *Ann Intern Med*. 2004;140:569–72.

107. U.S. Renal Data System. *USRDS 2006 Annual Data Report. Atlas of End-Stage Renal Disease in the United States*. Bethesda (MD): National Institutes of Health, National Institutes of Diabetes and Digestive and Kidney Diseases; 2006.

108. Van Drongelen S, Van der Woude LH, Janssen TW, Angenot EL, Chadwick EK, Veeger DH. Glenohumeral contact forces and muscle forces evaluated in wheelchair related activities of daily living in able-bodied subjects versus subjects with paraplegia and tetraplegia. *Arch Phys Med Rehabil*. 2005;86:1434–40.

109. Vanlandewijck YC, Theisen D, Daly D. Wheelchair propulsion biomechanics: implications for wheelchair sports. *Sports Med*. 2001;31:339–67.

110. Vinik A, Erbas T. Neuropathy. In: Ruderman N, Devlin JT, Schneider SH, Kriska A, editors. *Handbook of Exercise in Diabetes*. 2nd ed. Alexandria (VA): American Diabetes Association; 2002. p. 463–96.

111. Violan MA, Pomes T, Maldonado S, et al. Exercise capacity in hemodialysis and renal transplant patients. *Transplant Proc*. 2002;34:417–8.

112. Volberding PA, Murphy RL, Barbaro G, et al. The Pavia Consensus Statement. *AIDS* 2003; 17(Suppl):S170–9.

113. Wackers FJ, Young LH, Inzucchi SE, et al. Detection of ischemia in asymptomatic diabetics investigators: detection of silent myocardial ischemia in asymptomatic diabetic subjects: the DIAD study. *Diabetes Care*. 2004;27:1954–61.

114. Wing RR. Behavioral weight control. In: Wadden TA, Stunkard AJ, editors. *Handbook of Obesity Treatment*. New York (NY): Guilford Press; 2002. p. 301–16.

115. Womack CJ, Gardner AW. Peripheral arterial disease. In: Durstine JL, editor. *ACSM's Exercise Management for Persons with Chronic Diseases and Disabilities*. 2nd ed. Champaign (IL): Human Kinetics; 2003. p. 81–5.

116. Yarasheski KE, Roubenoff R. Exercise treatment for HIV-associated metabolic and anthropomorphic complications. *Exerc Sport Sci Rev*. 2001;29:170–4.

IV

Appendices

APPENDIX

A   Common Medications

β-BLOCKERS

Use or condition: Hypertension, angina, arrhythmias including supraventricular tachycardia, and increasing atrioventricular (AV) block to slow ventricular response in atrial fibrillation, acute myocardial infarction, migraine headaches, anxiety; mandatory as part of therapy for heart failure that is due to systolic dysfunction.

DRUG NAME	BRAND NAME[b]
Acebutolol[a]	Sectral[a]
Atenolol	Tenormin
Betaxolol	Kerlone
Bisoprolol	Zebeta
Esmolol	Brevibloc
Metoprolol	Lopressor SR, Toprol XL
Nadolol	Corgard
Penbutolol[a]	Levatol[a]
Pindolol[a]	Visken[a]
Propranolol	Inderal
Sotalol	Betapace
Timolol	Blocadren

[a]β-Blockers with intrinsic sympathomimetic activity.

[b]Represent selected brands; these are not necessarily all inclusive.

β-BLOCKERS IN COMBINATION WITH DIURETICS

Use or condition: Hypertension, diuretic, glaucoma.

DRUG NAME	BRAND NAME[b]
Atenolol, chlorthalidone	Tenoretic
Bendroflumethiazide, nadolol	Corzide
Bisoprolol, hydrochlorothiazide	Ziac
Metoprolol, hydrochlorothiazide	Lopressor HCT
Propranolol, hydrochlorothiazide	Inderide
Timolol, hydrochlorothiazide	Timolide

α- AND β-ADRENERGIC BLOCKING AGENTS

Use or condition: Hypertension, chronic heart failure, angina.

DRUG NAME	BRAND NAME[b]
Carvedilol	Coreg
Labetalol	Normodyne, Trandate

$α_1$-ADRENERGIC BLOCKING AGENTS

Use or condition: Hypertension, enlarged prostate.

DRUG NAME	BRAND NAME[b]
Cardura	Doxazosin
Flomax	Tamsulosin
Minipress	Prazosin
Terazosin	Hytrin

CENTRAL $α_2$-AGONISTS AND OTHER CENTRALLY ACTING DRUGS

Use or condition: Hypertension.

DRUG NAME	BRAND NAME[b]
Clonidine	Catapres, Catapres-TTS patch
Guanfacine	Tenex
Methyldopa	Aldomet
Reserpine	Serpasil

CENTRAL $α_2$-AGONISTS IN COMBINATION WITH DIURETICS

Use or condition: Hypertension.

DRUG NAME	BRAND NAME[b]
Methyldopa + hydrochlorothiazide	Aldoril
Reserpine + chlorothiazide	Diupres
Reserpine + hydrochlorothiazide	Hydropres

NITRATES AND NITROGLYCERIN

Use or condition: Angina, vasodilator in chronic heart failure.

DRUG NAME	BRAND NAME[b]
Amyl nitrite	Amyl Nitrite
Isosorbide mononitrate	Ismo, Imdur, Monoket
Isosorbide dinitrate	Dilatrate, Isordil, Sorbitrate
Nitroglycerin, sublingual	Nitrostat, NitroQuick
Nitroglycerin, translingual	Nitrolingual
Nitroglycerin, transmucosal	Nitrogard
Nitroglycerin, sustained release	Nitrong, Nitrocine, Nitroglyn, Nitro-Bid
Nitroglycerin, transdermal	Minitran, Nitro-Dur, Transderm-Nitro, Deponit, Nitrodisc, Nitro-Derm
Nitroglycerin, topical	Nitro-Bid, Nitrol

CALCIUM CHANNEL BLOCKERS (NONDIHYDROPYRIDINES)

Use or condition: Angina, hypertension, increasing AV block to slow ventricular response in atrial fibrillation, paroxysmal supraventricular tachycardia, headache.

DRUG NAME	BRAND NAME[b]
Diltiazem extended release	Cardizem CD, Cardizem LA, Dilacor XR, Tiazac
Verapamil immediate release	Calan, Isoptin
Verapamil long acting	Calan SR, Isoptin SR
Verapamil Coer 24	Covera HS, Verelan PM

CALCIUM CHANNEL BLOCKERS (DIHYDROPYRIDINES)

Use or condition: Hypertension, angina, neurologic deficits after subarachnoid hemorrhage.

DRUG NAME	BRAND NAME[b]
Amlodipine	Norvasc
Felodipine	Plendil
Isradipine	DynaCirc CR
Nicardipine sustained release	Cardene SR
Nifedipine long acting	Adalat, Procardia XL
Nimodipine	Nimotop
Nisoldipine	Sular

CARDIAC GLYCOSIDES

Use or condition: Chronic heart failure in the setting of dilated cardiomyopathy, increasing of AV block to slow ventricular response with atrial fibrillation.

DRUG NAME	BRAND NAME[b]
Digoxin	Lanoxin

DIRECT PERIPHERAL VASODILATORS

Use or condition: Hypertension, hair loss, vasodilation for heart failure.

DRUG NAME	BRAND NAME[b]
Hydralazine	Apresoline
Minoxidil	Loniten

ANGIOTENSIN-CONVERTING ENZYME (ACE) INHIBITORS

Use or condition: Hypertension, coronary artery disease, chronic heart failure that is due to systolic dysfunction, diabetes, chronic kidney disease, heart attacks, scleroderma, migraines.

DRUG NAME	BRAND NAME[b]
Benazepril	Lotensin
Captopril	Capoten
Cilazapril[a]	Inhibace
Enalapril	Vasotec
Fosinopril	Monopril
Lisinopril	Zestril, Prinivil
Moexipril	Univasc
Perindopril	Aceon
Quinapril	Accupril
Ramipril	Altace
Trandolapril	Mavik

[a]Available only in Canada.

ACE INHIBITORS IN COMBINATION WITH DIURETICS

Use or condition: Hypertension, chronic heart failure.

DRUG NAME	BRAND NAME[b]
Benazepril + hydrochlorothiazide	Lotensin
Captopril + hydrochlorothiazide	Capozide
Enalapril + hydrochlorothiazide	Vaseretic
Lisinopril + hydrochlorothiazide	Prinzide, Zestoretic
Moexipril + hydrochlorothiazide	Uniretic
Quinapril + hydrochlorothiazide	Accuretic

ACE INHIBITORS IN COMBINATION WITH CALCIUM CHANNEL BLOCKERS

Use or condition: Hypertension, chronic heart failure, angina.

DRUG NAME	BRAND NAME[b]
Benazepril + amlodipine	Lotrel
Enalapril + felodipine	Lexxel
Trandolapril + verapamil	Tarka

ANGIOTENSIN II RECEPTOR ANTAGONISTS

Use or condition: Hypertension.

DRUG NAME	BRAND NAME[b]
Candesartan	Atacand
Eprosartan	Teveten
Irbesartan	Avapro
Losartan	Cozaar
Olmesartan	Benicar
Telmisartan	Micardis
Valsartan	Diovan

ANGIOTENSIN II RECEPTOR ANTAGONISTS IN COMBINATION WITH DIURETICS

Use or condition: Hypertension, chronic heart failure, angina.

DRUG NAME	BRAND NAME[b]
Candesartan + hydrochlorothiazide	Atacand HCT
Eprosartan + hydrochlorothiazide	Teveten HCT
Irbesartan + hydrochlorothiazide	Avalide
Losartan + hydrochlorothiazide	Hyzaar
Telmisartan + hydrochlorothiazide	Micardis HCT
Valsartan + hydrochlorothiazide	Diovan HCT

DIURETICS

Use or condition: Edema, chronic heart failure, polycystic ovary syndrome, certain kidney disorders (i.e., kidney stones, diabetes insipidus, female hirsutism, osteoporosis).

THIAZIDES

DRUG NAME	BRAND NAME[b]
Chlorothiazide	Diuril
Hydrochlorothiazide (HCTZ)	Microzide, Hydrodiuril, Oretic
Indapamide	Lozol
Metolazone	Mykron, Zaroxolyn
Polythiazide	Renese

LOOP DIURETICS

DRUG NAME	BRAND NAME[b]
Bumetanide	Bumex
Ethacrynic acid	Edecrin
Furosemide	Lasix
Torsemide	Demadex

POTASSIUM-SPARING DIURETICS

DRUG NAME	BRAND NAME[b]
Amiloride	Midamor
Triamterene	Dyrenium

ALDOSTERONE RECEPTOR BLOCKERS

DRUG NAME	BRAND NAME[b]
Eplerenone	Inspra
Spironolactone	Aldactone

DIURETIC COMBINED WITH DIURETIC

DRUG NAME	BRAND NAME[b]
Amiloride + hydrochlorothiazide	Moduretic
Triamterene + hydrochlorothiazide	Dyazide, Maxide

ANTIARRHYTHMIC AGENTS

Use or condition: Specific for drug but include suppression of atrial fibrillation and maintenance of normal sinus rhythm (NSR), serious ventricular arrhythmias in certain clinical settings, increase in AV nodal block to slow ventricular response in atrial fibrillation.

DRUG NAME	BRAND NAME[b]
CLASS I	
IA	
Disopyramide	Norpace
Moricizine	Ethmozine
Procainamide	Pronestyl, Procan SR
Quinidine	Quinora, Quinidex, Quinaglute, Quinalan, Cardioquin
IB	
Lidocaine	Xylocaine, Xylocard
Mexiletine	Mexitil
Phenytoin	Dilantin
Tocainide	Tonocard
IC	
Flecainide	Tambocor
Propafenone	Rythmol
CLASS II	
β-Blockers	Refer to page 274
CLASS III	
Amiodarone	Cordarone, Pacerone
Bretylium	Bretylol
Sotalol	Betapace
Dofetilide	Tikosyn
CLASS IV	
Calcium channel blockers	Refer to page 276

ANTILIPEMIC AGENTS

Use or condition: Elevated blood cholesterol, low-density lipoproteins, triglycerides, low high-density lipoproteins, and metabolic syndrome.

CATEGORY	DRUG NAME	BRAND NAME[b]
A	Cholestyramine	Questran, Cholybar, Prevalite
A	Colesevelam	Welchol
A	Colestipol	Colestid
B	Clofibrate	Atromid
B	Fenofibrate	Tricor, Lofibra
B	Gemfibrozil	Lopid
C	Atorvastatin	Lipitor
C	Fluvastatin	Lescol
C	Lovastatin	Mevacor
C	Lovastatin + niacin	Advicor
C	Pravastatin	Pravachol
C	Rosuvastatin	Crestor
C	Simvastatin	Zocor
D	Atorvastatin + amlodipine	Caduet
E	Niacin	Niaspan, Nicobid, Slo-Niacin
F	Ezetimibe	Zeta
F	Ezetimibe + simvastatin	Vytorin

A, bile acid sequestrants; B, fibric acid sequestrants; C, HMG-CoA reductase inhibitors; D, HMG-CoA reductase inhibitors + calcium channel blocker; E, nicotinic acid; F, cholesterol absorption inhibitor.

BLOOD MODIFIERS (ANTICOAGULANT OR ANTIPLATELET)

Use or condition: To prevent blood clots, heart attack, stroke, intermittent claudication, or vascular death in patients with established peripheral arterial disease (PAD) or acute ST-segment elevation myocardial infarction. Also, used to reduce aching, tiredness and cramps in hands and feet. Plavix is critical to maintain for one year after percutaneous coronary intervention (PCI) for drug-eluting stents (DES) patency.

DRUG NAME	BRAND NAME[b]
Cilostazol	Pletal
Clopidogrel	Plavix
Dipyridamole	Persantine
Pentoxifylline	Trental
Ticlopidine	Ticlid
Warfarin	Coumadin

RESPIRATORY AGENTS

STEROIDAL ANTI-INFLAMMATORY AGENTS

Use or condition: Allergy symptoms including sneezing, itching, and runny or stuffed nose, shrink nasal polyps, various skin disorders, asthma.

DRUG NAME	BRAND NAME[b]
Beclomethasone	Beclovent, Qvar
Budesonide	Pulmicort
Flunisolide	AeroBid
Fluticasone	Flovent
Fluticasone and salmeterol (β_2 receptor agonist)	Advair Diskus
Triamcinolone	Azmacort

BRONCHODILATORS

Anticholinergics (Acetylcholine Receptor Antagonist)

Use or condition: To prevent wheezing, shortness of breath, and troubled breathing caused by asthma, chronic bronchitis, emphysema, and other lung diseases.

DRUG NAME	BRAND NAME[b]
Ipratropium	Atrovent

Anticholinergics with Sympathomimetics (β_2-Receptor Agonists)

Use or condition: Chronic obstructive pulmonary lung disease (COPD).

DRUG NAME	BRAND NAME[b]
Ipratropium and albuterol	Combivent

Sympathomimetics (β_2-Receptor Agonists)

Use or condition: To prevent wheezing, shortness of breath, and troubled breathing caused by asthma, chronic bronchitis, emphysema, and other lung diseases.

DRUG NAME	BRAND NAME[b]
Albuterol	Proventil, Ventolin
Metaproterenol	Alupent
Pirbuterol	Maxair
Salmeterol	Serevent
Salmeterol and fluticasone (steroid)	Advair
Terbutaline	Brethine

Xanthine Derivatives

Use or condition: To prevent wheezing, shortness of breath, and troubled breathing caused by asthma, chronic bronchitis, emphysema, and other lung diseases.

DRUG NAME	BRAND NAME[b]
Theophylline	Theo-Dur, Uniphyl

Leukotriene Antagonists and Formation Inhibitors

Use or condition: To prevent wheezing, shortness of breath, and troubled breathing caused by asthma, chronic bronchitis, emphysema, and other lung diseases.

DRUG NAME	BRAND NAME[b]
Montelukast	Singulair
Zafirlukast	Accolate
Zileuton	Zyflo

Mast Cell Stabilizers

Use or condition: To prevent wheezing, shortness of breath, and troubled breathing caused by asthma, chronic bronchitis, emphysema, and other lung diseases.

DRUG NAME	BRAND NAME[b]
Cromolyn inhaled	Intal
Nedocromil	Tilade
Omalizumab	Xolair

ANTIDIABETIC AGENTS

BIGUANIDES (DECREASES HEPATIC GLUCOSE PRODUCTION AND INTESTINAL GLUCOSE ABSORPTION)

Use or condition: Type 2 or adult onset diabetes.

DRUG NAME	BRAND NAME[b]
Metformin	Glucophage, Riomet
Metformin and glyburide	Glucovance

GLUCOSIDASE INHIBITORS (INHIBIT INTESTINAL GLUCOSE ABSORPTION)

Use or condition: Type 2 or adult onset diabetes.

DRUG NAME	BRAND NAME[b]
Miglitol	Glyset

INSULINS

Use or condition: Type 1, or sometimes Type 2 or adult onset diabetes.

RAPID-ACTING	INTERMEDIATE-ACTING	INTERMEDIATE- AND RAPID-ACTING COMBINATION	LONG-ACTING
Humalog	Humulin L	Humalog Mix	Humulin U
Humulin R	Humulin N	Humalog 50/50	Lantus injection
Novolin R	Iletin II Lente	Humalog 70/30	Levemir
Iletin II R	Iletin II NPH	Novolin 70/30	
	Novolin L		
	Nivalin N		

MEGLITINIDES (STIMULATE PANCREATIC ISLET β CELLs)

Use or condition: Type 2 or adult onset diabetes.

DRUG NAME	BRAND NAME[b]
Nateglinide	Starlix
Repaglinide	Prandin, Gluconorm

SULFONYLUREAS (STIMULATE PANCREATIC ISLET β CELLs)

Use or condition: Type 2 or adult onset diabetes.

DRUG NAME	BRAND NAME[b]
Chlorpropamide[a]	Diabinese
Gliclazide	Diamicron
Glimepiride[a]	Amaryl
Glipizide[a]	Glucotrol
Glyburide	DiaBeta, Glynase, Micronase
Tolazamide[a]	Tolinase
Tolbutamide[a]	Orinase

[a]These drugs have been associated with increased cardiovascular mortality.

THIAZOLIDINEDIONES (INCREASE INSULIN SENSITIVITY)

Use or condition: Type 2 or adult onset diabetes.

DRUG NAME	BRAND NAME[b]
Pioglitazone	Actos
Rosiglitazone	Avandia

INCRETIN MIMETICS (INCREASE INSULIN AND DECREASE GLUCAGON SECRETION)

Use or condition: Type 2 diabetes.

DRUG NAME	BRAND NAME[b]
Glucagon-like Peptide 1	Byetta

OBESITY MANAGEMENT

APPETITE SUPPRESSANTS

Use or condition: Morbid obesity and metabolic syndrome.

DRUG NAME	BRAND NAME[b]
Sibutramine	Meridia

LIPASE INHIBITORS

Use or condition: Morbid obesity and metabolic syndrome.

DRUG NAME	BRAND NAME[b]
Orlistat	Xenical

---

[b]Represent selected brands; these are not necessarily all inclusive.

TABLE A.2. EFFECTS OF MEDICATIONS ON HEART RATE, BLOOD PRESSURE, THE ELECTROCARDIOGRAM (ECG), AND EXERCISE CAPACITY

MEDICATIONS	HEART RATE	BLOOD PRESSURE	ECG	EXERCISE CAPACITY
I. β-Blockers (including carvedilol and labetalol)	↓[a] (R and E)	↓ (R and E)	↓ HR[a] (R) ↓ ischemia[b] (E)	↑ in patients with angina ↓ or ↔ in patients without angina
II. Nitrates	↑ (R) ↑ or ↔ (E)	↓ (R) ↓ or ↔ (E)	↑ HR (R) ↑ or ↔ HR (E) ↓ ischemia[b] (E)	↑ in patients with angina ↔ in patients without angina ↑ or ↔ in patients with chronic heart failure (CHF)
III. Calcium channel blockers				
Amlodipine Felodipine Isradipine Nicardipine Nifedipine Nimodipine Nisoldipine	↑ or ↔ (R and E)	↓ (R and E)	↑ or ↔ HR (R and E) ↓ ischemia[b] (E)	↑ in patients with angina ↔ in patients without angina
Diltiazem Verapamil	↓ (R and E) ↓ in patients with atrial fibrillation and possibly CHF Not significantly altered in patients with sinus rhythm		↓ HR (R and E) ↓ ischemia[b] (E)	
IV. Digitalis		↔ (R and E)	May produce non-specific ST-T wave changes (R) May produce ST segment depression (E)	Improved only in patients with atrial fibrillation or in patients with CHF

V. Diuretics	↔ (R and E)	↔ or ↓ (R and E)	↔ or PVCs (R) May cause PVCs and false-positive test results if hypokalemia occurs May cause PVCs if hypomagnesemia occurs (E)	↔, except possibly in patients with CHF
VI. Vasodilators, nonadrenergic	↑ or ↔ (R and E)	↓ (R and E)	↑ or ↔ HR (R and E)	↔, except ↑ or ↔ in patients with CHF
ACE inhibitors and angiotensin II receptor blockers	↔ (R and E)	↓ (R and E)	↔ (R and E)	↔, except ↑ or ↔ in patients with CHF
α-Adrenergic blockers	↔ (R and E)	↓ (R and E)	↔ (R and E)	↔
Antiadrenergic agents without selective blockade	↓ or ↔ (R and E)	↓ (R and E)	↓ or ↔ HR (R and E)	↔
VII. Antiarrhythmic agents	All antiarrhythmic agents may cause new or worsened arrhythmias (proarrhythmic effect)			
Class I				
Quinidine	↑ or ↔ (R and E)	↓ or ↔ (R)	↑ or ↔ HR (R) May prolong QRS and Quinidine may result in false-negative test results (E)	↔ QT intervals (R)
Disopyramide		↔ (E)		

(continued)

TABLE A.2. EFFECTS OF MEDICATIONS ON HEART RATE, BLOOD PRESSURE, THE ELECTROCARDIOGRAM (ECG), AND EXERCISE CAPACITY (*Continued*)

MEDICATIONS	HEART RATE	BLOOD PRESSURE	ECG	EXERCISE CAPACITY
Procainamide	↔ (R and E)	↔ (R and E)	May prolong QRS and QT intervals (R) May result in false-positive test results (E)	↔
Phenytoin Tocainide Mexiletine	↔ (R and E)	↔ (R and E)	↔ (R and E)	↔
Moricizine	↔ (R and E)	↔ (R and E)	May prolong QRS and QT intervals (R) ↔ (E)	↔
Propafenone	↓ (R) ↓ or ↔ (E)	↔ (R and E)	↓ HR (R) ↓ or ↔ HR (E)	↔
Class II β-Blockers (see I)				
Class III Amiodarone Sotalol	↓ (R and E)	↔ (R and E)	↓ HR (R) ↔ (E)	↔
Class IV Calcium channel blockers (see III)				
VIII. Bronchodilators	↔ (R and E)	↔ (R and E)	↔ (R and E)	Bronchodilators ↔ exercise capacity in patients limited by bronchospasm
Anticholinergic agents Xanthine derivatives	↑ or ↔ (R and E)	↔	↑ or ↔ HR May produce PVCs (R and E)	

Sympathomimetic agents	↑ or ↔ (R and E)	↑, ↔, or ↓ (R and E)	↑ or ↔ HR (R and E)	↔↑
Cromolyn sodium	↔ (R and E)	↔ (R and E)	↔ (R and E)	↔↑
Steroidal anti-inflammatory agents	↑ (R and E)	↔ (R and E)	↔ (R and E)	↔↑
IX. Antilipemic agents	Clofibrate may provoke arrhythmias, angina in patients with prior myocardial infarction Nicotinic acid may ↓ BP All other hyperlipidemic agents have no effect on HR, BP, and ECG			↔↑
X. Psychotropic medications				
Minor tranquilizers	May ↓ HR and BP by controlling anxiety; no other effects			
Antidepressants	↑ or ↔ (R and E)	↓ or ↔ (R and E)	Variable (R)	
Major tranquilizers	↑ or ↔ (R and E)	↓ or ↔ (R and E)	Variable (R)	
Lithium	↔ (R and E)	↔ (R and E)	May result in T-wave changes and arrhythmias (R and E)	
XI. Nicotine	↑ or ↔ (R and E)	↑ (R and E)	↑ or ↔ HR May provoke ischemia, arrhythmias (R and E)	↔, except ↓ or ↔ in patients with angina
XII. Antihistamines	↔ (R and E)	↔ (R and E)	↔ (R and E)	↔↑

(continued)

TABLE A.2. EFFECTS OF MEDICATIONS ON HEART RATE, BLOOD PRESSURE, THE ELECTROCARDIOGRAM (ECG), AND EXERCISE CAPACITY (*Continued*)

MEDICATIONS	HEART RATE	BLOOD PRESSURE	ECG	EXERCISE CAPACITY
XIII. Cold medications with sympathomimetic agents	Effects similar to those described in sympathomimetic agents, although magnitude of effects is usually smaller			↔
XIV. Thyroid medications	↑ (R and E)	↑ (R and E)	↑ HR May provoke arrhythmias ↑ ischemia (R and E)	↔, unless angina worsened
Only levothyroxine				
XV. Alcohol	↔ (R and E)	Chronic use may have role in ↑ BP (R and E)	May provoke arrhythmias (R and E)	↔
XVI. Hypoglycemic agents Insulin and oral agents	↔ (R and E)	↔ (R and E)	↔ (R and E)	↔
XVII. Blood modifiers (anticoagulants and antiplatelets)	↔ (R and E)	↔ (R and E)	↔ (R and E)	↔
XVIII. Pentoxifylline	↔ (R and E)	↔ (R and E)	↔ (R and E)	↑ or ↔ in patients limited by intermittent claudication (for cilostazol only)
XIX. Antigout medications	↔ (R and E)	↔ (R and E)	↔ (R and E)	↔ in patients limited by intermittent claudication
				↔

TABLE A.2. EFFECTS OF MEDICATIONS ON HEART RATE, BLOOD PRESSURE, THE ELECTROCARDIOGRAM (ECG) AND EXERCISE CAPACITY (*Continued*)

XX. Caffeine	Variable effects depending on previous use		
	Variable effects on exercise capacity		
	May provoke arrhythmias		
XXI. Anorexiants/diet pills	↑ or ↔ (R and E)	↑ or ↔ (R and E)	↑ or ↔ HR (R and E) Increased HR and BP common with norepinephrine reuptake inhibitors (e.g., sibutramine)

PVCs, premature ventricular contractions; ↑, increase; ↔, no effect; ↓, decrease; R, rest; E, exercise; HR, heart rate; BP, blood pressure.

^{a}β-Blockers with intrinsic sympathomimetic activity (ISA) lower resting heart rate only slightly.

^{b}May prevent or delay myocardial ischemia (see text).

B

Medical Emergency Management

The following key points are essential components of all medical emergency plans:

1. All personnel involved with exercise testing and supervision should be trained in basic cardiopulmonary resuscitation (CPR) and preferably advanced cardiac life support (ACLS).
2. All personnel should be trained in the proper handling of blood and bodily fluids and familiar with the risks of bloodborne pathogens according to the OSHA Guidelines For Healthcare Workers.
3. There should be at least one and preferably two trained ACLS personnel and a physician immediately available at all times when maximal sign- or symptom-limited exercise testing is performed.
4. Telephone numbers for emergency assistance should be posted clearly on or near all telephones. Emergency communication devices must be readily available and working properly.
5. Medical emergency plans should be available in writing, approved by the medical director, and easily accessible to all personnel. Regular review and training procedures should be provided to all personnel at the beginning of employment for relevant emergency procedures.
6. Regular rehearsal of emergency plans and scenarios should be conducted and documented specifying rehearsal dates, attendees, and emergency performance markers.
   a. Regular drills should be conducted at least quarterly for all personnel, including support staff as well as the medical emergency response team and/or paramedics (if exercise testing and/or training is performed outside of a hospital setting).
   b. Designated personnel should be assigned to the regular maintenance of the emergency equipment and regular surveillance of all pharmacologic substances (i.e., monthly and/or as determined by hospital and/or facility protocol).
   c. Records should be kept documenting proper functioning of medical emergency equipment, such as defibrillator, automated external defibrillator (AED), oxygen supply, and suction (i.e., daily for all days of operations). All malfunctioning medical emergency equipment should be locked out/tagged out and dealt with immediately with operations suspended until repaired and/or replaced. In addition, expiration dates for pharmacologic agents and other supportive supplies (e.g., intravenous equipment and intravenous fluids) should be kept on file and readily available for review.

d. Medical emergency response teams and other sources of support such as paramedics (if exercise testing and/or training is performed outside of a hospital setting) should be advised as to the location of the exercise area as well as the usual times of operation.

e. Incident reports should clearly be documented, including the event time and date, witnesses present, and a detailed report of the medical emergency care provided. Copies of all documentation should be preserved onsite, maintaining the injuried personnel's confidentiality; a corresponding follow-up postincident report is highly recommended.

If a medical emergency occurs during exercise testing and/or training, the nearest available physician and/or other trained ACLS provider should be solicited along with the medical emergency response team and/or paramedic (if exercise is conducted outside of the hospital setting). The physician or lead medical responder should decide whether to evacuate to the emergency department based on whether the medical emergency is life-threatening. If a physician is not available and there is any likelihood of decompensation, then transportation to the emergency department should be made immediately.

Emergency equipment and drugs that should be available in any area where maximal exercise testing is performed are listed in Table B-1. Only personnel authorized by law and policy to use certain medical emergency equipment (e.g., defibrillators, syringes, needles) and dispense drugs can lawfully do so. It is expected that such personnel be immediately available during maximal exercise testing of persons with known coronary artery disease.

AUTOMATED EXTERNAL DEFIBRILLATORS

Automated external defibrillators are computerized, sophisticated devices that provide voice and visual cues to guide lay and healthcare providers to safely defibrillate pulseless ventricular tachycardia/fibrillation (VF) sudden cardiac arrest (SCA). Early defibrillation plays a critical role for successful survival of SCA for the following reasons:

1. VF is the most frequent SCA witnessed.
2. Electrical defibrillation is the treatment for VF.
3. With delayed electrical defibrillation, the probability of success diminishes rapidly.
4. VF deteriorates to asystole within minutes.

According to the American Heart Association 2005 Guidelines for Cardiopulmonary Resuscitation (CPR) and Emergency Cardiovascular Care, "rescuers must be able to rapidly integrate CPR with use of the AED" (1,2). Three key components must occur within the initial moments of a cardiac arrest:

1. Activation of the emergency medical services
2. CPR
3. Operation of an AED

TABLE B.1. MEDICAL EMERGENCY EQUIPMENT AND DRUGS

EQUIPMENT

- Portable, battery-operated defibrillator-monitor with hardcopy printout or memory, cardioversion capability, direct-current capability in case of battery failure (equipment must have battery low-light indicator). Defibrillator should be able to perform hard-wire monitoring in case of exercise testing monitor failure. An automated external defibrillator (AED) is an acceptable alternative to a manual defibrillator in most settings.
- Sphygmomanometer, including aneroid cuff and stethoscope
- Airway supplies, including oral, nasopharyngeal, and/or intubation equipment (only in situations in which trained personnel are available for use)
- Oxygen, available by nasal cannula and mask
- Ambu bag with pressure-release valve
- Suction equipment
- Intravenous fluids and stand
- Intravenous access equipment in varying sizes, including butterfly intravenous supplies
- Syringes and needles in multiple sizes
- Tourniquets
- Adhesive tape, alcohol wipes, gauze pads
- Emergency documentation forms (incident/accident form or code charting form)

DRUGS (IV FORM UNLESS OTHERWISE INDICATED)[a]

- Pharmacologic agents used to treat ventricular fibrillation/pulseless ventricular tachycardia: epinephrine, vasopressin
- Asystole and pulseless electrical activity: vasopressin, epinephrine, atropine
- Antiarrhythmics for VF and pulseless VT: amiodarone, lidocaine, procainamide, and magnesium
- Pharmacologic agents used to treat acute coronary syndromes: acute ischemia chest pain:
  - Oxygen (mask or nasal cannula), aspirin (oral), nitroglycerin (oral or IV), morphine (if pain not relieved with nitroglycerin)
  - β-Adrenergic blockers (see Appendix A for list), heparin, ACE inhibitors (see Appendix A for list), glycoprotein IIb/IIIa receptor inhibitors, fibrinolytic agents
  - Tissue plasminogen activator (tPA): alteplase
    - □ Streptokinase
    - □ Reteplase: Retavase
    - □ Anisoylated plasminogen activator complex (APSAC): Eminase
    - □ TNKase: Tenecteplase
- Pharmacologic agents used to treat bradycardias: atropine, dopamine, epinephrine, isoproterenol
- Pharmacologic agents used to treat unstable and stable tachycardias:
  Most commonly used: adenosine, β-adrenergic blockers (esmolol, atenolol, metoprolol), calcium channel blockers (diltiazem, verapamil), digoxin, procainamide, amiodarone, lidocaine, ibutilide, magnesium sulfate
  Less commonly used: flecainide, propafenone, sotalol (not approved for use in United States)

[a]American Heart Association, 2005. Drugs in parentheses are used most frequently for tachycardias within a class of agents.

The reader is encouraged to review ACLS algorithms, where the pharmacologic agents described in this table are used in the context of the ABCDs (airway—opening and maintaining the airway; breathing—providing positive-pressure ventilations; circulation—chest compressions; defibrillation/transcutaneous electrical pacing or synchronized cardioversion).

Delays in CPR or defibrillation reduces SCA survival. Use of both CPR and AED units have shown survival rates between 49% and 75% for out-of-hospital SCA events. Thus, there is growing use and support for AEDs in medical and nonmedical settings (e.g., airports, airplanes, casinos). Recent guidelines from the American Heart Association indicate that for a witnessed cardiac arrest, immediate bystander CPR and early use of an AED can achieve outcomes equivalent to those achieved with the full ACLS armamentarium.

AED GENERAL GUIDELINES

1. In hospital settings, CPR and an AED should be used immediately for cardiac arrest incidents.
2. For out-of-hospital events when an AED is available, the AED should be used as soon as possible. Survival rate is improved when AED use is proceeded by five CPR cycles at a rate of 100 compressions per minute for approximately two minutes. One CPR cycle consists of 30 compressions and two breaths.
3. When ventricular fibrillation/pulseless ventricular tachycardia (VT) is present, one AED shock treatment should be administered and CPR resumed for an additional five cycles. Following five cycles of CPR, the rescuer should allow the AED to reanalyze the cardiac rhythm and deliver another shock if indicated. For nonshockable rhythms (asystole, pulseless electrical activity), CPR should be resumed immediately as the AED indicates.

AED USE SPECIAL CONSIDERATIONS

1. Use a standard AED for a patient who is unresponsive, not breathing, pulseless, and 8 years of age or older ≥25 kilograms or 55 pounds of body weight. If the patient is between 1 and 8 years of age, use a pediatric pad-cable system. If the pediatric system is not available, use a standard AED unit.
2. For individuals with pacemakers or implanted cardioverter defibrillators (ICDs), an AED may be used; pads should be placed one inch from the implanted device. If an ICD is active, allow about 30 to 60 seconds to complete its cycle.
3. If a transdermal medication patch is present, be certain to remove it, wipe the the area clean, and dry the area before placing the AED pads.
4. If the patient's chest is dirty or wet, clean and dry the areas where the AED pads will be placed.
5. In patients with excessive chest hair, the AED pads may not adhere well, resulting in a "check electrode warning." If pressing down firmly on the pads does correct the problem, *quickly* remove and apply a new set of pads. If the problem continues, remove the pads again and *quickly* shave the areas of the chest where a new set of pads will be placed.
6. Do not use the AED on a patient while standing in water or other conditions where potential electrical shock can occur.

TABLE B.2. PLAN FOR MEDICAL INCIDENTS/
NONEMERGENCY SITUATIONS

LEVEL: BASIC	INTERMEDIATE	HIGH
At a field, pool, or park without emergency equipment	At a gymnasium or outside facility with basic equipment plus manual defibrillator (or automated external defibrillator [AED]) and possibly a small start-up kit with drugs	Hospital or hospital adjunct with all the equipment of intermediate level plus a code cart containing emergency drugs and equipment for intravenous drug administration, intubation, drawing arterial blood gas samples, and suctioning Victim may be inpatient or outpatient

LEVEL: BASIC FIRST RESCUER	INTERMEDIATE FIRST RESCUER	HIGH FIRST RESCUER

1. Instruct victim to stop activity
2. Remain with victim until symptoms subside.
  a. If symptoms worsen, use basic first aid.
  b. If symptoms do not subside, victim should be transported by ambulance to ER or physician's office for evaluation immediately.
3. Advise victim to seek medical advice before further activity.
4. Document event.
	Same as basic level nos. 1 to 4
	Add:
	5. Take vital signs.
	6. Monitor and record ECG rhythm (or apply AED).
	7. Bring record of vital signs and ECG rhythm strip to ER/physician's office if symptoms do not subside and visit is necessary.
		Inpatient facility
		
		Same as intermediate level nos. 1 to 6
		Add:
		7. Call for medical personnel on duty.
		8. Notify primary physician.
		9. Request new consult from physician to resume exercise if more than three consecutive exercise sessions are interrupted for same symptom.

LEVEL: BASIC SECOND RESCUER	INTERMEDIATE SECOND RESCUER	HIGH SECOND RESCUER
1. Assist first rescuer, drive victim to ER or physician's office, if necessary.	Same as Basic Level No. 1 Add: 2. Bring blood pressure cuff and ECG monitor to site. 3. Assist with taking and monitoring vital signs.	Same as intermediate level nos. 1 to 3

ECG, electrocardiogram; ER, emergency room; IV, intravenous; AED, automated external defibrillator.

For more detailed explanations on the expanding role of AEDs and management of various cardiovascular emergencies, refer to the 2005 American Heart Association Guidelines for Cardiopulmonary Resuscitation and Emergency Cardiovascular Care or any American Heart Association updates.

Tables B-2 through B-4 provide sample plans for medical incidents/nonemergency situations (see Table B-2) and emergency situations (see Tables B-3 and B-4, respectively). These plans are provided only as examples. Specific plans must be customized to individual program needs and local standards. Pay particular attention to local, state, and federal laws governing the use of these guidelines or defibrillation devices.

TABLE B.3. PLAN FOR MEDICAL EMERGENCY—POTENTIALLY LIFE-THREATENING SITUATIONS (i.e., CARDIAC ARREST)

LEVEL: BASIC	INTERMEDIATE	HIGH
At a field, pool, or park without emergency equipment	At a gymnasium or outside facility with basic equipment plus manual defibrillator (or AED) and possibly a small start-up kit with drugs	Hospital or hospital adjunct with all the equipment of intermediate level plus a code cart containing emergency drugs and equipment for oxygen, intravenous drug administration, intubation, drawing arterial blood gas samples, and suctioning Victim may be inpatient or outpatient

LEVEL: BASIC FIRST RESCUER	INTERMEDIATE FIRST RESCUER	HIGH FIRST RESCUER
1. Establish responsiveness. a. Responsive: Instruct victim to sit or lay down, assuming a position of comfort. Activate EMS. Direct second rescuer to call EMS. Stay with victim until EMS team arrives. Note time of incident. Apply pressure to any bleeding. Note if victim takes any medication (i.e., nitroglycerin).	Same as basic level nos. 1 and 2 Add: 3. Apply monitor to victim and record rhythm (or apply AED). Monitor continuously. 4. Take vital signs every 1 to 5 minutes. 5. Document vital signs and rhythm. Note time and victim signs and symptoms.	Same as intermediate level nos. 1 to 5 Also may adapt/add: 1. Call nurse on ward. 2. Call nurse if physician is off ward. 3. Notify primary physician as soon as possible.

(continued)

TABLE B.3. PLAN FOR MEDICAL EMERGENCY—POTENTIALLY LIFE-THREATENING SITUATIONS (I.E., CARDIAC ARREST) (*Continued*)

LEVEL: BASIC FIRST RESCUER	INTERMEDIATE FIRST RESCUER	HIGH FIRST RESCUER
Take pulse.		

Take pulse.
  b. Unresponsive:
  Activate EMS.
  Place victim supine.
  Open airway.
  Check respiration. If absent, follow directions in Table B-4. Maintain open airway.
  Check pulse. If absent, follow directions in Table B-4. Direct second rescuer to call EMS. Stay with victim; continue to monitor respiration and pulse.
2. Other considerations
  a. If bleeding, compress area to decrease/stop bleeding.
  b. Suspected neck fracture: open airway with a jaw-thrust maneuver; do not hyperextend neck.
  c. If seizing, prevent injury by removing harmful objects; place something under head if possible.
  d. Turn victim on side, once seizure activity stops, to help drain secretions.

LEVEL: BASIC SECOND RESCUER	INTERMEDIATE SECOND RESCUER	HIGH SECOND RESCUER
1. Call EMS. 2. Wait to direct emergency team to scene. 3. Return to scene to assist.	Same as basic level nos. 1 to 3 Add:	Same as intermediate level nos. 1 to 4

TABLE B.3. PLAN FOR MEDICAL EMERGENCY—POTENTIALLY LIFE-THREATENING SITUATIONS (I.E., CARDIAC ARREST) (*Continued*)

4. Bring all emergency equipment and
   a. Place victim on monitor.
   b. Run ECG rhythm strips (or apply AED).
   c. Take vital signs.

LEVEL: BASIC THIRD RESCUER	INTERMEDIATE THIRD RESCUER	HIGH THIRD RESCUER
1. Direct emergency team to scene or 2. Assist first rescuer.	Same as basic level	Same as basic level

AED, automated external defibrillator; ECG, electrocardiogram; EMS, emergency medical services.

TABLE B.4. PLAN FOR LIFE-THREATENING SITUATIONS

LEVEL: BASIC	INTERMEDIATE	HIGH
At a field, pool, or park without emergency equipment	At a gymnasium or outside facility with basic equipment plus manual defibrillator (or AED) and possibly a small start-up kit with drugs	Hospital or hospital adjunct with all the equipment of intermediate level plus a code cart containing emergency drugs and equipment for intravenous drug administration, intubation, oxygenation, drawing arterial blood gas samples, and suctioning Victim may be inpatient or outpatient

LEVEL: BASIC FIRST RESCUER	INTERMEDIATE FIRST RESCUER	HIGH FIRST RESCUER
1. Position victim (pull from pool if necessary) and place supine; determine unresponsiveness. 2. Activate EMS 3. Open airway; look, listen, and feel for the air. 4. Give two ventilations if no respirations. 5. Check pulse (carotid artery).	Step nos. 1 to 7 for basic level	Step nos. 1 to 7 for basic level

(*continued*)

LEVEL: BASIC FIRST RESCUER	INTERMEDIATE FIRST RESCUER	HIGH FIRST RESCUER
6. Administer 15:2 compression/ventilation if no pulse. 7. Continue ventilation if no respiration.		

LEVEL: BASIC SECOND RESCUER	INTERMEDIATE SECOND RESCUER	HIGH SECOND RESCUER

1. Locate nearest phone and call EMS.
2. Return to scene and help with two-person CPR, or
3. Remain at designated area and direct emergency team to location.
	Step basic level nos. 1 to 3
	
	Add:
	
	4. Return to scene, bringing defibrillator: take quick look at rhythm. Document rhythm (do not defibrillate unless certified to do so and this activity is part of your clinical privileges for the facility in which the work is being completed) or apply AED.
	5. Place monitor leads on patient and monitor rhythm during CPR.
	6. Bring emergency drug kit if available.
	  a. Open oxygen equipment and use Ambu bag with oxygen at 10 L/min (i.e., 100%) (if trained to do so).
	  b. Open drug kit and prepare intravenous line and drug administration (must only be done by trained, licensed professionals).
	  c. Keep equipment at scene for use by emergency personnel
		Step intermediate level nos. 1 to 6

LEVEL: BASIC THIRD RESCUER	INTERMEDIATE THIRD RESCUER	HIGH THIRD RESCUER
1. Assist with two-person CPR or 2. Help direct emergency team to site. 3. Help clear area.	Same as basic level	Same as basic level

AED, automated external defibrillator; EMS, emergency medical service; CPR, cardiopulmonary resuscitation.

REFERENCES

1. American Heart Association's 2005 Guidelines for Cardiopulmonary Resuscitation (CPR) and Emergency Cardiovascular Care. *Circulation.* 2005;112(24):1–211.
2. American Heart Association. Basic Life Support for Health Care Providers. Greenville (TX): American Heart Association; 2001.

Electrocardiogram
Interpretation

The tables in this appendix provide a quick reference source for electrocardiogram (ECG) recording and interpretation. Each of these tables should be used as part of the overall clinical picture when making diagnostic decisions about an individual.

TABLE C.1. LIMB AND AUGMENTED LEAD ELECTRODE PLACEMENT[a]

LEAD	ELECTRODE PLACEMENT	HEART SURFACE VIEWED
Lead I	Left arm (+), right arm (−)	Lateral
Lead II	Left leg (+), right arm (−)	Inferior
Lead III	Left leg (+), left arm (−)	Inferior
aVR	Right arm (+)	None
aVL	Left arm (+)	Lateral
aVF	Left leg (+)	Inferior

[a]Exercise modifications: The limb leads are positioned over the left and right superior clavicular region for the arm leads, and over the left and right lower quadrants of the abdomen for the leg leads. This ECG configuration minimizes motion artifacts during exercise. However, torso-placed limb leads should be noted for all ECG tracings to avoid misdiagnosis of an ECG tracing. The most common changes observed are produced by right axis deviation and standing that may obscure or produce Q waves inferiorly or anteriorly and T-wave or frontal QRS axis changes even in normal people. From Jowett NI, Turner AM, Cole A, Jones PA. Modified electrode placement must be recorded when perfomring 12-lead elecrocardiograms. *Postgrad Med J.* 2005;81:122–5, and Gamble P, McManus H, Jensen D, Froelicher VF. A comparison of the standard 12-lead electrocardiogram to exercise electrode placement. *Chest.* 1984;85:616–22.

TABLE C.2. PRECORDIAL (CHEST LEAD) ELECTRODE PLACEMENT

LEAD	ELECTRODE PLACEMENT	HEART SURFACE VIEWED
V_1	Fourth intercostal space just to the right of the sternal border	Septum
V_2	Fourth intercostal space just to the left of the sternal border	Septum
V_3	At the midpoint of a straight line between V_2 and V_4	Anterior
V_4	On the midclavicular line in the fifth intercostal space	Anterior
V_5	On the anterior axillary line and on a horizontal plane through V_4	Lateral
V_6	On the midaxillary line and on a horizontal plane through V_4 and V_5	Lateral

Adapted from Goldberger AL. *Clinical Electrocardiography: A Simplified Approach.* 7th Ed. Philadelphia (PA): Mosby-Elsevier; 2006. p. 14–6.

TABLE C.3. ELECTROCARDIOGRAM INTERPRETATION STEPS

1. Check for correct calibration (1 mV = 10 mm) and paper speed (25 mm/s).
2. Verify the heart rate and determine the heart rhythm. (Computers do this very accurately. However, when there is unusual tracing noise or atrial flutter in people with low amplitude on their QRS wave, it is important to double-check a specific tracing segment.)
3. Measure intervals and durations (PR, QRS, QT).
4. Determine the mean QRS axis and mean T-wave axis in the limb leads.
5. Look for morphologic abnormalities of the P wave, QRS complex, ST segments, T waves, and U waves (e.g., chamber enlargement, conduction delays, infarction, repolarization changes).
6. Interpret the present electrocardiogram (ECG).
7. Compare the present ECG with previous available ECGs.[a]
8. Offer conclusion, clinical correlation, and recommendations.

[a]Baseline ECG comparisons before exercise should be compared with the previous ECGs if available. The supine ECG before the test rather than the standing ECG is the most appropriate for comparing with the prior ECGs because these are usually recorded in the supine position. Abnormal serial changes along with or without symptoms can result in canceling the test. Certain patterns negate the value of ST analysis during the exercise test (LBBB, IVCD, WPW, 2 mm or more of ST depression). If a treadmill test is being performed, the standing ECG before exercise is the most appropriate resting tracing for ST analyses comparisons during and after the exercise test.

TABLE C.4. RESTING 12-LEAD ELECTROCARDIOGRAM: NORMAL VERSUS ABNORMAL LIMITS

PARAMETER	NORMAL LIMITS	ABNORMAL IF:	POSSIBLE INTERPRETATION(S)[a]
Heart rate	60–100 beats·min^{-1}	<60	Bradycardia
		>100	Tachycardia
PR interval	0.12–0.20 s	<0.12 s	Preexcitation (i.e., WPW, LGL)
		>0.20 s	First-degree AV block
QRS duration	Up to 0.10 s	If ≥0.11 s	Conduction abnormality (i.e., incomplete or complete bundle-branch block, WPW, IVCD, PVCs, VT, or electronic pacer)
QT interval*	Rate dependent Normal QT= K$\sqrt{RR}$, where K = 0.37 for men and children and 0.40 for women	QTc long QTc short	Drug effects, electrolyte abnormalities, congenital ion channel abnormalities, ischemia Digitalis effect, hypercalcemia, hypermagnesia There is controversy over the correct equation for correcting QT for rate, and there are studies suggesting that this relationship is different for everyone.[b]
QRS axis	0 to +90 degrees	<0 degrees	Left axis deviation (i.e., chamber enlargement, hemiblock, infarction)
		>+90 degrees	Right axis deviation (i.e., RVH, pulmonary disease, infarction)
		Indeterminate	All limb leads transitional
T axis	Generally same direction as QRS axis	The T axis (vector) is typically deviated away from the area of "mischief" (i.e., ischemia, bundle-branch block, hypertrophy)	Chamber enlargement, ischemia, drug effects, electrolyte disturbances

ST segments	Generally at isoelectric line (PR segment) or within 1 mm	Elevation of ST segment	Injury, ischemia, pericarditis, electrolyte abnormality, normal variant (early repolarization)
	The ST may be elevated up to 1–2 mm in leads V_1–V_4.[c]	Depression of ST segment	Injury, ischemia, electrolyte abnormality, drug effects, normal variant
Q waves	<0.04 s and <25% of R-wave amplitude (exceptions lead III and V_1)	>0.04 s and/or >25% of R-wave amplitude except lead III (the lead of exceptions) and V_1	Infarction or pseudoinfarction (as from chamber enlargement, conduction abnormalities, WPW, chronic obstructive pulmonary disease cardiomyopathy)
Transition zone	Usually between V_2–V_4	Before V_2	Counterclockwise rotation
		After V_4	Clockwise rotation

WPW, Wolff-Parkinson-White syndrome; LGL, Lown-Ganong-Levine syndrome; QTc, QT corrected for heart rate; AV, atrioventricular; IVCD, intraventricular conduction delay; PVC, premature ventricular contraction; VT, ventilatory threshold; RVH, right ventricular hypertrophy.

[a]If supported by other electrocardiograms (ECGs) and related clinical criteria.

[b]Malik M. Problems of heart rate correction in assessment of drug-induced QT interval prolongation. *J Cardiovasc Electrophys.* 2001;12(4):411–20; Malik V, Farbom P, Batchvarov V, Hnatkova K, Camm AJ. Relation between QT and RR intervals is highly individua among healthy subjects: implications for heart rate correction of the QT interval. *Heart.* 2002;87:220–8.

[c]Menown, IB, Mackenzie G, Adgey AA. Optimizing the initial 12-lead electrocardiographic diagnosis of acute myocardial infarction. *Eur Heart J.* 2000;21 275–83.

TABLE C.5. LOCALIZATION OF TRANSMURAL INFARCTS[a] (LOCATION OF DIAGNOSTIC Q-WAVE)

TYPICAL ECG LEADS	INFARCT LOCATION
V_1-V_3	Anteroseptal
V_3-V_4	Localized anterior
V_4-V_6, I, aVL	Anterolateral
V_1-V_6	Extensive anterior
I, aVL	High lateral
II, III, aVF	Inferior
V_1-V_2	Septal
V_1, V_{3R}, V_{4R}	Right ventricular

ECG, electrocardiogram.

[a]When diagnostic Q waves are present in the inferior leads and the R wave is greater than the S wave in V_1 or V_2, this can reflect the presence of posterior extension of the inferior myocardial infarction.

TABLE C.6. SUPRAVENTRICULAR VERSUS VENTRICULAR ECTOPIC BEATS[a]

PARAMETER		SUPRAVENTRICULAR (NORMAL CONDUCTION)	SUPRAVENTRICULAR (ABERRANT CONDUCTION)	VENTRICULAR
QRS complex	Duration	Up to 0.11 s	≥0.12 s	≥0.12 s
	Configuration	Normal	Widened QRS usually with unchanged initial vector P wave precedes QRS	Widened QRS often with abnormal initial vector QRS not preceded by a P wave
P wave		Present or absent but with relationship to QRS	Present or absent but with relationship to QRS	Present or absent but without relationship to QRS
Rhythm		Usually less than compensatory pause	Usually less than compensatory pause	Usually compensatory pause

[a]Numerous ECG criteria exist to try to distinguish premature ventricular contractions (PVCs) from aberrant conduction. Standard electrocardiogram (ECG) texts review these. A major clinical problem is the patient with a wide QRS tachycardia. Such tachycardias can be ventricular or supraventricular with aberrant conduction. A good rule of thumb is that any wide QRS tachycardia in a patient with heart disease or a history of heart failure is likely to be ventricular tachycardia, especially if atrioventricular (AV) dissociation is identified.

TABLE C.7. ATRIOVENTRICULAR BLOCK

INTERPRETATION	P WAVE RELATIONSHIP TO QRS	PR INTERVAL	R-R INTERVAL
First-degree atrioventricular (AV) block	1:1	>0.20 s	Regular or follows P-P interval
Second-degree AV block: Mobitz I (Wenckebach)	>1:1	Progressively lengthens until a P wave fails to conduct	Progressively shortens; pause less than two other cycles
Second-degree AV block: Mobitz II	>1:1	Constant but with sudden dropping of QRS	Regular except for pause, which usually equals two other cycles
Third-degree AV block	None	Variable but P-P interval constant	Usually regular (escape rhythm)

TABLE C.8. ATRIOVENTRICULAR DISSOCIATION[a]

TYPE OF ATRIOVENTRICULAR (AV) DISSOCIATION	ELECTROPHYSIOLOGY	EXAMPLE	SIGNIFICANCE	COMMENT
AV dissociation resulting from complete AV block	AV block	Sinus rhythm with complete AV block	Pathologic	Unrelated P wave and QRS complexes PP interval is shorter than RR interval
AV dissociation by default causing interference	Slowing of the primary or dominant pacemaker with escape of a subsidiary pacemaker	Sinus bradycardia with junctional escape rhythm	Physiologic	Unrelated P wave and QRS complexes PP interval is longer than RR interval
AV dissociation by usurpation	Acceleration of a subsidiary pacemaker usurping control of the ventricles	Sinus rhythm with either AV junctional or ventricular tachycardia	Physiologic	Unrelated P wave and QRS complexes PP interval is longer than RR interval
Combination	AV block and interference	Atrial fibrillation with accelerated AV junctional pacemaker and block below this pacemaker	Pathologic	Unrelated P wave and QRS complexes

[a]What is meant by AV *dissociation*? When the atria and ventricles beat independently, their contractions are "dissociated," and AV dissociation exists. Thus, P waves and QRS complexes in the ECG are unrelated. AV dissociation may be complete or incomplete, transient or permanent. The causes of AV dissociation are block and interference, and both may be present in the same electrocardiogram (ECG). *Block* is associated with a pathologic state of refractoriness, preventing the primary pacemaker's impulse from reaching the lower chamber. An example of this is sinus rhythm with complete AV block. *Interference* results from slowing of the primary pacemaker or acceleration of a subsidiary pacemaker. The lower chamber's impulse "interferes" with conduction by producing physiologic refractoriness, and AV dissociation results. An example of this is sinus rhythm with AV junctional or ventricular tachycardia and no retrograde conduction into the atria. A clear distinction must be made between block and interference. This table describes the four types of AV dissociation.

D

American College of Sports Medicine Certifications

This appendix details information about American College of Sports Medicine (ACSM) Certification and Registry Programs and gives a complete listing of the current knowledge, skills, and abilities (KSAs) that compose the foundations of these certification and registry examinations. The mission of the ACSM Committee on Certification and Registry Boards is to develop and provide high-quality, accessible, and affordable credentials and continuing education programs for health and exercise professionals who are responsible for preventive and rehabilitative programs that influence the health and well-being of all individuals.

ACSM CERTIFICATIONS AND THE PUBLIC

The first of the ACSM clinical certifications was initiated more than 30 years ago in conjunction with publication of the first edition of *Guidelines for Exercise Testing and Prescription*. That era was marked by rapid development of exercise programs for patients with stable coronary artery disease (CAD). ACSM sought a means to disseminate accurate information on this healthcare initiative through expression of consensus from its members in basic science, clinical practice, and education. Thus, these early clinical certifications were viewed as an aid to the establishment of safe and scientifically based exercise services within the framework of cardiac rehabilitation.

Over the past 30 years, exercise has gained widespread favor as an important component in programs of rehabilitative care or health maintenance for an expanding list of chronic diseases and disabling conditions. The growth of public interest in the role of exercise in health promotion has been equally impressive. In addition, federal government policy makers have revisited questions of medical efficacy and financing for exercise services in rehabilitative care of selected patients. Over the past several years, recommendations from the U.S. Public Health Service and the U.S. Surgeon General have acknowledged the central role for regular physical activity in the prevention of disease and promotion of health.

The development of the health/fitness certifications in the 1980s reflected ACSM's intent to increase the availability of qualified professionals to provide scientifically sound advice and supervision regarding appropriate physical activities for health maintenance in the apparently healthy adult population. Since 1975, more than 35,000 certificates have been awarded. With this consistent growth, ACSM has taken steps to ensure that its competency-based certifications will continue to be regarded as the premier program in the exercise field.

The ACSM Committee on Certification and Registry Boards (CCRB) Publications Sub-Committee publishes *ACSM's Certified News*, a periodical addressing professional practice issues; its target audience is those who are certified. The CCRB Continuing Professional Education Sub-Committee has oversight of the continuing education requirements for maintenance of certification and auditing renewal candidates. Continuing education credits can be accrued through ACSM-sponsored educational programs, such as ACSM workshops (ACSM Certified Personal Trainer[SM], ACSM Certified Health Fitness Specialist, ACSM Certified Clinical Exercise Specialist, ACSM Registered Clinical Exercise Physiologist[®]), regional chapter and annual meetings, and other educational programs approved by the ACSM Professional Education Committee. These enhancements are intended to support the continued professional growth of those who have made a commitment to service in this rapidly growing health and fitness field.

In 2004, ACSM was a founding member of the multiorganizational Committee on Accreditation for the Exercise Sciences (CoAES) and assisted with the development of standards and guidelines for educational programs seeking accreditation under the auspices of the Commission on Accreditation of Allied Health Education Programs (CAAHEP). Additional information on outcomes-based, programmatic accreditation can be obtained by visiting www.caahep.org, and specific information regarding the standards and guidelines can be obtained by visiting www.coaes.org. Because the standards and guidelines refer to the KSAs that follow, reference to specific KSAs as they relate to given sets of standards and guidelines will be noted when appropriate.

ACSM also acknowledges the expectation from successful candidates that the public will be informed of the high standards, values, and professionalism implicit in meeting these certification requirements. The college has formally organized its volunteer committee structure and national office staff to give added emphasis to informing the public, professionals, and government agencies about issues of critical importance to ACSM. Informing these constituencies about the meaning and value of ACSM certification is one important priority that will be given attention in this initiative.

ACSM CERTIFICATION PROGRAMS

The ACSM Certified Personal Trainer[SM] is a fitness professional involved in developing and implementing an individualized approach to exercise leadership in healthy populations and/or those individuals with medical clearance to exercise. Using a variety of teaching techniques, the CPT is proficient in leading and demonstrating safe and effective methods of exercise by applying the fundamental principles of exercise science. The CPT is familiar with forms of exercise used to improve, maintain, and/or optimize health-related components of physical fitness and performance. The CPT is proficient in writing appropriate exercise recommendations, leading and demonstrating safe and effective methods of exercise, and motivating individuals to begin and to continue with their healthy behaviors.

The ACSM Certified Health Fitness Specialist (HFS) is a degreed health and fitness professional qualified for career pursuits in the university, corporate, commercial, hospital, and community settings. The HFS has knowledge and skills in management, administration, training, and in supervising entry-level personnel. The HFS is skilled in conducting risk stratification, conducting physical fitness assessments and interpreting results, constructing appropriate exercise prescriptions, and motivating apparently healthy individuals and individuals with medically controlled diseases to adopt and maintain healthy lifestyle behaviors.

The ACSM Certified Clinical Exercise Specialist (CES) is a healthcare professional certified by ACSM to deliver a variety of exercise assessment, training, rehabilitation, risk-factor identification, and lifestyle management services to individuals with or at risk for cardiovascular, pulmonary, and metabolic disease(s). These services are typically delivered in cardiovascular/pulmonary rehabilitation programs, physicians' offices, or medical fitness centers. The ACSM Certified Clinical Exercise Specialist is also competent to provide exercise-related consulting for research, public health, and other clinical and nonclinical services and programs.

The ACSM Registered Clinical Exercise Physiologist® (RCEP) is an allied health professional who works in the application of physical activity and behavioral interventions for those clinical conditions for which they have been shown to provide therapeutic and/or functional benefit. Persons for whom RCEP services are appropriate may include, but are not limited to, those individuals with cardiovascular, pulmonary, metabolic, orthopedic, musculoskeletal, neuromuscular, neoplastic, immunologic, or hematologic disease. The RCEP provides primary and secondary prevention strategies designed to improve fitness and health in populations ranging from children to older adults. The RCEP performs exercise screening, exercise and fitness testing, exercise prescription, exercise and physical activity counseling, exercise supervision, exercise and health education/promotion, and measurement and evaluation of exercise and physical activity related outcome measures. The RCEP works individually or as part of an interdisciplinary team in a clinical, community, or public health setting. The practice and supervision of the RCEP is guided by published professional guidelines, standards, and applicable state and federal regulations.

Certification at a given level requires the candidate to have a knowledge and skills base commensurate with that specific level of certification. In addition, the HFS level of certification incorporates the KSAs associated with the ACSM Certified Personal Trainer[SM] certification, the CES level of certification incorporates the KSAs associated with the CPT and HFS certification, and the RCEP level of certification incorporates the KSAs associated with the CPT, HFS, and CES levels of certification, as illustrated in Figure D.1. In addition, each level of certification has minimum requirements for experience, level of education, or other certifications.

FIGURE D.1.

LEVEL	REQUIREMENTS	RECOMMENDED COMPETENCIES
ACSM Certified Personal Trainer[SM]	• 18 years of age or older • High school diploma or equivalent (GED) • Possess current adult CPR certification that has a practical skills examination component (such as the American Heart Association or the American Red Cross)	• Demonstrate competence in the KSAs required of the ACSM Certified Personal Trainer™ as listed in the current edition of the *ACSM's Guidelines for Exercise Testing and Prescription* • Adequate knowledge of and skill in risk-factor and health-status identification, fitness appraisal, and exercise prescription • Demonstrate ability to incorporate suitable and innovative activities that will improve an individual's functional capacity Demonstrate the ability to effectively educate and/or communicate with individuals regarding lifestyle modification
ACSM Certified Health Fitness Specialist	• Associate's degree or a bachelor's degree in a health-related field from a regionally accredited college or university (one is eligible to sit for the exam if the candidate is in the last term of their degree program); AND • Possess current adult CPR certification that has a practical skills examination component (such as the American Heart Association or the American Red Cross)	• Demonstrate competence in the KSAs required of the ACSM Certified Health Fitness Specialist In as listed in the current edition of the *ACSM's Guidelines for Exercise Testing and Prescription* • Work-related experience within the health and fitness field • Adequate knowledge of, and skill in, risk-factor and health-status identification, fitness appraisal, and exercise prescription • Demonstrate ability to incorporate suitable and innovative activities that will improve an individual's functional capacity • Demonstrate the ability to effectively educate and/or counsel individuals regarding lifestyle modification • Knowledge of exercise science including kinesiology, functional anatomy, exercise physiology, nutrition, program administration, psychology, and injury prevention
ACSM Certified Clinical Exercise Specialist	• Bachelor's degree in an allied health field from a regionally accredited college of university (one is eligible to sit for the exam if the candidate is in the last term of their degree program); AND	• Demonstrate competence in the KSAs required of the ACSM Certified Clinical Exercise Specialist and Certified Health Fitness Specialist, as listed in the current edition of *ACSM's Guidelines for Exercise Testing and Prescription* • Ability to demonstrate extensive knowledge of functional anatomy,

LEVEL	REQUIREMENTS	RECOMMENDED COMPETENCIES
	• Minimum of 600 hours of observational and active patient/client care in a clinical exercise program (e.g., cardiac/pulmonary rehabilitation programs; exercise testing; exercise prescription; electrocardiography; patient education and counseling; disease management of cardiac, pulmonary, and metabolic diseases; and emergency management); AND • Current certification as a basic life support provider or CPR for the professional rescuer (available through the American Heart Association or the American Red Cross)	exercise physiology, pathophysiology, electrocardiography, human behavior/psychology, gerontology, graded exercise testing for healthy and diseased populations, exercise supervision/leadership, patient counseling, and emergency procedures related to exercise testing and training situations
ACSM Registered Clinical Exercise Physiologist®	• Master's degree in exercise science, exercise physiology, or kinesiology from a regionally accredited college or university • Current certification as a basic life support provider or CPR for the professional rescuer (available through the American Heart Association or the American Red Cross) • Minimum of 600 clinical hours or alternatives as described in the current issue of ACSM's *Certification Resource Guide* (hours may be completed as part of a formal degree program) • Recommendation of hours in clinical practice areas: cardiovascular—200; pulmonary—100 ; metabolic—120; orthopedic/ musculoskeletal—100; neuromuscular—40; immunologic/hematologic—40	• Demonstrate competence in the KSAs required of the ACSM Registered Clinical Exercise Physiologist®, ACSM Certified Clinical Excercise Specialist, ACSM Certified Health Fitness Specialist, and ACSM Certified Personal Trainer[SM] as listed in the current edition of *ACSM's Guidelines for Exercise Testing and Prescription*

ACSM also develops specialty certifications to enhance the breadth of knowledge for individuals working in a health, fitness, or clinical setting. For information on KSAs, eligibility, and scope of practice for ACSM specialty certifications, visit www.acsm.org/certification or call 1-800-486-5643.

HOW TO OBTAIN INFORMATION AND APPLICATION MATERIALS

The certification programs of ACSM are subject to continuous review and revision. Content development is entrusted to a diverse committee of professional volunteers with expertise in exercise science, medicine, and program management. Expertise in design and procedures for competency assessment is also represented on this committee. The administration of certification exams is conducted through Pearson VUE authorized testing centers. Inquiries regarding exam registration can be made to Pearson VUE at 1-888-883-2276 or online at www.pearsonvue.com/acsm.

For general certification questions, contact the ACSM Certification Resource Center:

1-800-486-5643
Web site: www.acsm.org/certification
E-mail: certification@acsm.org

KNOWLEDGE, SKILLS, AND ABILITIES (KSAs) UNDERLINING ACSM CERTIFICATIONS

Minimal competencies for each certification level are outlined below. Certification examinations are constructed based on these KSAs. For the ACSM Certified Health Fitness Specialist and the ACSM Certified Clinical Exercise Specialist credentials, two companion ACSM publications, *ACSM's Resource Manual for Guidelines for Exercise Testing and Prescription*, sixth edition, and *ACSM's Certification Review Book*, third edition, may also be used to gain further insight pertaining to the topics identified here. For the ACSM Certified Personal Trainer[SM], candidates should refer to *ACSM's Resources for the Personal Trainer*, current edition, and *ACSM's Certification Review Book*, third edition. For the ACSM Registered Clinical Exercise Physiologist[®], candidates should refer to ACSM's *Resources for Clinical Exercise Physiology*, current edition, and *ACSM's Resource Manual for Guidelines for Exercise Testing and Prescription*, sixth edition. However, neither the *ACSM's Guidelines for Exercise Testing and Prescription* nor any of the above-mentioned resource manuals provides all of the information upon which the ACSM Certification examinations are based. Each may prove to be beneficial as a review of specific topics and as a general outline of many of the integral concepts to be mastered by those seeking certification.

CLASSIFICATION/NUMBERING SYSTEM FOR KNOWLEDGE, SKILLS, AND ABILITIES (KSAs)

All the KSAs for a given certification/credential are listed in their entirety across a given practice area and/or content matter area for each level of certification.

Within each certification's/credential's KSA set, the numbering of individual KSAs uses a three-part number as follows:

- First number: denotes practice area (1.x.x)
- Second number: denotes content area (x.1.x)
- Third number: denotes the sequential number of each KSA (x.x.1) within each content area. If there is a break in numeric sequence, it indicates that a KSA was deleted in response to the recent job-task analysis from the prior version of the KSAs. From this edition forward, new KSAs will acquire a new KSA number.

The practice areas (the first number) are numbered as follows:

1.x.x	General population/core
2.x.x	Cardiovascular
3.x.x	Pulmonary
4.x.x	Metabolic
5.x.x	Orthopedic/musculoskeletal
6.x.x	Neuromuscular
7.x.x	Neoplastic, immunologic, and hematologic

The content matter areas (the second number) are numbered as follows:

x.1.x	Exercise physiology and related exercise science
x.2.x	Pathophysiology and risk factors
x.3.x	Health appraisal, fitness, and clinical exercise testing
x.4.x	Electrocardiography and diagnostic techniques
x.5.x	Patient management and medications
x.6.x	Medical and surgical management
x.7.x	Exercise prescription and programming
x.8.x	Nutrition and weight management
x.9.x	Human behavior and counseling
x.10.x	Safety, injury prevention, and emergency procedures
x.11.x	Program administration, quality assurance, and outcome assessment
x.12.x	Clinical and medical considerations (ACSM Certified Personal Trainer^{SM} only)

EXAMPLES BY LEVEL OF CERTIFICATION/CREDENTIAL

ACSM CERTIFIED PERSONAL TRAINER^{SM} KSAs

1.1.10 Knowledge to describe the normal acute responses to cardiovascular exercise.

In this example, the practice area is *general population/core*; the content matter area is *exercise physiology and related exercise science*; and this KSA is the tenth KSA within this content matter area.

ACSM CERTIFIED HEALTH FITNESS SPECIALIST KSAs

1.3.8 Skill in accurately measuring heart rate, blood pressure, and obtaining rating of perceived exertion (RPE) at rest and during exercise according to established guidelines.

In this example, the practice area is *general population/core*; the content matter area is *health appraisal, fitness, and clinical exercise testing*; and this KSA is the eighth KSA within this content matter area.

ACSM CERTIFIED CLINICAL EXERCISE SPECIALIST KSAs[a]

1.7.17   Design strength and flexibility programs for individuals with cardiovascular, pulmonary, and/or metabolic diseases; the elderly; and children.

In this example, the practice area is *general population/core*; the content matter area is *exercise prescription and programming*; and this KSA is the seventeenth KSA within this content matter area. Furthermore, because this specific KSA appears in bold, it covers multiple practice areas and content areas.

ACSM REGISTERED CLINICAL EXERCISE PHYSIOLOGIST® KSAs

7.6.1   List the drug classifications commonly used in the treatment of patients with a neoplastic, immunologic, and hematologic (NIH) disease, name common generic and brand-name drugs within each class, and explain the purposes, indications, major side effects, and the effects, if any, on the exercising individual.

The practice area is *neoplastic, immunologic, and hematologic*; the content matter area is *medical and surgical management*; and this KSA is the first KSA within this content matter area.

---

[a] *A special note about ACSM Certified Clinical Exercise Specialist KSAs*

Like the other certifications presented thus far, the ACSM Certified Clinical Exercise Specialist KSAs are categorized by content area. However, some CES KSAs cover multiple practices areas within each area of content. For example, several of them describe a specific topic with respect to both exercise testing and training, which are two distinct content areas. Rather than write out each separately (which would have greatly expanded the KSA list length), they have been listed under a single content area. When reviewing these KSAs, please note that KSAs in bold text cover multiple content areas. Each CES KSA begins with a 1 as the practice area. However, where appropriate, some KSAs mention specific patient populations (i.e., practice area). If a specific practice area is not mentioned within a given KSA, then it applies equally to each of the general population, cardiovascular, pulmonary, and metabolic practice areas. Note that "metabolic patients" are defined as those with at least one of the following: overweight or obese, diabetes (type I or II), or metabolic syndrome. Each KSA describes either a single or multiple knowledge (K), skill (S), or ability (A)—or a combination of K, S, or A—that an individual should have mastery of to be considered a competent ACSM Certified Clinical Exercise Specialist.

ACSM CERTIFIED PERSONAL TRAINER[SM] KNOWLEDGE, SKILLS, AND ABILITIES (KSAs)

GENERAL POPULATION/CORE: EXERCISE PHYSIOLOGY AND RELATED EXERCISE SCIENCE

1.1.1   Knowledge of the basic structures of bone, skeletal muscle, and connective tissue.

1.1.2   Knowledge of the basic anatomy of the cardiovascular system and respiratory system.

1.1.3   Knowledge of the definition of the following terms: inferior, superior, medial, lateral, supination, pronation, flexion, extension, adduction, abduction, hyperextension, rotation, circumduction, agonist, antagonist, and stabilizer.

1.1.4   Knowledge of the plane in which each muscle action occurs.

1.1.5   Knowledge of the interrelationships among center of gravity, base of support, balance, stability, and proper spinal alignment.

1.1.6   Knowledge of the following curvatures of the spine: lordosis, scoliosis, and kyphosis.

1.1.8   Knowledge of the biomechanical principles for the performance of common physical activities (e.g., walking, running, swimming, cycling, resistance training, yoga, Pilates, functional training).

1.1.9   Ability to distinguish between aerobic and anaerobic metabolism.

1.1.10   Knowledge to describe the normal acute responses to cardiovascular exercise.

1.1.11   Knowledge to describe the normal acute responses to resistance training.

1.1.12   Knowledge of the normal chronic physiologic adaptations associated with cardiovascular exercise.

1.1.13   Knowledge of the normal chronic physiologic adaptations associated with resistance training.

1.1.14   Knowledge of the physiologic principles related to warm-up and cool-down.

1.1.15   Knowledge of the common theories of muscle fatigue and delayed onset muscle soreness (DOMS).

1.1.16   Knowledge of the physiologic adaptations that occur at rest and during submaximal and maximal exercise following chronic aerobic and anaerobic exercise training.

1.1.17   Knowledge of the physiologic principles involved in promoting gains in muscular strength and endurance.

1.1.18   Knowledge of blood pressure responses associated with acute exercise, including changes in body position.

1.1.19   Knowledge of how the principle of specificity relates to the components of fitness.

1.1.20   Knowledge of the concept of detraining or reversibility of conditioning and its implications in fitness programs.

1.1.21   Knowledge of the physical and psychological signs of overtraining and to provide recommendations for these problems.

1.1.22   Knowledge of muscle actions, such as isotonic, isometric (static), iso-kinetic, concentric, eccentric.

1.1.23   Ability to identify the major muscles. Major muscles include, but are not limited to, the following: trapezius, pectoralis major, latissimus dorsi, biceps, triceps, rectus abdominis, internal and external obliques, erector spinae, gluteus maximus, quadriceps, hamstrings, adductors, abductors, and gastrocnemius.

1.1.24   Ability to identify the major bones. Major bones include, but are not limited to, the clavicle, scapula, sternum, humerus, carpals, ulna, radius, femur, fibula, tibia, and tarsals.

1.1.25   Ability to identify the various types of joints of the body (e.g., hinge, ball, and socket).

1.1.26   Knowledge of the primary action and joint range of motion for each major muscle group.

1.1.27   Ability to locate the anatomic landmarks for palpation of peripheral pulses.

1.1.28   Knowledge of the unique physiologic considerations of children, older adults, persons with diabetes (type 2), pregnant women, and persons who are overweight and/or obese.

1.1.29   Knowledge of the following related terms: hypertrophy, atrophy, and hyperplasia.

GENERAL POPULATION/CORE: HEALTH APPRAISAL, FITNESS, AND CLINICAL EXERCISE TESTING

1.3.1   Knowledge of and ability to discuss the physiologic basis of the major components of physical fitness: flexibility, cardiovascular fitness, muscular strength, muscular endurance, and body composition.

1.3.2   Knowledge of the components of a health/medical history.

1.3.3   Knowledge of the value of a medical clearance before exercise participation.

1.3.4   Knowledge of the categories of participants who should receive medical clearance before administration of an exercise test or participation in an exercise program.

1.3.5   Knowledge of relative and absolute contraindications to exercise testing or participation.

1.3.6   Knowledge of the limitations of informed consent and medical clearance.

1.3.7   Knowledge of the advantages/disadvantages and limitations of the various body composition techniques including, but not limited to, skinfolds, plethysmography (BOD POD®), bioelectrical impedance, infrared, dual-energy x-ray absorptiometry (DEXA), and circumference measurements.

1.3.8   Skill in accurately measuring heart rate and obtaining rating of perceived exertion (RPE) at rest and during exercise according to established guidelines.

1.3.9   Ability to locate body sites for circumference (girth) measurements.

1.3.10   Ability to obtain a basic health history and risk appraisal and to stratify risk in accordance with ACSM Guidelines.

1.3.11   Ability to explain and obtain informed consent.

1.3.13   Knowledge of preactivity fitness testing, including assessments of cardiovascular fitness, muscular strength, muscular endurance, flexibility, and body composition.

1.3.14   Knowledge of criteria for terminating a fitness evaluation and proper procedures to be followed after discontinuing such a test.

1.3.15   Knowledge of and ability to prepare for the initial client consultation.

1.3.16   Ability to recognize postural abnormalities that may affect exercise performance.

1.3.17   Skill in assessing body alignment.

GENERAL POPULATION/CORE: EXERCISE PRESCRIPTION AND PROGRAMMING

1.7.1   Knowledge of the benefits and risks associated with exercise training and recommendations for exercise programming in children and adolescents.

1.7.2   Knowledge of the benefits and precautions associated with resistance and endurance training in older adults and recommendations for exercise programming.

1.7.3   Knowledge of specific leadership techniques appropriate for working with participants of all ages.

1.7.4   Knowledge of how to modify cardiovascular and resistance exercises based on age and physical condition.

1.7.5   Knowledge of and ability to describe the unique adaptations to exercise training with regard to strength, functional capacity, and motor skills.

1.7.6   Knowledge of common orthopedic and cardiovascular considerations for older participants and the ability to describe modifications in exercise prescription that are indicated.

1.7.7   Knowledge of selecting appropriate training modalities according to the age and functional capacity of the individual.

1.7.8   Knowledge of the recommended intensity, duration, frequency, and type of physical activity necessary for development of cardiorespiratory fitness in an apparently healthy population.

1.7.9   Knowledge to describe and the ability to safely demonstrate exercises designed to enhance muscular strength and/or endurance.

1.7.10   Knowledge of the principles of overload, specificity, and progression and how they relate to exercise programming.

1.7.11   Knowledge of how to conduct and the ability to teach/demonstrate exercises during a comprehensive session that would include pre-exercise evaluation, warm-up, aerobic exercise, cool-down, muscular fitness training, and flexibility exercise.

1.7.12   Knowledge of special precautions and modifications of exercise programming for participation at altitude, different ambient temperatures, humidity, and environmental pollution.

1.7.13   Knowledge of the importance and ability to record exercise sessions and performing periodic evaluations to assess changes in fitness status.

1.7.14   Knowledge of the advantages and disadvantages of implementation of interval, continuous, and circuit training programs.

1.7.15   Knowledge of the concept of activities of daily living (ADLs) and its importance in the overall health of the individual.

1.7.16   Knowledge of progressive adaptation in resistance training and its implications on program design and periodization.

1.7.17   Knowledge of interpersonal limitations when working with clients one on one.

1.7.19   Skill to teach and demonstrate appropriate modifications in specific exercises and make recommendations for exercise programming for the following groups: children, older adults, persons with diabetes (type 2), pregnant women, persons with arthritis, persons who are overweight and/or obese, and persons with chronic back pain.

1.7.20   Skill to teach and demonstrate appropriate exercises for improving range of motion of all major joints.

1.7.21   Skill in the use of various methods for establishing and monitoring levels of exercise intensity, including heart rate, RPE, and metabolic equivalents (METs).

1.7.22   Knowledge of and ability to apply methods used to monitor exercise intensity, including heart rate and rating of perceived exertion.

1.7.24   Ability to differentiate between the amount of physical activity required for health benefits and the amount of exercise required for fitness development.

1.7.25   Ability to determine training heart rates using two methods: percent of age-predicted maximum heart rate and heart rate reserve (Karvonen).

1.7.26   Ability to identify proper and improper technique in the use of resistive equipment, such as stability balls, weights, bands, resistance bars, and water exercise equipment.

1.7.27   Ability to identify proper and improper technique in the use of cardiovascular conditioning equipment (e.g., stair-climbers, stationary cycles, treadmills, and elliptical trainers).

1.7.28   Ability to teach a progression of exercises for all major muscle groups to improve muscular fitness.

1.7.29   Ability to modify exercises based on age and physical condition.

1.7.30   Ability to explain and implement exercise prescription guidelines for apparently healthy clients or those who have medical clearance to exercise.

1.7.31   Ability to adapt frequency, intensity, duration, mode, progression, level of supervision, and monitoring techniques in exercise programs for apparently healthy clients or those who have medical clearance to exercise.

1.7.34   Ability to evaluate, prescribe, and demonstrate appropriate flexibility exercises for all major muscle groups.

1.7.35   Ability to design training programs using interval, continuous, and circuit training programs.

1.7.36   Ability to describe the advantages and disadvantages of various types of commercial exercise equipment in developing cardiorespiratory and muscular fitness.

1.7.37   Ability to safely demonstrate a wide variety of conditioning exercises involving equipment, such as stability balls, BOSU® balls, elastic bands, medicine balls, and foam rollers.

1.7.38   Ability to safely demonstrate a wide range of resistance-training modalities, including variable resistance devices, dynamic constant external resistance devices, static resistance devices, and other resistance devices.

1.7.39   Ability to safely demonstrate a wide variety of conditioning exercises that promote improvements in agility, balance, coordination, reaction time, speed, and power.

1.7.40   Knowledge of training principles, such as progressive overload, variation, and specificity.

1.7.41   Knowledge of the Valsalva maneuver and the associated risks.

1.7.42   Knowledge of the appropriate repetitions, sets, volume, repetition maximum, and rest periods necessary for desired outcome goals.

1.7.43   Ability to safely demonstrate a wide variety of plyometric exercises and be able to determine when such exercises would be inappropriate to perform.

1.7.44   Ability to apply training principles so as to distinguish goals between an athlete and an individual exercising for general health.

1.7.45   Knowledge of periodization in exercise in aerobic and resistance-training program design.

GENERAL POPULATION/CORE: NUTRITION AND WEIGHT MANAGEMENT

1.8.1   Knowledge of the role of carbohydrates, fats, and proteins as fuels.

1.8.2   Knowledge to define the following terms: obesity, overweight, percent fat, body mass index (BMI), lean body mass, anorexia nervosa, bulimia nervosa, and body fat distribution.

1.8.3   Knowledge of the relationship between body composition and health.

1.8.4   Knowledge of the effects of diet plus exercise, diet alone, and exercise alone as methods for modifying body composition.

1.8.5   Knowledge of the importance of an adequate daily energy intake for healthy weight management.

1.8.6   Knowledge of the importance of maintaining normal hydration before, during, and after exercise.

1.8.7   Knowledge and understanding of the current Dietary Guidelines for Americans, including the USDA Food Pyramid.

1.8.8   Knowledge of the female athlete triad.

1.8.9   Knowledge of the myths and consequences associated with inappropriate weight loss methods (e.g., saunas, vibrating belts, body wraps, electric simulators, sweat suits, fad diets).

1.8.10   Knowledge of the number of kilocalories in one gram of carbohydrate, fat, protein, and alcohol.

1.8.11   Knowledge of the number of kilocalories equivalent to losing one pound of body fat.

1.8.12   Knowledge of the guidelines for caloric intake for an individual desiring to lose or gain weight.

1.8.13   Knowledge of common ergogenic aids, the purported mechanism of action, and potential risks and/or benefits (e.g., anabolic steroids, caffeine, amino acids, vitamins, minerals, creatine monohydrate, adrostenedione, DHEA).

1.8.14 Ability to describe the health implications of variation in body-fat distribution patterns and the significance of the waist-to-hip ratio.

1.8.15 Ability to describe the health implications of commonly used herbs (e.g., echinacea, St. John's wort, ginseng).

GENERAL POPULATION/CORE: HUMAN BEHAVIOR AND COUNSELING

1.9.1 Knowledge of behavioral strategies to enhance exercise and health behavior change (e.g., reinforcement, goal setting, social support).

1.9.2 Knowledge of the stages of motivational readiness and effective strategies that support and facilitate behavioral change.

1.9.3 Knowledge of the three stages of learning: cognitive, associative, autonomous.

1.9.4 Knowledge of specific techniques to enhance motivation (e.g., posters, recognition, bulletin boards, games, competitions). Define extrinsic and intrinsic reinforcement and give examples of each.

1.9.5 Knowledge of the different types of learners (auditory, visual, kinesthetic) and how to apply teaching and training techniques to optimize a client's training session.

1.9.6 Knowledge of the types of feedback and ability to use communication skills to optimize a client's training session.

1.9.7 Knowledge of common obstacles that interfere with adherence to an exercise program and strategies to overcome these obstacles.

1.9.8 Ability to identify, clarify, and set behavioral and realistic goals with the client (i.e., SMART goals).

1.9.9 Knowledge of basic communication and coaching techniques that foster and facilitate behavioral changes.

1.9.10 Knowledge of various learning theories (e.g., motivation theory, attribution theory, transfer theory, retention theory, and goal theory).

1.9.11 Knowledge of attributes or characteristics necessary for effective teaching.

GENERAL POPULATION/CORE: SAFETY, INJURY PREVENTION, AND EMERGENCY PROCEDURES

1.10.1 Knowledge of and skill in obtaining basic life support, automated external defibrillators (AEDs), and cardiopulmonary resuscitation certification.

1.10.2 Knowledge of appropriate emergency procedures (i.e., telephone procedures, written emergency procedures, personnel responsibilities) in a health and fitness setting.

1.10.3 Knowledge of basic first-aid procedures for exercise-related injuries, such as bleeding, strains/sprains, fractures, and exercise intolerance (dizziness, syncope, heat injury).

1.10.4 Knowledge of basic precautions taken in an exercise setting to ensure participant safety.

1.10.5   Knowledge of the physical and physiologic signs and symptoms of overtraining.

1.10.6   Knowledge of the effects of temperature, humidity, altitude, and pollution on the physiologic response to exercise.

1.10.7   Knowledge of the following terms: shin splints, sprain, strain, tennis elbow, bursitis, stress fracture, tendonitis, patello-femoral pain syndrome, low back pain, plantar fasciitis, and rotator cuff tendonitis.

1.10.8   Knowledge of hypothetical concerns and potential risks that may be associated with the use of exercises such as straight-leg sit-ups, double leg raises, full squats, hurdler's stretch, yoga plow, forceful back hyperextension, and standing bent-over toe touch.

1.10.10   Knowledge of the Certified Personal Trainer's^{SM} responsibilities, limitations, and the legal implications of carrying out emergency procedures.

1.10.11   Knowledge of potential musculoskeletal injuries (e.g., contusions, sprains, strains, fractures), cardiovascular/pulmonary complications (e.g., tachycardia, bradycardia, hypotension/hypertension, tachypnea), and metabolic abnormalities (e.g., fainting/syncope, hypoglycemia/hyperglycemia, hypothermia/hyperthermia).

1.10.12   Knowledge of the initial management and first-aid techniques associated with open wounds, musculoskeletal injuries, cardiovascular/pulmonary complications, and metabolic disorders.

1.10.13   Knowledge of the components of an equipment service plan/agreement and how it may be used to evaluate the condition of exercise equipment to reduce the potential risk of injury.

1.10.14   Knowledge of the legal implications of documented safety procedures, the use of incident documents, and ongoing safety training.

1.10.15   Skill in demonstrating appropriate emergency procedures during exercise testing and/or training.

1.10.16   Ability to identify the components that contribute to the maintenance of a safe exercise environment.

1.10.17   Ability to assist or spot a client in a safe and effective manner during resistance exercise.

GENERAL POPULATION/CORE: PROGRAM ADMINISTRATION, QUALITY ASSURANCE, AND OUTCOME ASSESSMENT

1.11.1   Knowledge of the Certified Personal Trainer's^{SM} scope of practice and role in the administration/program management within a health/fitness facility.

1.11.2   Knowledge of and the ability to use the documentation required when a client shows abnormal signs or symptoms during an exercise session and should be referred to a physician.

1.11.3   Knowledge of professional liability and most common types of negligence seen in training environments.

1.11.4   Understanding of the practical and legal ramifications of the employee versus independent contractor classifications as they relate to the Certified Personal Trainer^{SM}.

1.11.5   Knowledge of appropriate professional responsibilities, practice standards, and ethics in relationships dealing with clients, employers, and other allied health/medical/fitness professionals.

1.11.6   Knowledge of the types of exercise programs available in the community and how these programs are appropriate for various populations.

1.11.7   Knowledge of and ability to implement effective, professional business practices and ethical promotion of personal training services.

1.11.8   Ability to develop a basic business plan, which includes establishing a budget, developing management policies, marketing, sales, and pricing.

GENERAL POPULATION/CORE: CLINICAL AND MEDICAL CONSIDERATIONS

1.12.1   Knowledge of cardiovascular, respiratory, metabolic, and musculoskeletal risk factors that may require further evaluation by medical or allied health professionals before participation in physical activity.

1.12.2   Knowledge of risk factors that may be favorably modified by physical activity habits.

1.12.3   Knowledge of the risk-factor concept of coronary artery disease (CAD) and the influence of heredity and lifestyle on the development of CAD.

1.12.4   Knowledge of how lifestyle factors—including nutrition, physical activity, and heredity—influence blood lipid and lipoprotein (i.e., cholesterol: high-density lipoprotein and low-density lipoprotein) profiles.

1.12.5   Knowledge of cardiovascular risk factors or conditions that may require consultation with medical personnel before testing or training, including inappropriate changes of resting or exercise heart rate and blood pressure; new onset discomfort in chest, neck, shoulder, or arm; changes in the pattern of discomfort during rest or exercise; fainting or dizzy spells; and claudication.

1.12.6   Knowledge of respiratory risk factors or conditions that may require consultation with medical personnel before testing or training, including asthma, exercise-induced bronchospasm, extreme breathlessness at rest or during exercise, bronchitis, and emphysema.

1.12.7   Knowledge of metabolic risk factors or conditions that may require consultation with medical personnel before testing or training, including body weight more than 20% above optimal, BMI >30, thyroid disease, diabetes or glucose intolerance, and hypoglycemia.

1.12.8   Knowledge of musculoskeletal risk factors or conditions that may require consultation with medical personnel before testing or training, including acute or chronic back pain, arthritis, osteoporosis, and joint inflammation.

1.12.10 Knowledge of common drugs from each of the following classes of medications and ability to describe their effects on exercise: antianginals, anticoagulants, antihypertensives, antiarrhythmics, bronchodilators, hypoglycemics, psychotropics, vasodilators, and over-the-counter medications such as pseudoephedrine.

1.12.11   Knowledge of the effects of the following substances on exercise: antihistamines, tranquilizers, alcohol, diet pills, cold tablets, caffeine, and nicotine.

The ACSM Certified Health Fitness Specialist is responsible for the mastery of
the ACSM Certified Personal Trainer[SM] KSAs and the following ACSM Certified
Health Fitness Specialist KSAs.

GENERAL POPULATION/CORE: EXERCISE PHYSIOLOGY AND RELATED EXERCISE SCIENCE

1.1.1   Knowledge of the structures of bone, skeletal muscle, and connective
tissues.

1.1.2   Knowledge of the anatomy and physiology of the cardiovascular system
and pulmonary system.

1.1.3   Knowledge of the following muscle action terms: inferior, superior,
medial, lateral, supination, pronation, flexion, extension, adduction,
abduction, hyperextension, rotation, circumduction, agonist, antagonist, and stabilizer.

1.1.4   Knowledge of the plane in which each movement action occurs and the
responsible muscles.

1.1.5   Knowledge of the interrelationships among center of gravity, base of
support, balance, stability, posture, and proper spinal alignment.

1.1.6   Knowledge of the curvatures of the spine including lordosis, scoliosis,
and kyphosis.

1.1.7   Knowledge of the stretch reflex and how it relates to flexibility.

1.1.8   Knowledge of biomechanical principles that underlie performance of
the following activities: walking, jogging, running, swimming, cycling,
weight lifting, and carrying or moving objects.

1.1.9   Ability to describe the systems for the production of energy.

1.1.10   Knowledge of the role of aerobic and anaerobic energy systems in the
performance of various physical activities.

1.1.11   Knowledge of the following cardiorespiratory terms: ischemia, angina
pectoris, tachycardia, bradycardia, arrhythmia, myocardial infarction,
claudication, dyspnea, and hyperventilation.

1.1.12   Ability to describe normal cardiorespiratory responses to static and
dynamic exercise in terms of heart rate, stroke volume, cardiac output,
blood pressure, and oxygen consumption.

1.1.13   Knowledge of the heart rate, stroke volume, cardiac output, blood pressure, and oxygen consumption responses to exercise.

1.1.14   Knowledge of the anatomic and physiologic adaptations associated
with strength training.

1.1.15   Knowledge of the physiologic principles related to warm-up and cool-
down.

1.1.16   Knowledge of the common theories of muscle fatigue and delayed
onset muscle soreness (DOMS).

1.1.17   Knowledge of the physiologic adaptations that occur at rest and during
submaximal and maximal exercise following chronic aerobic and
anaerobic exercise training.

1.1.18   Knowledge of the differences in cardiorespiratory response to acute graded exercise between conditioned and unconditioned individuals.

1.1.19   Knowledge of the structure and function of the skeletal muscle fiber.

1.1.20   Knowledge of the characteristics of fast- and slow-twitch muscle fibers.

1.1.21   Knowledge of the sliding filament theory of muscle contraction.

1.1.22   Knowledge of twitch, summation, and tetanus with respect to muscle contraction.

1.1.23   Knowledge of the principles involved in promoting gains in muscular strength and endurance.

1.1.24   Knowledge of muscle fatigue as it relates to mode, intensity, duration, and the accumulative effects of exercise.

1.1.26   Knowledge of the response of the following variables to acute static and dynamic exercise: heart rate, stroke volume, cardiac output, pulmonary ventilation, tidal volume, respiratory rate, and arteriovenous oxygen difference.

1.1.27   Knowledge of blood pressure responses associated with acute exercise, including changes in body position.

1.1.28   Knowledge of and ability to describe the implications of ventilatory threshold (anaerobic threshold) as it relates to exercise training and cardiorespiratory assessment.

1.1.29   Knowledge of and ability to describe the physiologic adaptations of the pulmonary system that occur at rest and during submaximal and maximal exercise following chronic aerobic and anaerobic training.

1.1.30   Knowledge of how each of the following differs from the normal condition: dyspnea, hypoxia, and hyperventilation.

1.1.31   Knowledge of how the principles of specificity and progressive overload relate to the components of exercise programming.

1.1.32   Knowledge of the concept of detraining or reversibility of conditioning and its implications in exercise programs.

1.1.33   Knowledge of the physical and psychological signs of overreaching/overtraining and to provide recommendations for these problems.

1.1.34   Knowledge of and ability to describe the changes that occur in maturation from childhood to adulthood for the following: skeletal muscle, bone, reaction time, coordination, posture, heat and cold tolerance, maximal oxygen consumption, strength, flexibility, body composition, resting and maximal heart rate, and resting and maximal blood pressure.

1.1.35   Knowledge of the effect of the aging process on the musculoskeletal and cardiovascular structure and function at rest, during exercise, and during recovery.

1.1.36   Knowledge of the following terms: progressive resistance, isotonic/isometric, concentric, eccentric, atrophy, hyperplasia, hypertrophy, sets, repetitions, plyometrics, Valsalva maneuver.

1.1.37   Knowledge of and skill to demonstrate exercises designed to enhance muscular strength and/or endurance of specific major muscle groups.

1.1.38   Knowledge of and skill to demonstrate exercises for enhancing musculoskeletal flexibility.

1.1.39   Ability to identify the major muscles. Major muscles include, but are not limited to, the following: trapezius, pectoralis major, latissimus dorsi, biceps, triceps, rectus abdominis, internal and external obliques, erector spinae, gluteus maximus, quadriceps, hamstrings, adductors, abductors, and gastrocnemius.

1.1.40   Ability to identify the major bones. Major bones include, but are not limited to, the clavicle, scapula, strernum, humerus, carpals, ulna, radius, femur, fibia, tibia, and tarsals.

1.1.41   Ability to identify the joints of the body.

1.1.42   Knowledge of the primary action and joint range of motion for each major muscle group.

1.1.43   Ability to locate the anatomic landmarks for palpation of peripheral pulses and blood pressure.

GENERAL POPULATION/CORE: PATHOPHYSIOLOGY AND RISK FACTORS

1.2.1   Knowledge of the physiologic and metabolic responses to exercise associated with chronic disease (heart disease, hypertension, diabetes mellitus, and pulmonary disease).

1.2.2   Knowledge of cardiovascular, pulmonary, metabolic, and musculoskeletal risk factors that may require further evaluation by medical or allied health professionals before participation in physical activity.

1.2.3   Knowledge of risk factors that may be favorably modified by physical activity habits.

1.2.4   Knowledge to define the following terms: total cholesterol (TC), high-density lipoprotein cholesterol (HDL-C), TC/HDL-C ratio, low-density lipoprotein cholesterol (LDL-C), triglycerides, hypertension, and atherosclerosis.

1.2.5   Knowledge of plasma cholesterol levels for adults as recommended by the National Cholesterol Education Program.

1.2.6   Knowledge of the risk-factor thresholds for ACSM risk stratification, which includes genetic and lifestyle factors related to the development of CAD.

1.2.7   Knowledge of the atherosclerotic process, the factors involved in its genesis and progression, and the potential role of exercise in treatment.

1.2.8   Knowledge of how lifestyle factors, including nutrition and physical activity, influence lipid and lipoprotein profiles.

GENERAL POPULATION/CORE: HEALTH APPRAISAL, FITNESS, AND CLINICAL EXERCISE TESTING

1.3.1   Knowledge of and ability to discuss the physiologic basis of the major components of physical fitness: flexibility, cardiovascular fitness, muscular strength, muscular endurance, and body composition.

1.3.2   Knowledge of the value of the health/medical history.

1.3.3   Knowledge of the value of a medical clearance before exercise participation.

1.3.4   Knowledge of and the ability to perform risk stratification and its implications toward medical clearance before administration of an exercise test or participation in an exercise program.

1.3.5   Knowledge of relative and absolute contraindications to exercise testing or participation.

1.3.6   Knowledge of the limitations of informed consent and medical clearance before exercise testing.

1.3.7   Knowledge of the advantages/disadvantages and limitations of the various body-composition techniques, including but not limited to, air displacement plethysmography (BOD POD®), dual-energy x-ray absorptiometry (DEXA), hydrostatic weighing, skinfolds, and bioelectrical impedence.

1.3.8   Skill in accurately measuring heart rate and blood pressure, and obtaining rating of perceived exertion (RPE) at rest and during exercise according to established guidelines.

1.3.9   Skill in measuring skinfold sites, skeletal diameters, and girth measurements used for estimating body composition.

1.3.10 Knowledge of calibration of a cycle ergometer and a motor-driven treadmill.

1.3.11 Ability to locate the brachial artery and correctly place the cuff and stethoscope in position for blood-pressure measurement.

1.3.12 Ability to locate common sites for measurement of skinfold thicknesses and circumferences (for determination of body composition and waist-hip ratio).

1.3.13 Ability to obtain a health history and risk appraisal that includes past and current medical history, family history of cardiac disease, orthopedic limitations, prescribed medications, activity patterns, nutritional habits, stress and anxiety levels, and smoking and alcohol use.

1.3.14 Ability to obtain informed consent.

1.3.15 Ability to explain the purpose and procedures and perform the monitoring (heart rate, RPE, and blood pressure) of clients before, during, and after cardiorespiratory fitness testing.

1.3.16 Ability to instruct participants in the use of equipment and test procedures.

1.3.17 Ability to explain purpose of testing, determine an appropriate submaximal or maximal protocol, and perform an assessment of cardiovascular fitness on the treadmill or the cycle ergometer.

1.3.18 Ability to describe the purpose of testing, determine appropriate protocols, and perform assessments of muscular strength, muscular endurance, and flexibility.

1.3.19 Ability to perform various techniques of assessing body composition.

1.3.20 Ability to analyze and interpret information obtained from the cardiorespiratory fitness test and the muscular strength and endurance, flexibility, and body-composition assessments for apparently healthy individuals and those with controlled chronic disease.

1.3.21 Ability to identify appropriate criteria for terminating a fitness evaluation and demonstrate proper procedures to be followed after discontinuing such a test.

1.3.22   Ability to modify protocols and procedures for cardiorespiratory fitness tests in children, adolescents, and older adults.

1.3.23   Ability to identify individuals for whom physician supervision is recommended during maximal and submaximal exercise testing.

GENERAL POPULATION/CORE: ELECTROCARDIOGRAPHY AND DIAGNOSTIC TECHNIQUES

1.4.1   Knowledge of how each of the following arrhythmias differs from the normal condition: premature atrial contractions and premature ventricular contractions.

1.4.3   Knowledge of the basic properties of cardiac muscle and the normal pathways of conduction in the heart.

GENERAL POPULATION/CORE: PATIENT MANAGEMENT AND MEDICATIONS

1.5.1   Knowledge of common drugs from each of the following classes of medications and ability to describe the principal action and the effects on exercise testing and prescription: antianginals, antihypertensives, antiarrhythmics, anticoagulants, bronchodilators, hypoglycemics, psychotropics, and vasodilators.

1.5.2   Knowledge of the effects of the following substances on the exercise response: antihistamines, tranquilizers, alcohol, diet pills, cold tablets, caffeine, and nicotine.

GENERAL POPULATION/CORE: EXERCISE PRESCRIPTION AND PROGRAMMING

1.7.1   Knowledge of the relationship between the number of repetitions, intensity, number of sets, and rest with regard to strength training.

1.7.2   Knowledge of the benefits and precautions associated with exercise training in apparently healthy and controlled disease.

1.7.3   Knowledge of the benefits and precautions associated with exercise training across the life span (from youth to the elderly).

1.7.4   Knowledge of specific group exercise leadership techniques appropriate for working with participants of all ages.

1.7.5   Knowledge of how to select and/or modify appropriate exercise programs according to the age, functional capacity, and limitations of the individual.

1.7.6   Knowledge of the differences in the development of an exercise prescription for children, adolescents, and older participants.

1.7.7   Knowledge of and ability to describe the unique adaptations to exercise training in children, adolescents, and older participants with regard to strength, functional capacity, and motor skills.

1.7.8   Knowledge of common orthopedic and cardiovascular considerations for older participants and the ability to describe modifications in exercise prescription that are indicated.

1.7.10   Knowledge of the recommended intensity, duration, frequency, and type of physical activity necessary for development of cardiorespiratory fitness in an apparently healthy population.

1.7.11   Knowledge of and the ability to describe exercises designed to enhance muscular strength and/or endurance of specific major muscle groups.

1.7.12   Knowledge of the principles of overload, specificity, and progression and how they relate to exercise programming.

1.7.13   Knowledge of the various types of interval, continuous, and circuit training programs.

1.7.14   Knowledge of approximate METs for various sport, recreational, and work tasks.

1.7.15   Knowledge of the components incorporated into an exercise session and the proper sequence (i.e., pre-exercise evaluation, warm-up, aerobic stimulus phase, cool-down, muscular strength and/or endurance, and flexibility).

1.7.16   Knowledge of special precautions and modifications of exercise programming for participation at altitude, different ambient temperatures, humidity, and environmental pollution.

1.7.17   Knowledge of the importance of recording exercise sessions and performing periodic evaluations to assess changes in fitness status.

1.7.18   Knowledge of the advantages and disadvantages of implementation of interval, continuous, and circuit training programs.

1.7.19   Knowledge of the exercise programs that are available in the community and how these programs are appropriate for various populations.

1.7.20   Knowledge of and ability to describe activities of daily living (ADLs) and its importance in the overall health of the individual.

1.7.21   Skill to teach and demonstrate the components of an exercise session (i.e., warm-up, aerobic stimulus phase, cool-down, muscular strength/endurance, flexibility).

1.7.22   Skill to teach and demonstrate appropriate modifications in specific exercises for groups such as older adults, pregnant and postnatal women, obese persons, and persons with low back pain.

1.7.23   Skill to teach and demonstrate appropriate exercises for improving range of motion of all major joints.

1.7.24   Skill in the use of various methods for establishing and monitoring levels of exercise intensity, including heart rate, RPE, and oxygen cost.

1.7.25   Ability to identify and apply methods used to monitor exercise intensity, including heart rate and RPE.

1.7.26   Ability to describe modifications in exercise prescriptions for individuals with functional disabilities and musculoskeletal injuries.

1.7.27   Ability to differentiate between the amount of physical activity required for health benefits and/or for fitness development.

1.7.28   Knowledge of and ability to determine target heart rates using two methods: percent of age-predicted maximum heart rate and heart rate reserve (Karvonen).

1.7.29   Ability to identify proper and improper technique in the use of resistive equipment, such as stability balls, weights, bands, resistance bars, and water exercise equipment.

1.7.30   Ability to identify proper and improper technique in the use of cardio-vascular conditioning equipment (e.g., stair-climbers, stationary cycles, treadmills, elliptical trainers, rowing machines).

1.7.31   Ability to teach a progression of exercises for all major muscle groups to improve muscular strength and endurance.

1.7.32   Ability to communicate appropriately with exercise participants during initial screening and exercise programming.

1.7.33   Ability to design, implement, and evaluate individualized and group exercise programs based on health history and physical fitness assessments.

1.7.34   Ability to modify exercises based on age, physical condition, and cognitive status.

1.7.35   Ability to apply energy cost, $\dot{V}O_2$, METs, and target heart rates to an exercise prescription.

1.7.36   Ability to convert between the U.S. and metric systems for length/height (inches to centimeters), weight (pounds to kilograms), and speed (miles per hour to meters per minute).

1.7.37   Ability to convert between absolute ($mL \cdot kg^{-1} \cdot min^{-1}$ or $L \cdot min^{-1}$) and relative ($mL \cdot kg^{-1} \cdot min^{-1}$, and/or METs) oxygen costs.

1.7.38   Ability to determine the energy cost for given exercise intensities during horizontal and graded walking and running stepping exercise, cycle ergometry, arm ergometry, and stepping.

1.7.39   Ability to prescribe exercise intensity based on $\dot{V}O_2$ data for different modes of exercise, including graded and horizontal running and walking, cycling, and stepping exercise.

1.7.40   Ability to explain and implement exercise prescription guidelines for apparently healthy clients, increased risk clients, and clients with controlled disease.

1.7.41   Ability to adapt frequency, intensity, duration, mode, progression, level of supervision, and monitoring techniques in exercise programs for patients with controlled chronic disease (e.g., heart disease, diabetes mellitus, obesity, hypertension), musculoskeletal problems (including fatigue), pregnancy and/or postpartum, and exercise-induced asthma.

1.7.42   Ability to design resistive exercise programs to increase or maintain muscular strength and/or endurance.

1.7.43   Ability to evaluate flexibility and prescribe appropriate flexibility exercises for all major muscle groups.

1.7.44   Ability to design training programs using interval, continuous, and circuit training programs.

1.7.45   Ability to describe the advantages and disadvantages of various commercial exercise equipment in developing cardiorespiratory fitness, muscular strength, and muscular endurance.

1.7.46   Ability to modify exercise programs based on age, physical condition, and current health status.

1.7.47   Ability to assess postural alignment and recommend appropriate exercise to meet individual needs and refer as necessary.

GENERAL POPULATION/CORE: NUTRITION AND WEIGHT MANAGEMENT

1.8.1   Knowledge of the role of carbohydrates, fats, and proteins as fuels for aerobic and anaerobic metabolism.

1.8.2   Knowledge of the following terms: obesity, overweight, percent fat, BMI, lean body mass, anorexia nervosa, bulimia nervosa, metabolic syndrome, and body-fat distribution.

1.8.3   Knowledge of the relationship between body composition and health.

1.8.4   Knowledge of the effects of diet, exercise, and behavior modification as methods for modifying body composition.

1.8.5   Knowledge of the importance of an adequate daily energy intake for healthy weight management.

1.8.6   Knowledge of the difference between fat-soluble and water-soluble vitamins.

1.8.7   Knowledge of the importance of maintaining normal hydration before, during, and after exercise.

1.8.8   Knowledge of the USDA Food Pyramid and Dietary Guidelines for Americans.

1.8.9   Knowledge of the importance of calcium and iron in women's health.

1.8.10 Knowledge of the myths and consequences associated with inappropriate weight loss methods (e.g., fad diets, dietary supplements, overexercising, starvation diets).

1.8.11 Knowledge of the number of kilocalories in one gram of carbohydrate, fat, protein, and alcohol.

1.8.12 Knowledge of the number of kilocalories equivalent to losing one pound (0.45 kg) of body fat and the ability to prescribe appropriate amount of exercise to achieve weight-loss goals.

1.8.13 Knowledge of the guidelines for caloric intake for an individual desiring to lose or gain weight.

1.8.14 Knowledge of common nutritional ergogenic aids, the purported mechanism of action, and any risk and/or benefits (e.g., carbohydrates, protein/amino acids, vitamins, minerals, herbal products, creatine, steroids, caffeine).

1.8.15 Knowledge of nutritional factors related to the female athlete triad syndrome (i.e., eating disorders, menstrual cycle abnormalities, and osteoporosis).

1.8.16 Knowledge of the NIH consensus statement regarding health risks of obesity, Nutrition for Physical Fitness Position Paper of the American Dietetic Association, and the ACSM position stand on proper and improper weight loss programs.

1.8.17 Ability to describe the health implications of variation in body-fat distribution patterns and the significance of the waist-to-hip ratio.

1.8.18 Knowledge of the nutrition and exercise effects on blood glucose levels in diabetes.

GENERAL POPULATION/CORE: HUMAN BEHAVIOR AND COUNSELING

1.9.1   Knowledge of behavioral strategies to enhance exercise and health behavior change (e.g., reinforcement, goal setting, social support).

1.9.2   Knowledge of the important elements that should be included in each behavior-modification session.

1.9.3   Knowledge of specific techniques to enhance motivation (e.g., posters, recognition, bulletin boards, games, competitions).

1.9.4   Knowledge of extrinsic and intrinsic reinforcement and ability to give examples of each.

1.9.5   Knowledge of the stages of motivational readiness.

1.9.6   Knowledge of approaches that may assist less motivated clients to increase their physical activity.

1.9.7   Knowledge of signs and symptoms of mental health states (e.g., anxiety, depression, eating disorders) that may necessitate referral to a medical or mental health professional.

1.9.8   Knowledge of the potential symptoms and causal factors of test anxiety (i.e., performance, appraisal threat during exercise testing) and how it may affect physiologic responses to testing.

1.9.9   Ability to coach clients to set achievable goals and overcome obstacles through a variety of methods (e.g., in person, on phone, and on Internet).

GENERAL POPULATION/CORE: SAFETY, INJURY PREVENTION, AND EMERGENCY PROCEDURES

1.10.1   Knowledge of and skill in obtaining basic life support, first aid, cardiopulmonary resuscitation, and automated external defibrillator certifications.

1.10.2   Knowledge of appropriate emergency procedures (i.e., telephone procedures, written emergency procedures, personnel responsibilities) in a health and fitness setting.

1.10.3   Knowledge of and skill in performing basic first-aid procedures for exercise-related injuries, such as bleeding, strains/sprains, fractures, and exercise intolerance (dizziness, syncope, heat and cold injuries).

1.10.4   Knowledge of basic precautions taken in an exercise setting to ensure participant safety.

1.10.5   Knowledge of the physical and physiologic signs and symptoms of overtraining and the ability to modify a program to accommodate this condition.

1.10.6   Knowledge of the effects of temperature, humidity, altitude, and pollution on the physiologic response to exercise and the ability to modify the exercise prescription to accommodate for these environmental conditions.

1.10.7   Knowledge of the signs and symptoms of the following conditions: shin splints, sprain, strain, tennis elbow, bursitis, stress fracture, tendonitis, patellar femoral pain syndrome, low back pain, plantar fasciitis, and rotator cuff tendonitis; the ability to recommend exercises to prevent these injuries.

1.10.8   Knowledge of hypothetical concerns and potential risks that may be associated with the use of exercises such as straight-leg sit-ups, double leg raises, full squats, hurdler's stretch, yoga plow, forceful back hyperextension, and standing bent-over toe touch.

1.10.9   Knowledge of safety plans, emergency procedures, and first-aid techniques needed during fitness evaluations, exercise testing, and exercise training.

1.10.10   Knowledge of the Health Fitness Specialist's responsibilities and limitations, and the legal implications of carrying out emergency procedures.

1.10.11   Knowledge of potential musculoskeletal injuries (e.g., contusions, sprains, strains, fractures), cardiovascular/pulmonary complications (e.g., tachycardia, bradycardia, hypotension/hypertension, tachypnea), and metabolic abnormalities (e.g., fainting/syncope, hypoglycemia/hyperglycemia, hypothermia/hyperthermia).

1.10.12   Knowledge of the initial management and first-aid techniques associated with open wounds, musculoskeletal injuries, cardiovascular/pulmonary complications, and metabolic disorders.

1.10.13   Knowledge of the components of an equipment maintenance/repair program and how it may be used to evaluate the condition of exercise equipment to reduce the potential risk of injury.

1.10.14   Knowledge of the legal implications of documented safety procedures, the use of incident documents, and ongoing safety training documentation for the purposes of safety and risk management.

1.10.15   Skill to demonstrate exercises used for people with low back pain; neck, shoulder, elbow, wrist, hip, knee and/or ankle pain; and the ability to modify a program for people with these conditions.

1.10.16   Skill in demonstrating appropriate emergency procedures during exercise testing and/or training.

1.10.17   Ability to identify the components that contribute to the maintenance of a safe environment, including equipment operation and maintenance, proper sanitation, safety and maintenance of exercise areas, and overall facility maintenance.

1.10.18   Knowledge of basic ergonomics to address daily activities that may cause musculoskeletal problems in the workplace and the ability to recommend exercises to alleviate symptoms caused by repetitive movements.

GENERAL POPULATION/CORE: PROGRAM ADMINISTRATION, QUALITY ASSURANCE, AND OUTCOME ASSESSMENT

1.11.1   Knowledge of the Health Fitness Specialist's role in administration and program management within a health/fitness facility.

1.11.2   Knowledge of and the ability to use the documentation required when a client shows signs or symptoms during an exercise session and should be referred to a physician.

1.11.3   Knowledge of how to manage a fitness department (e.g., working within a budget, interviewing and training staff, scheduling, running staff meetings, staff development).

1.11.4   Knowledge of the importance of tracking and evaluating member retention.

1.11.6   Ability to administer fitness-related programs within established budgetary guidelines.

1.11.7   Ability to develop marketing materials for the purpose of promoting fitness-related programs.

1.11.8   Ability to create and maintain records pertaining to participant exercise adherence, retention, and goal setting.

1.11.9   Ability to develop and administer educational programs (e.g., lectures, workshops) and educational materials.

1.11.10   Knowledge of basic sales techniques to promote health, fitness, and wellness services.

1.11.11   Knowledge of networking techniques with other healthcare professionals for referral purposes.

1.11.12   Ability to provide and administer appropriate customer service.

1.11.13   Knowledge of the importance of tracking and evaluating health promotion program results.

CARDIOVASCULAR: PATHOPHYSIOLOGY AND RISK FACTORS

2.2.1   Knowledge of cardiovascular risk factors or conditions that may require consultation with medical personnel before testing or training, including inappropriate changes of resting or exercise heart rate and blood pressure; new onset discomfort in chest, neck, shoulder, or arm; changes in the pattern of discomfort during rest or exercise; fainting or dizzy spells; and claudication.

2.2.2   Knowledge of the pathophysiology of myocardial ischemia and infarction.

2.2.3   Knowledge of the pathophysiology of stroke, hypertension, and hyperlipidemia.

2.2.4   Knowledge of the effects of the above diseases and conditions on the cardiorespiratory responses at rest and during exercise.

PULMONARY: PATHOPHYSIOLOGY AND RISK FACTORS

3.2.1   Knowledge of pulmonary risk factors or conditions that may require consultation with medical personnel before testing or training, including asthma, exercise-induced asthma/bronchospasm, extreme breathlessness at rest or during exercise, bronchitis, and emphysema.

METABOLIC: PATHOPHYSIOLOGY AND RISK FACTORS

4.2.1   Knowledge of metabolic risk factors or conditions that may require consultation with medical personnel before testing or training, including obesity, metabolic syndrome, thyroid disease, kidney disease, diabetes or glucose intolerance, and hypoglycemia.

ORTHOPEDIC/MUSCULOSKELETAL: PATHOPHYSIOLOGY AND RISK FACTORS

5.2.1   Knowledge of musculoskeletal risk factors or conditions that may require consultation with medical personnel before testing or training, including acute or chronic back pain, osteoarthritis, rheumatoid arthritis, osteoporosis, inflammation/pain, and low back pain.

NEUROMUSCULAR: PATHOPHYSIOLOGY AND RISK FACTORS

6.2.1   Knowledge of neuromuscular risk factors or conditions that may require consultation with medical personnel before testing or training, including spinal cord injuries and multiple sclerosis.

IMMUNOLOGIC: PATHOPHYSIOLOGY AND RISK FACTORS

7.2.1   Knowledge of immunologic risk factors or conditions that may require consultation with medical personnel before testing or training, including AIDS and cancer.

NOTE: The KSAs listed above for the ACSM Certified Health Fitness Specialist are the same KSAs for educational programs in Exercise Science seeking undergraduate (Bachelor's) academic accreditation through the CoAES. For more information, please visit www.coaes.org.

The ACSM Certified Clinical Exercise Specialist is responsible for the mastery of the ACSM Certified Personal Trainer[SM] KSAs, the ACSM Certified Health Fitness Specialist KSAs, and the following ACSM Certified Clinical Exercise Specialist KSAs.

GENERAL POPULATION/CORE: EXERCISE PHYSIOLOGY AND RELATED EXERCISE SCIENCE

1.1.1   Describe and illustrate the normal cardiovascular anatomy.

1.1.2   Describe the physiologic effects of bed rest, and discuss the appropriate physical activities that might be used to counteract these changes.

1.1.3   Identify the cardiorespiratory responses associated with postural changes.

1.1.5   Identify the metabolic equivalent (MET) requirements of various occupational, household, sport/exercise, and leisure-time activities.

1.1.6   Demonstrate knowledge of the unique hemodynamic responses of arm versus leg exercise, combined arm and leg exercise, and of static versus dynamic exercise.

1.1.7   Define the determinants of myocardial oxygen consumption (i.e., heart rate $\times$ systolic blood pressure = double product OR rate-pressure product) and the effects of acute exercise and exercise training on those determinants.

1.1.8   Describe the methodology for measuring peak oxygen consumption ($\dot{V}O_{2peak}$).

1.1.9   Plot the normal resting and exercise values associated with increasing exercise intensity (and how they may differ for cardiac, pulmonary, and metabolic diseased populations) for the following: heart rate, stroke volume, cardiac output, double product, arteriovenous O_2 difference, O_2 consumption, systolic and diastolic blood pressure, minute ventilation, tidal volume, breathing frequency, Vd/Vt, $\dot{V}_E/\dot{V}O_2$, $\dot{V}_E/\dot{V}CO_2$, $FEV_{1.0}$, SaO_2, and blood glucose.

1.1.10   Discuss the effects of isometric exercise in individuals with cardiovascular, pulmonary, and/or metabolic diseases.

1.1.11   Demonstrate knowledge of acute and chronic adaptations to exercise for those with cardiovascular, pulmonary, and metabolic diseases.

1.1.12   Describe the effects of variation in environmental factors (e.g., temperature, humidity, altitude) for normal individuals and those with cardiovascular, pulmonary, and metabolic diseases.

1.1.13   Understand the hormonal (i.e., insulin, glucagon, epinephrine, norepinephrine, angiotensin, aldosterone, renin, erythropoieten) responses to acute and chronic exercise.

1.1.14   Identify normal and abnormal respiratory responses during rest and exercise as assessed during a pulmonary function test (i.e., FVC, MVV, $FEV_{1.0}$, flow volume loop).

GENERAL POPULATION/CORE: PATHOPHYSIOLOGY AND RISK FACTORS

1.2.1   Summarize the atherosclerotic process, including current hypotheses regarding onset and rate of progression and/or regression.

1.2.2   Compare and contrast the differences between typical, atypical, and vasospastic angina and how these may differ in specific subgroups (i.e., men, women, people with diabetes).

1.2.3   Describe the pathophysiology of the healing myocardium and the potential complications after acute myocardial infarction (MI) (remodeling, rupture).

1.2.5   Examine the role of lifestyle on cardiovascular risk factors, such as hypertension, blood lipids, glucose tolerance, and body weight.

1.2.6   Describe the lipoprotein classifications, and define their relationship to atherosclerosis.

1.2.7   Describe the resting and exercise cardiorespiratory and metabolic responses in those with pulmonary disease.

1.2.8   Describe the influence of exercise on cardiovascular, pulmonary, and metabolic risk factors.

1.2.11   Describe the cardiorespiratory and metabolic responses in myocardial dysfunction and ischemia at rest and during exercise.

1.2.12   Recognize and describe the pathophysiology of the differing severities (e.g., NYHA classification) of heart failure, including cardiac output, heart rate, blood pressure, cardiac dimensions, and basic echocardiography parameters (ejection fraction, wall motion, left ventricular dimension).

1.2.13 Recognize and describe the pathophysiology of diabetes mellitus (prediabetes, types 1 and 2, gestational), including blood glucose, Hb_{A1c}, insulin sensitivity, and the risk and affect on comorbid conditions.

1.2.14 Identify the contributing factors to metabolic syndrome, their pathologic sequelae, and their affect on the primary or secondary risk of cardiovascular disease.

1.2.15 Recognize the pathologic process that various risk factors contribute for the development of cardiac, pulmonary, and metabolic diseases (e.g., smoking, hypertension, abnormal blood lipid values, obesity, inactivity, sex, genetics, diabetes).

GENERAL POPULATION/CORE: HEALTH APPRAISAL, FITNESS, AND CLINICAL EXERCISE TESTING

1.3.1 Describe common procedures and apply knowledge of results from radionuclide imaging (e.g., thallium, technetium, sestamibi, tetrafosmin, single-photon emission computed tomography [SPECT]), stress echocardiography, and pharmacologic testing (e.g., dobutamine, adenosine, persantine).

1.3.2 Demonstrate knowledge of exercise testing procedures for various clinical populations, including those individuals with cardiovascular, pulmonary, and metabolic diseases in terms of exercise modality, protocol, physiologic measurements, and expected outcomes.

1.3.3 Describe anatomic landmarks as they relate to exercise testing and programming (e.g., electrode placement, blood pressure).

1.3.4 Locate and palpate anatomic landmarks of radial, brachial, carotid, femoral, popliteal, and tibialis arteries.

1.3.5 Select an appropriate test protocol according to the age, functional capacity, physical ability, and health status of the individual.

1.3.6 Identify individuals for whom physician supervision is recommended during maximal and submaximal exercise testing.

1.3.7 Conduct pre-exercise test procedures.

1.3.8 Describe basic equipment and facility requirements for exercise testing.

1.3.9 Instruct the test participant in the use of the RPE scale and other appropriate subjective rating scales, such as the dyspnea, pain, claudication, and angina scales.

1.3.11 Describe the importance of accurate and calibrated testing equipment (e.g., treadmill, ergometers, electrocardiograph [ECG], gas analysis systems, and sphygmomanometers) and demonstrate the ability to recognize and remediate equipment that is no longer properly calibrated.

1.3.12 Obtain and recognize normal and abnormal physiologic and subjective responses (e.g., symptoms, ECG, blood pressure, heart rate, RPE and other scales, oxygen saturation, and oxygen consumption) at appropriate intervals during the test.

1.3.15   Demonstrate the ability to provide testing procedures and protocol for children and the elderly with or without various clinical conditions.

1.3.16   Evaluate medical history and physical examination findings as they relate to health appraisal and exercise testing.

1.3.17   Accurately record and interpret right and left arm pre-exercise blood pressures in the supine and upright positions.

1.3.18   Describe and analyze the importance of the absolute and relative contraindications and test termination indicators of an exercise test.

1.3.19   Select and perform appropriate procedures and protocols for the exercise test, including modes of exercise, starting levels, increments of work, ramping versus incremental protocols, length of stages, and frequency of data collection.

1.3.20   Describe and conduct immediate postexercise procedures and various approaches to cool-down and recognize normal and abnormal responses.

1.3.21   Record, organize, perform, and interpret necessary calculations of test data.

1.3.22   Describe the differences in the physiologic responses to various modes of ergometry (e.g., treadmill, cycle and arm ergometers) as they relate to exercise testing and training.

1.3.23   Describe normal and abnormal chronotropic and inotropic responses to exercise testing and training.

1.3.24   Understand and apply pretest likelihood of CAD, the positive and negative predictive values of various types of stress tests (e.g., ECG only, stress echo, radionuclide), and the potential of false positive/negative and true positive/negative results.

1.3.25   Compare and contrast obstructive and restrictive lung diseases and their effect on exercise testing and training.

1.3.26   Identify orthopedic limitations (e.g., gout, foot drop, specific joint problems, amputation, prosthesis) as they relate to modifications of exercise testing and programming.

1.3.27   Identify basic neuromuscular disorders (e.g., Parkinson's disease, multiple sclerosis) as they relate to modifications of exercise testing and programming.

1.3.28   Describe the aerobic and anaerobic metabolic demands of exercise testing and training in individuals with cardiovascular, pulmonary, and/or metabolic diseases undergoing exercise testing or training.

1.3.29   Identify the variables measured during cardiopulmonary exercise testing (e.g., heart rate, blood pressure, rate of perceived exertion, ventilation, oxygen consumption, ventilatory threshold, pulmonary circulation) and their potential relationship to cardiovascular, pulmonary, and metabolic disease.

1.3.31   Understand the basic principle and methods of coronary calcium scoring using computed-tomography (CT) methods.

1.3.32   Recognize the emergence of new imaging techniques for the assessment of heart disease (e.g., CT angiography).

1.3.33   Recognize the value of heart and lung sounds in the assessment of patients with cardiovascular and/or pulmonary disease.

1.3.34   Demonstrate the ability to perform a six-minute walk test and appropriately use the results to assess prognosis, fitness, and/or improvement.

GENERAL POPULATION/CORE: ELECTROCARDIOGRAPHY AND DIAGNOSTIC TECHNIQUES

1.4.1   Summarize the purpose of coronary angiography.

1.4.2   Describe myocardial ischemia and identify ischemic indicators of various cardiovascular diagnostic tests.

1.4.3   Describe the differences between Q-wave and non-Q-wave infarction, and ST elevation (STEMI) and non-ST elevation myocardial infarction (non-STEMI).

1.4.4   Identify the ECG patterns at rest and responses to exercise in patients with pacemakers and implantable cardiac defibrillators (ICDs). In addition, recognize the ability of biventricular pacing and possibility of pacemaker malfunction (e.g., failure to sense and failure to pace).

1.4.5   Identify resting and exercise ECG changes associated with the following abnormalities: axis; bundle-branch blocks and bifascicular blocks; atrioventricular blocks; sinus bradycardia and tachycardia; sinus arrest; supraventricular premature contractions and tachycardia; ventricular premature contractions (including frequency, form, couplets, salvos, tachycardia); atrial flutter and fibrillation; ventricular fibrillation; myocardial ischemia, injury, and infarction.

1.4.6   Define the ECG criteria for initiating and/or terminating exercise testing or training.

1.4.7   Identify ECG changes that correspond to ischemia in various myocardial regions.

1.4.8   Describe potential causes and pathophysiology of various cardiac arrhythmias.

1.4.9   Identify potentially hazardous arrhythmias or conduction defects observed on the ECG at rest, during exercise, and recovery.

1.4.10   Describe the diagnostic and prognostic significance of ischemic ECG responses and arrhythmias at rest, during exercise, or recovery.

1.4.11   Identify resting and exercise ECG changes associated with cardiovascular disease, hypertensive heart disease, cardiac chamber enlargement, pericarditis, pulmonary disease, and metabolic disorders.

1.4.12   Administer and interpret basic resting spirometric tests and measures, including $FEV_{1.0}$, FVC, and MVV.

1.4.13   Locate the appropriate sites for the limb and chest leads for resting, standard, and exercise (Mason Likar) ECGs, as well as commonly used bipolar systems (e.g., CM-5).

1.4.14   Obtain and interpret a pre-exercise standard and modified (Mason-Likar) 12-lead ECG on a participant in the supine and upright position.
1.4.15   Demonstrate the ability to minimize ECG artifact.
1.4.16   Describe the diagnostic and prognostic implications of the exercise test ECG and hemodynamic responses.
1.4.17   Identify ECG changes that typically occur as a result of hyperventilation, electrolyte abnormalities, and drug therapy.
1.4.18   Identify the causes of false-positive and false-negative exercise ECG responses and methods for optimizing sensitivity and specificity.
1.4.19   Identify and describe the significance of ECG abnormalities in designing the exercise prescription and in making activity recommendations.

GENERAL POPULATION/CORE: PATIENT MANAGEMENT AND MEDICATIONS

1.5.2   Describe mechanisms and actions of medications that may affect exercise testing and prescription (i.e., β-blockers, nitrates, calcium channel blockers, digitalis, diuretics, vasodilators, antiarrhythmic agents, bronchodilators, antilipemics, psychotropics, nicotine, antihistamines, over-the-counter [OTC] cold medications, thyroid medications, alcohol, hypoglycemic agents, blood modifiers, pentoxifylline, antigout medications, and anorexiants/diet pills).
1.5.3   Recognize medications associated in the clinical setting, their indications for care, and their effects at rest and during exercise (i.e., β-blockers, nitrates, calcium channel blockers, digitalis, diuretics, vasodilators, anitarrhythmic agents, bronchodilators, antilipemics, psychotropics, nicotine, antihistamines, OTC cold medications, thyroid medications, alcohol, hypoglycemic agents, blood modifiers, pentoxifylline, antigout medications, and anorexiants/diet pills).
1.5.4   Recognize the use of herbal and nutritional supplements, OTC medications, homeopathic remedies, and other alternative therapies often used by patients with chronic diseases.
1.5.5   Practice disease/case management responsibilities, including daily follow-up concerning patient needs, signs and symptoms, physician appointments, and medication changes for patients with chronic diseases, including cardiovascular, pulmonary, and metabolic diseases; comorbid conditions; arthritis; osteoporosis; and renal dysfunction/transplant/dialysis.
1.5.6   Direct patients actively attempting to lose weight in a formal or informal setting using behavioral, diet, exercise, or surgical methods.
1.5.7   Manage patients on oxygen therapy as needed during exercise testing or training.
1.5.8   Recognize patient clinical need for referral to other (non-ES) allied health professionals (e.g., behavioralist, physical therapist, diabetes educator, nurse).
1.5.9   Recognize patients with chronic pain who may be in a chronic pain management treatment program and who may require special adaptations during exercise testing and training.

1.5.10 Recognize exercise testing and training needs of patients with joint replacement or prosthesis.

1.5.11 Address exercise testing and training needs of elderly and young patients.

1.5.12 Recognize treatment goals and guidelines for hypertension using the most recent JNC report and other relevant evidence-based guidelines.

1.5.13 Recognize treatment goals and guidelines for dyslipidemia using the most recent NCEP report and other relevant evidence-based guidelines.

1.5.14 Demonstrate the ability to perform pulse-oximetry and blood glucose evaluations and appropriately interpret the data in a given clinical situation.

1.5.15 Demonstrate the ability to assess for peripheral edema and other indicators of fluid retention and respond appropriately in a given clinical setting.

GENERAL POPULATION/CORE: MEDICAL AND SURGICAL MANAGEMENT

1.6.1 Describe percutaneous coronary interventions (PCI) and peripheral interventions as an alternative to medical management or bypass surgery.

1.6.2 Describe indications and limitations for medical management and interventional techniques in different subsets of individuals with CAD and peripheral arterial disease (PAD).

1.6.3 Identify risk, benefit, and unique management issues of patients with mechanical, prosthetic valve replacement and valve repair.

1.6.4 Describe and recognize bariatric surgery as a therapy for obesity.

1.6.5 Recognize external counterpulsation (ECP) as a method of treating severe, difficult-to-treat chest pain (i.e., angina).

GENERAL POPULATION/CORE: EXERCISE PRESCRIPTION AND PROGRAMMING

1.7.2 Compare and contrast benefits and risks of exercise for individuals with risk factors for or established cardiovascular, pulmonary, and/or metabolic diseases.

1.7.3 Design appropriate exercise prescription in environmental extremes for those with cardiovascular, pulmonary, and metabolic diseases.

1.7.4 Design, implement, and supervise individualized exercise prescriptions for people with chronic disease and disabling conditions or for people who are young or elderly.

1.7.5 Design a supervised exercise program beginning at hospital discharge and continuing for up to six months for the following conditions: MI; angina: left ventricular assist device (LVAD); congestive heart failure; PCI; coronary artery bypass graft (surgery) (CABG[S]); medical management of CAD; chronic pulmonary disease; weight management; diabetes; metabolic syndrome; and cardiac transplants.

1.7.6   Demonstrate knowledge of the concept of activities of daily living (ADLs) and its importance in the overall rehabilitation of the individual.

1.7.7   Prescribe exercise using nontraditional modalities (e.g., bench stepping, elastic bands, isodynamic exercise, water aerobics, yoga, tai chi) for individuals with cardiovascular, pulmonary, or metabolic diseases.

1.7.8   Demonstrate exercise equipment adaptations necessary for different age groups, physical abilities, and other potential contributing factors.

1.7.9   Identify patients who require a symptom-limited exercise test before exercise training.

1.7.10   Organize graded exercise tests and clinical data to counsel patients regarding issues such as ADL, return to work, and physical activity.

1.7.11   Describe relative and absolute contraindications to exercise training.

1.7.12   Identify characteristics that correlate or predict poor compliance to exercise programs and strategies to increase exercise adherence.

1.7.13   Describe the importance of warm-up and cool-down sessions with specific reference to angina and ischemic ECG changes, and for overall patient safety.

1.7.14   Identify and explain the mechanisms by which exercise may contribute to reducing disease risk or rehabilitating individuals with cardiovascular, pulmonary, and metabolic diseases.

1.7.15   Describe common gait, movement, and coordination abnormalities as they relate to exercise testing and programming.

1.7.16   Describe the principle of specificity as it relates to the mode of exercise testing and training.

1.7.17   Design strength and flexibility programs for individuals with cardiovascular, pulmonary, and/or metabolic diseases; the elderly; and children.

1.7.18   Determine appropriate testing and training modalities according to the age, functional capacity, physical ability, and health status of the individual.

1.7.19   Describe the indications and methods for ECG monitoring during exercise testing and training.

1.7.20   Discuss the appropriate use of static and dynamic resistance exercise for individuals with cardiovascular, pulmonary, and metabolic disease.

1.7.21   Demonstrate the ability to modify exercise testing and training to the limitations of PAD.

1.7.22   Design, describe, and demonstrate specific resistance exercises for major muscle groups for patients with cardiovascular, pulmonary, and metabolic diseases and conditions.

1.7.23   Identify procedures for pre-exercise assessment of blood glucose, determining safety for exercise, and avoidance of exercise-induced hypoglycemia in patients with diabetes. Manage postexercise hypoglycemia when it occurs.

GENERAL POPULATION/CORE: NUTRITION AND WEIGHT MANAGEMENT

1.8.1 Describe and discuss dietary considerations for cardiovascular and pulmonary diseases, chronic heart failure, and diabetes that are recommended to minimize disease progression and optimize disease management.

1.8.2 Compare and contrast dietary practices used for weight reduction, and address the benefits, risks, and scientific support for each practice. Examples of dietary practices are high-protein/low-carbohydrate diets, Mediterranean diet, and low-fat diets, such as the American Heart Association recommended diet.

1.8.3 Calculate the effect of caloric intake and energy expenditure on weight management.

1.8.4 Describe the hypotheses related to diet, weight gain, and weight loss.

1.8.5 Demonstrate the ability to differentiate and educate patients between nutritionally sound diets versus fad diets and scientifically supported supplements and anecdotally supported supplements.

1.8.6 Differentiate among and understand the value of the various vegetarian diets (i.e., Ovo-lacto, vegan).

GENERAL POPULATION/CORE: HUMAN BEHAVIOR AND COUNSELING

1.9.1 List and apply behavioral strategies that apply to lifestyle modifications, such as exercise, diet, stress, and medication management.

1.9.2 Describe signs and symptoms of maladjustment and/or failure to cope during an illness crisis and/or personal adjustment crisis (e.g., job loss) that might prompt a psychological consult or referral to other professional services.

1.9.3 Describe the general principles of crisis management and factors influencing coping and learning in illness states.

1.9.4 Identify the psychological stages involved with the acceptance of death and dying and demonstrate the ability to recognize when it is necessary for a psychological consult or referral to a professional resource.

1.9.5 Recognize observable signs and symptoms of anxiety or depressive symptoms and the need for a psychiatric referral.

1.9.6 Describe the psychological issues to be confronted by the patient and by family members of patients who have cardiovascular or pulmonary disease or diseases of the metabolic syndrome.

1.9.7 Identify the psychological issues associated with an acute cardiac event versus those associated with chronic cardiac conditions.

1.9.8 Recognize and implement methods of stress management for patients with chronic disease.

1.9.9 Use common assessment tools to access behavioral change, such as the Transtheoretical Model.

1.9.10 Facilitate effective and contemporary motivational and behavior modification techniques to promote behavioral change.

1.9.11   Demonstrate the ability to conduct effective and informative group and individual education sessions directed at primary or secondary prevention of chronic disease.

GENERAL POPULATION/CORE: SAFETY, INJURY PREVENTION, AND EMERGENCY PROCEDURES

1.10.1   Respond appropriately to emergency situations (e.g., cardiac arrest, hypoglycemia and hyperglycemia; bronchospasm; sudden onset hypotension; severe hypertensive response; angina; serious cardiac arrhythmias; ICD discharge; transient ischemic attack [TIA] or stroke; MI) that might arise before, during, and after administration of an exercise test and/or exercise session.

1.10.2   List medications that should be available for emergency situations in exercise testing and training sessions.

1.10.3   Describe the emergency equipment and personnel that should be present in an exercise testing laboratory and rehabilitative exercise training setting.

1.10.4   Describe the appropriate procedures for maintaining emergency equipment and supplies.

1.10.5   Describe the effects of cardiovascular and pulmonary disease and the diseases of the metabolic syndrome on performance of and safety during exercise testing and training.

1.10.6   Stratify individuals with cardiovascular, pulmonary, and metabolic diseases, using appropriate risk-stratification methods and understanding the prognostic indicators for high-risk individuals.

1.10.7   Describe the process for developing and updating emergency policies and procedures (e.g., call 911, call code team, call medical director, transport and use defibrillator).

1.10.8   Be aware of the current CPR, AED, and ACLS standards to be able to assist with emergency situations.

GENERAL POPULATION/CORE: PROGRAM ADMINISTRATION, QUALITY ASSURANCE, AND OUTCOME ASSESSMENT

1.11.1   Discuss the role of outcome measures in chronic disease management programs, such as cardiovascular and pulmonary rehabilitation programs.

1.11.2   Identify and discuss various outcome measurements used in a cardiac or pulmonary rehabilitation program.

1.11.3   Use specific outcome collection instruments to collect outcome data in a cardiac or pulmonary rehabilitation program.

1.11.4   Understand the most recent cardiac and pulmonary rehabilitation Centers for Medicare Services (CMS) rules for patient enrollment and reimbursement (e.g., diagnostic current procedure terminology [CPT] codes, diagnostic related groups [DRG]).

The Registered Clinical Exercise Physiologist® is responsible for the mastery of the ACSM Certified Personal Trainer^SM KSAs, the ACSM Certified Health Fitness

Specialist KSAs, the ACSM Certified Clinical Exercise Specialist KSAs, and the following ACSM Registered Clinical Exercise Physiologist® KSAs:

GENERAL POPULATION/CORE: EXERCISE PHYSIOLOGY AND RELATED EXERCISE SCIENCE

1.1.1   Describe the acute responses to aerobic, resistance, and flexibility training on the function of the cardiovascular, respiratory, musculoskeletal, neuromuscular, metabolic, endocrine, and immune systems.

1.1.2   Describe the chronic effects of aerobic, resistance, and flexibility training on the structure and function of the cardiovascular, respiratory, musculoskeletal, neuromuscular, metabolic, endocrine, and immune systems.

1.1.3   Explain differences in typical values between sedentary and trained persons in those with chronic diseases for oxygen uptake, heart rate, mean arterial pressure, systolic and diastolic blood pressure, cardiac output, stroke volume, rate pressure product, minute ventilation, respiratory rate, and tidal volume at rest and during submaximal and maximal exercise.

1.1.4   Describe the physiologic determinants of $\dot{V}O_2$, $m\dot{V}O_2$, and mean arterial pressure and explain how these determinants may be altered with aerobic and resistance exercise training.

1.1.5   Describe appropriate modifications in the exercise prescription that are due to environmental conditions in individuals with chronic disease.

1.1.6   Explain the health benefits of a physically active lifestyle, the hazards of sedentary behavior, and summarize key recommendations of U.S. national reports of physical activity (e.g., U.S. Surgeon General, Institute of Medicine, ACSM, AHA).

1.1.7   Explain the physiologic adaptations to exercise training that may result in improvement in or maintenance of health, including cardiovascular, pulmonary, metabolic, orthopedic/musculoskeletal, neuromuscular, and immune system health.

1.1.8   Explain the mechanisms underlying the physiologic adaptations to aerobic and resistance training, including those resulting in changes in or maintenance of maximal and submaximal oxygen consumption, lactate and ventilatory (anaerobic) threshold, myocardial oxygen consumption, heart rate, blood pressure, ventilation (including ventilatory threshold), muscle structure, bioenergetics, and immune function.

1.1.9   Explain the physiologic effects of physical inactivity, including bed rest, and methods that may counteract these effects.

1.1.10 Recognize and respond to abnormal signs and symptoms during exercise.

GENERAL POPULATION/CORE: PATHOPHYSIOLOGY AND RISK FACTORS

1.2.1   Describe the epidemiology, pathophysiology, risk factors, and key clinical findings of cardiovascular, pulmonary, metabolic, orthopedic/musculoskeletal, neuromuscular, and NIH diseases.

GENERAL POPULATION/CORE: HEALTH APPRAISAL, FITNESS, AND CLINICAL EXERCISE TESTING

1.3.1   Conduct pretest procedures, including explaining test procedures, obtaining informed consent, obtaining a focused medical history, reviewing results of prior tests and physical exam, assessing disease-specific risk factors, and presenting concise information to other healthcare providers and third-party payers.

1.3.2   Conduct a brief physical examination including evaluation of peripheral edema, measuring blood pressure, peripheral pulses, respiratory rate, and ausculating heart and lung sounds.

1.3.3   Calibrate lab equipment used frequently in the practice of clinical exercise physiology (e.g., motorized/computerized treadmill, mechanical cycle ergometer and arm ergometer), electrocardiograph, spirometer, respiratory gas analyzer (metabolic cart).

1.3.4   Administer exercise tests consistent with U.S. nationally accepted standards for testing.

1.3.5   Evaluate contraindications to exercise testing.

1.3.6   Appropriately select and administer functional tests to measure individual outcomes and functional status, including the six-minute walk, Get Up and Go, Berg Balance Scale, and the Physical Performance Test.

1.3.8   Interpret the variables that may be assessed during clinical exercise testing, including maximal oxygen consumption, resting metabolic rate, ventilatory volumes and capacities, respiratory exchange ratio, ratings of perceived exertion and discomfort (chest pain, dyspnea, claudication), ECG, heart rate, blood pressure, rate pressure product, ventilatory (anaerobic) threshold, oxygen saturation, breathing reserve, muscular strength, muscular endurance, and other common measures employed for diagnosis and prognosis of disease.

1.3.9   Determine atrial and ventricular rate from rhythm strip and 12-lead ECG and explain the clinical significance of abnormal atrial or ventricular rate (e.g., tachycardia, bradycardia).

1.3.10   Identify ECG changes associated with drug therapy, electrolyte abnormalities, subendocardial and transmural ischemia, myocardial injury, and infarction, and explain the clinical significance of each.

1.3.11   Identify SA, AV, and bundle-branch blocks from a rhythm strip and 12-lead ECG, and explain the clinical significance of each.

1.3.12   Identify sinus, atrial, junctional, and ventricular dysrhythmias from a rhythm strip and 12-lead ECG, and explain the clinical significance of each.

1.3.14   Determine an individual's pretest and posttest probability of coronary heart disease, identify factors associated with test complications, and apply appropriate precautions to reduce risks to the individual.

1.3.16   Identify probable disease-specific endpoints for testing in an individual with cardiovascular, pulmonary, metabolic, orthopedic/musculoskeletal, neuromuscular, and NIH disease.

1.3.17   Select and employ appropriate techniques for preparation and measurement of ECG, heart rate, blood pressure, oxygen saturation, RPE, symptoms, expired gases, and other measures as needed before, during, and following exercise testing.

1.3.18   Select and administer appropriate exercise tests to evaluate functional capacity, strength, and flexibility in individuals with cardiovascular, pulmonary, metabolic, orthopedic/musculoskeletal, neuromuscular, and NIH disease.

1.3.19   Discuss strengths and limitations of various methods of measures and indices of body composition.

1.3.20   Appropriately select, apply, and interpret body-composition tests and indices.

1.3.21   Discuss pertinent test results with other healthcare professionals.

GENERAL POPULATION/CORE: EXERCISE PRESCRIPTION AND PROGRAMMING

1.7.3   Determine the appropriate level of supervision and monitoring recommended for individuals with known disease based on disease-specific risk-stratification guidelines and current health status.

1.7.4   Develop, adapt, and supervise appropriate aerobic, resistance, and flexibility training for individuals with cardiovascular, pulmonary, metabolic, orthopedic/musculoskeletal, neuromuscular, and NIH disease.

1.7.6   Instruct individuals with cardiovascular, pulmonary, metabolic, orthopedic/musculoskeletal, neuromuscular, and NIH disease in techniques for performing physical activities safely and effectively in an unsupervised exercise setting.

1.7.7   Modify the exercise prescription or discontinue exercise based on individual symptoms, current health status, musculoskeletal limitations, and environmental considerations.

1.7.8   Extract and interpret clinical information needed for safe exercise management of individuals with cardiovascular, pulmonary, metabolic, orthopedic/musculoskeletal, neuromuscular, and NIH disease.

1.7.9   Evaluate individual outcomes from serial outcome data collected before, during, and after exercise interventions.

GENERAL POPULATION/CORE: HUMAN BEHAVIOR AND COUNSELING

1.9.1   Summarize contemporary theories of health behavior change, including social cognitive theory, theory of reasoned action, theory of planned behavior, transtheoretical model, and health belief model. Apply techniques to promote healthy behaviors, including physical activity.

1.9.2   Describe characteristics associated with poor adherence to exercise programs.

1.9.3   Describe the psychological issues associated with acute and chronic illness, such as anxiety, depression, social isolation, hostility, aggression, and suicidal ideation.

1.9.4   Counsel individuals with cardiovascular, pulmonary, metabolic, ortho-pedic/musculoskeletal, neuromuscular, and NIH disease on topics such as disease processes, treatments, diagnostic techniques, and lifestyle management.

1.9.6   Explain factors that may increase anxiety before or during exercise testing, and describe methods to reduce anxiety.

1.9.7   Recognize signs and symptoms of failure to cope during personal crises such as job loss, bereavement, and illness.

GENERAL POPULATION/CORE: SAFETY, INJURY PREVENTION, AND EMERGENCY PROCEDURES

1.10.1   List routine emergency equipment, drugs, and supplies present in an exercise testing laboratory and therapeutic exercise session area.

1.10.2   Provide immediate responses to emergencies, including basic cardiac life support, AED, activation of emergency medical services, and joint immobilization.

1.10.3   Verify operating status of emergency equipment, including defibrillator, laryngoscope, and oxygen.

1.10.4   Explain universal precautions procedures and apply as appropriate.

1.10.5   Develop and implement a plan for responding to emergencies.

1.10.6   Demonstrate knowledge of advanced cardiac life support procedures.

GENERAL POPULATION/CORE: PROGRAM ADMINISTRATION, QUALITY ASSURANCE, AND OUTCOME ASSESSMENT

1.11.1   Describe appropriate staffing for exercise testing and programming based on factors such as individual health status, facilities, and program goals.

1.11.2   List necessary equipment and supplies for exercise testing and programs.

1.11.3   Select, evaluate, and report treatment outcomes using individual-relevant results of tests and surveys.

1.11.4   Explain legal issues pertinent to healthcare delivery by licensed and nonlicensed healthcare professionals providing rehabilitative services and exercise testing and legal risk-management techniques .

1.11.5   Identify individuals requiring referral to a physician or allied health services such as physical therapy, dietary counseling, stress management, weight management, and psychological and social services.

1.11.6   Develop a plan for individual discharge from therapeutic exercise program, including community referrals.

CARDIOVASCULAR: EXERCISE PHYSIOLOGY AND RELATED EXERCISE SCIENCE

2.1.2   Describe the potential benefits and hazards of aerobic, resistance, and flexibility training in individuals with cardiovascular diseases.

2.1.4   Explain how cardiovascular diseases may affect the physiologic responses to aerobic and resistance training.

2.1.5   Describe the immediate and long-term influence of medical therapies for cardiovascular diseases on the responses to aerobic and resistance training.

CARDIOVASCULAR: PATHOPHYSIOLOGY AND RISK FACTORS

2.2.1   Describe the epidemiology, pathophysiology, rate of progression of disease, risk factors, and key clinical findings of cardiovascular diseases.

2.2.2   Explain the ischemic cascade and its effect on myocardial function.

2.2.4   Explain methods of reducing risk in individuals with cardiovascular diseases.

CARDIOVASCULAR: HEALTH APPRAISAL, FITNESS, AND CLINICAL EXERCISE TESTING

2.3.1   Describe common techniques used to diagnose cardiovascular disease, including graded exercise testing, echocardiography, radionuclide imaging, angiography, pharmacologic testing, and biomarkers (e.g., troponin, CK), and explain the indications, limitations, risks, and normal and abnormal results for each.

2.3.2   Explain how cardiovascular disease may affect physical examination findings.

2.3.4   Recognize and respond to abnormal signs and symptoms—such as pain, peripheral edema, dyspnea, and fatigue—in individuals with cardiovascular diseases.

2.3.5   Conduct and interpret appropriate exercise testing methods for individuals with cardiovascular diseases.

CARDIOVASCULAR: MEDICAL AND SURGICAL MANAGEMENT

2.6.2   Explain the common medical and surgical treatments of cardiovascular diseases.

2.6.3   Apply key recommendations of current U.S. clinical practice guidelines for the prevention, treatment, and management of cardiovascular diseases (e.g., AHA, ACC, NHLBI).

2.6.4   List the commonly used drugs (generic and brand names) in the treatment of individuals with cardiovascular diseases, and explain the indications, mechanisms of actions, major side effects, and the effects on the exercising individual.

2.6.5   Explain how treatments for cardiovascular disease, including preventive care, may affect the rate of progression of disease.

CARDIOVASCULAR: EXERCISE PRESCRIPTION AND PROGRAMMING

2.7.2   Design, adapt, and supervise an appropriate Exercise Prescription (e.g., aerobic, resistance, and flexibility training) for individuals with cardiovascular diseases.

2.7.4   Instruct an individual with cardiovascular disease in techniques for performing physical activities safely and effectively in an unsupervised setting.

2.7.5   Counsel individuals with cardiovascular disease on the proper uses of sublingual nitroglycerin.

PULMONARY (e.g., OBSTRUCTIVE AND RESTRICTIVE LUNG DISEASES): EXERCISE PHYSIOLOGY AND RELATED EXERCISE SCIENCE

3.1.1   Describe the potential benefits and hazards of aerobic, resistance, and flexibility training in individuals with pulmonary diseases.

3.1.2   Explain how pulmonary diseases may affect the physiologic responses to aerobic, resistance, and flexibility training.

3.1.3   Explain how scheduling of exercise relative to meals can affect dyspnea.

3.1.5   Describe the immediate and long-term influence of medical therapies for pulmonary diseases on the responses to aerobic, resistance, and flexibility training.

PULMONARY: PATHOPHYSIOLOGY AND RISK FACTORS

3.2.1   Describe the epidemiology, pathophysiology, rate of progression of disease, risk factors, and key clinical findings of pulmonary diseases.

3.2.3   Explain methods of reducing risk in individuals with pulmonary diseases.

PULMONARY: HEALTH APPRAISAL, FITNESS, AND CLINICAL EXERCISE TESTING

3.3.1   Explain how pulmonary disease may affect physical examination findings.

3.3.3   Demonstrate knowledge of lung volumes and capacities (e.g., tidal volume, residual volume, inspiratory volume, expiratory volume, total lung capacity, vital capacity, functional residual capacity, peak flow rate, diffusion capacity) and how they may differ between normals and individuals with pulmonary disease.

3.3.4   Recognize and respond to abnormal signs and symptoms to exercise in individuals with pulmonary diseases.

3.3.5   Describe common techniques and tests used to diagnose pulmonary diseases, and explain the indications, limitations, risks, and normal and abnormal results for each.

3.3.6   Conduct and interpret appropriate exercise testing methods for individuals with pulmonary diseases.

PULMONARY: MEDICAL AND SURGICAL MANAGEMENT

3.6.3   Explain how treatments for pulmonary disease, including preventive care, may affect the rate of progression of disease.

3.6.5   Explain the common medical and surgical treatments of pulmonary diseases.

3.6.6   List the commonly used drugs (generic and brand names) in the treatment of individuals with pulmonary diseases, and explain the indications, mechanisms of actions, major side effects, and the effects on the exercising individual.

3.6.7   Apply key recommendations of current U.S. clinical practice guidelines (e.g., ALA, NIH, NHLBI) for the prevention, treatment, and management of pulmonary diseases.

PULMONARY: EXERCISE PRESCRIPTION AND PROGRAMMING

3.7.2   Design, adapt, and supervise an appropriate exercise prescription (e.g., aerobic, resistance, and flexibility training) for individuals with pulmonary diseases.

3.7.4   Instruct an individual with pulmonary diseases in proper breathing techniques and exercises and methods for performing physical activities safely and effectively.

3.7.5   Demonstrate knowledge of the use of supplemental oxygen during exercise and its influences on exercise tolerance.

METABOLIC (e.g., DIABETES, HYPERLIPIDEMIA, OBESITY, FRAILTY, CHRONIC RENAL FAILURE, METABOLIC SYNDROME): EXERCISE PHYSIOLOGY AND RELATED EXERCISE SCIENCE

4.1.1   Explain how metabolic diseases may affect aerobic endurance, muscular strength and endurance, flexibility, and balance.

4.1.2   Describe the immediate and long-term influence of medical therapies for metabolic diseases on the responses to aerobic, resistance, and flexibility training.

4.1.3   Describe the potential benefits and hazards of aerobic, resistance, and flexibility training in individuals with metabolic diseases.

METABOLIC: PATHOPHYSIOLOGY AND RISK FACTORS

4.2.1   Describe the epidemiology, pathophysiology, rate of progression of disease, risk factors, and key clinical findings of metabolic diseases.

4.2.5   Describe the probable effects of dialysis treatment on exercise performance, functional capacity, and safety, and explain methods for preventing adverse effects.

4.2.6   Describe the probable effects of hypo/hyperglycemia on exercise performance, functional capacity, and safety, and explain methods for preventing adverse effects.

4.2.7   Explain methods of reducing risk in individuals with metabolic diseases.

METABOLIC: HEALTH APPRAISAL, FITNESS, AND CLINICAL EXERCISE TESTING

4.3.1   Describe common techniques and tests used to diagnose metabolic diseases, and explain the indications, limitations, risks, and normal and abnormal results for each.

4.3.3   Explain appropriate techniques for monitoring blood glucose before, during, and after an exercise session.

4.3.4   Recognize and respond to abnormal signs and symptoms in individuals with metabolic diseases.

4.3.5   Conduct and interpret appropriate exercise testing methods for individuals with metabolic diseases.

METABOLIC: MEDICAL AND SURGICAL MANAGEMENT

4.6.2   Apply key recommendations of current U.S. clinical practice guidelines (e.g., ADA, NIH, NHLBI) for the prevention, treatment, and management of metabolic diseases.

4.6.3   Explain the common medical and surgical treatments of metabolic diseases.

4.6.4   List the commonly used drugs (generic and brand names) in the treatment of individuals with metabolic diseases, and explain the indications, mechanisms of actions, major side effects, and the effects on the exercising individual.

4.6.5   Explain how treatments for metabolic diseases, including preventive care, may affect the rate of progression of disease.

METABOLIC: EXERCISE PRESCRIPTION AND PROGRAMMING

4.7.2   Design, adapt, and supervise an appropriate exercise prescription (e.g., aerobic, resistance, and flexibility training) for individuals with metabolic diseases.

4.7.4   Instruct individuals with metabolic diseases in techniques for performing physical activities safely and effectively in an unsupervised exercise setting.

4.7.5   Adapt the exercise prescription based on the functional limits and benefits of assistive devices (e.g., wheelchairs, crutches, and canes).

ORTHOPEDIC/MUSCULOSKELETAL (e.g., LOW BACK PAIN, OSTEOARTHRITIS, RHEUMATOID ARTHRITIS, OSTEOPOROSIS, AMPUTATIONS, VERTEBRAL DISORDERS): EXERCISE PHYSIOLOGY AND RELATED EXERCISE SCIENCE

5.1.1   Describe the potential benefits and hazards of aerobic, resistance, and flexibility training in individuals with orthopedic/musculoskeletal diseases.

5.1.4   Explain how orthopedic/musculoskeletal diseases may affect aerobic endurance, muscular strength and endurance, flexibility, balance, and agility.

5.1.5   Describe the immediate and long-term influence of medical therapies for orthopedic/musculoskeletal diseases on the responses to aerobic, resistance, and flexibility training.

ORTHOPEDIC/MUSCULOSKELETAL: PATHOPHYSIOLOGY AND RISK FACTORS

5.2.1 Describe the epidemiology, pathophysiology, risk factors, and key clinical findings of orthopedic/musculoskeletal diseases.

ORTHOPEDIC/MUSCULOSKELETAL: HEALTH APPRAISAL, FITNESS, AND CLINICAL EXERCISE TESTING

5.3.1 Recognize and respond to abnormal signs and symptoms to exercise in individuals with orthopedic/musculoskeletal diseases.

5.3.2 Describe common techniques and tests used to diagnose orthopedic/musculoskeletal diseases.

5.3.3 Conduct and interpret appropriate exercise testing methods for individuals with orthopedic/musculoskeletal diseases.

ORTHOPEDIC/MUSCULOSKELETAL: MEDICAL AND SURGICAL MANAGEMENT

5.6.1 List the commonly used drugs (generic and brand names) in the treatment of individuals with orthopedic/musculoskeletal diseases, and explain the indications, mechanisms of actions, major side effects, and the effects on the exercising individual.

5.6.2 Explain the common medical and surgical treatments of orthopedic/musculoskeletal diseases.

5.6.3 Apply key recommendations of current U.S. clinical practice guidelines (e.g., NIH, National Osteoporosis Foundation, Arthritis Foundation) for the prevention, treatment, and management of orthopedic/musculoskeletal diseases.

5.6.4 Explain how treatments for orthopedic/musculoskeletal disease may affect the rate of progression of disease.

ORTHOPEDIC/MUSCULOSKELETAL: EXERCISE PRESCRIPTION AND PROGRAMMING

5.7.1 Explain exercise training concepts specific to industrial or occupational rehabilitation, which includes work hardening, work conditioning, work fitness, and job coaching.

5.7.2 Design, adapt, and supervise an appropriate exercise prescription (e.g., aerobic, resistance, and flexibility training) for individuals with orthopedic/musculoskeletal diseases.

5.7.3 Instruct an individual with orthopedic/musculoskeletal disease in techniques for performing physical activities safely and effectively in an unsupervised exercise setting.

5.7.4 Adapt the exercise prescription based on the functional limits and benefits of assistive devices (e.g., wheelchairs, crutches, and canes).

NEUROMUSCULAR (e.g., MULTIPLE SCLEROSIS, MUSCULAR DYSTROPHY AND OTHER MYOPATHIES, ALZHEIMER DISEASE, PARKINSON DISEASE, POLIO AND POSTPOLIO SYNDROME, STROKE AND BRAIN INJURY, CEREBRAL PALSY, PERIPHERAL NEUROPATHIES): EXERCISE PHYSIOLOGY AND RELATED EXERCISE SCIENCE

6.1.1   Describe the potential benefits and hazards of aerobic, resistance, and flexibility training in individuals with neuromuscular diseases.

6.1.4   Explain how neuromuscular diseases may affect aerobic endurance, muscular strength and endurance, flexibility, balance, and agility.

6.1.5   Describe the immediate and long-term influence of medical therapies for neuromuscular diseases on the responses to aerobic, resistance, and flexibility training.

NEUROMUSCULAR: PATHOPHYSIOLOGY AND RISK FACTORS

6.2.1   Describe the epidemiology, pathophysiology, risk factors, and key clinical findings of neuromuscular diseases.

NEUROMUSCULAR: HEALTH APPRAISAL, FITNESS, AND CLINICAL EXERCISE TESTING

6.3.1   Recognize and respond to abnormal signs and symptoms to exercise in individuals with neuromuscular diseases.

6.3.2   Describe common techniques and tests used to diagnose neuromuscular diseases.

6.3.3   Conduct and interpret appropriate exercise testing methods for individuals with neuromuscular diseases.

NEUROMUSCULAR: MEDICAL AND SURGICAL MANAGEMENT

6.6.1   Explain the common medical and surgical treatments of neuromuscular diseases.

6.6.2   List the commonly used drugs (generic and brand names) in the treatment of individuals with neuromuscular disease, and explain the indications, mechanisms of actions, major side effects, and the effects on the exercising individual.

6.6.3   Apply key recommendations of current U.S. clinical practice guidelines (e.g., NIH) for the prevention, treatment, and management of neuromuscular diseases.

6.6.4   Explain how treatments for neuromuscular disease may affect the rate of progression of disease.

NEUROMUSCULAR: EXERCISE PRESCRIPTION AND PROGRAMMING

6.7.1   Adapt the exercise prescription based on the functional limits and benefits of assistive devices (e.g., wheelchairs, crutches, and canes).

6.7.3 Design, adapt, and supervise an appropriate exercise prescription (e.g., aerobic, resistance, and flexibility training) for individuals with neuro muscular diseases.

6.7.4 Instruct an individual with neuromuscular diseases in techniques for performing physical activities safely and effectively in an unsupervised exercise setting.

NEOPLASTIC, IMMUNOLOGIC, AND HEMATOLOGIC (e.g., CANCER, ANEMIA, BLEEDING DISORDERS, HIV, AIDS, ORGAN TRANSPLANT, CHRONIC FATIGUE SYNDROME, FIBROMYALGIA): EXERCISE PHYSIOLOGY AND RELATED EXERCISE SCIENCE

7.1.1 Explain how NIH diseases may affect the physiologic responses to aerobic, resistance, and flexibility training.

7.1.2 Describe the immediate and long-term influence of medical therapies for NIH on the responses to aerobic, resistance, and flexibility training.

7.1.3 Describe the potential benefits and hazards of aerobic, resistance, and flexibility training in individuals with NIH diseases.

NEOPLASTIC, IMMUNOLOGIC, AND HEMATOLOGIC: PATHOPHYSIOLOGY AND RISK FACTORS

7.2.1 Describe the epidemiology, pathophysiology, risk factors, and key clinical findings of NIH diseases.

NEOPLASTIC, IMMUNOLOGIC, AND HEMATOLOGIC: HEALTH APPRAISAL, FITNESS, AND CLINICAL EXERCISE TESTING

7.3.1 Recognize and respond to abnormal signs and symptoms to exercise in individuals with NIH diseases.

7.3.2 Describe common techniques and tests used to diagnose NIH diseases.

7.3.3 Conduct and interpret appropriate exercise testing methods for individuals with NIH diseases.

NEOPLASTIC, IMMUNOLOGIC, AND HEMATOLOGIC: MEDICAL AND SURGICAL MANAGEMENT

7.6.1 List the commonly used drugs (generic and brand names) in the treatment of individuals with NIH disease, and explain the indications, mechanisms of actions, major side effects, and the effects on the exercising individual.

7.6.2 Apply key recommendations of current U.S. clinical practice guidelines (e.g., ACS, NIH) for the prevention, treatment, and management of NIH diseases.

7.6.3 Explain the common medical and surgical treatments of NIH diseases.

7.6.4 Explain how treatments for NIH disease may affect the rate of progression of disease.

NEOPLASTIC, IMMUNOLOGIC, AND HEMATOLOGIC: EXERCISE PRESCRIPTION AND PROGRAMMING

7.7.1   Design, adapt, and supervise an appropriate exercise prescription (e.g., aerobic, resistance, and flexibility training) for individuals with NIH diseases.

7.7.4   Instruct an individual with NIH diseases in techniques for performing physical activities safely and effectively in an unsupervised exercise setting.

NOTE: The KSAs listed above for the ACSM Registered Clinical Exercise Physiologist® are the same KSAs for educational programs in clinical exercise physiology seeking graduate (master's degree) academic accreditation through the CoAES. For more information, please visit www.coaes.org.

Additional KSAs required (in addition to the ACSM Certified Health Fitness Specialist KSAs) for programs seeking academic accreditation in applied exercise physiology. The KSAs that follow, IN ADDITION TO the ACSM Certified Health Fitness Specialist KSAs above, represent the KSAs for educational programs in applied exercise physiology seeking graduate (master's degree) academic accreditation through the CoAES. For more information, please visit www.coaes.org.

GENERAL POPULATION/CORE: EXERCISE PHYSIOLOGY AND RELATED EXERCISE SCIENCE

1.1.1   Ability to describe modifications in exercise prescription for individuals with functional disabilities and musculoskeletal injuries.

1.1.2   Ability to describe the relationship between biomechanical efficiency, oxygen cost of activity (economy), and performance of physical activity.

1.1.3   Knowledge of the muscular, cardiorespiratory, and metabolic responses to decreased exercise intensity.

GENERAL POPULATION/CORE: PATHOPHYSIOLOGY AND RISK FACTORS

1.2.1   Ability to define atherosclerosis, the factors causing it, and the interventions that may potentially delay or reverse the atherosclerotic process.

1.2.2   Ability to describe the causes of myocardial ischemia and infarction.

1.2.3   Ability to describe the pathophysiology of hypertension, obesity, hyperlipidemia, diabetes, chronic obstructive pulmonary diseases, arthritis, osteoporosis, chronic diseases, and immunosuppressive disease.

1.2.4   Ability to describe the effects of the above diseases and conditions on cardiorespiratory and metabolic function at rest and during exercise.

GENERAL POPULATION/CORE: HEALTH APPRAISAL, FITNESS, AND CLINICAL EXERCISE TESTING

1.3.1   Knowledge of the selection of an appropriate behavioral goal and the suggested method to evaluate goal achievement for each stage of change.

1.3.2   Knowledge of the use and value of the results of the fitness evaluation and exercise test for various populations.

1.3.3   Ability to design and implement a fitness testing/health appraisal program that includes, but is not limited to, staffing needs, physician interaction, documentation, equipment, marketing, and program evaluation.

1.3.4   Ability to recruit, train, and evaluate appropriate staff personnel for performing exercise tests, fitness evaluations, and health appraisals.

GENERAL POPULATION/CORE: PATIENT MANAGEMENT AND MEDICATIONS

1.5.1   Ability to identify and describe the principal action, mechanisms of action, and major side effects from each of the following classes of medications: antianginals, antihypertensives, antiarrhythmics, bronchodilators, hypoglycemics, psychotropics, and vasodilators.

GENERAL POPULATION/CORE: HUMAN BEHAVIOR AND COUNSELING

1.9.1   Knowledge of and ability to apply basic cognitive-behavioral intervention, such as shaping, goal setting, motivation, cueing, problem solving, reinforcement strategies, and self-monitoring.

1.9.2   Knowledge of the selection of an appropriate behavioral goal and the suggested method to evaluate goal achievement for each stage of change.

GENERAL POPULATION/CORE: SAFETY, INJURY PREVENTION, AND EMERGENCY PROCEDURES

1.10.1   Ability to identify the process to train the exercise staff in cardiopulmonary resuscitation.

1.10.2   Ability to design and evaluate emergency procedures for a preventive exercise program and an exercise testing facility.

1.10.3   Ability to train staff in safety procedures, risk-reduction strategies, and injury-care techniques.

1.10.4   Knowledge of the legal implications of documented safety procedures, the use of incident documents, and ongoing safety training.

GENERAL POPULATION/CORE: PROGRAM ADMINISTRATION, QUALITY ASSURANCE, AND OUTCOME ASSESSMENT

1.11.1   Ability to manage personnel effectively.

1.11.2   Ability to describe a management plan for the development of staff, continuing education, marketing and promotion, documentation, billing, facility management, and financial planning.

1.11.3   Ability to describe the decision-making process related to budgets, market analysis, program evaluation, facility management, staff allocation, and community development.

1.11.4   Ability to describe the development, evaluation, and revision of policies and procedures for programming and facility management.

1.11.5   Ability to describe how the computer can assist in data analysis, spreadsheet report development, and daily tracking of customer utilization.

1.11.6   Ability to define and describe the total quality management (TQM) and continuous quality improvement (CQI) approaches to management.

1.11.7   Ability to interpret applied research in the areas of exercise testing, exercise programming, and educational programs to maintain a comprehensive and current state-of-the-art program.

1.11.8   Ability to develop a risk factor screening program, including procedures, staff training, feedback, and follow-up.

1.11.9   Knowledge of administration, management, and supervision of personnel.

1.11.10   Ability to describe effective interviewing, hiring, and employee termination procedures.

1.11.11   Ability to describe and diagram an organizational chart and show the relationships between a health/fitness director, owner, medical advisor, and staff.

1.11.12   Knowledge of and ability to describe various staff training techniques.

1.11.13   Knowledge of and ability to describe performance reviews and their role in evaluating staff.

1.11.14   Knowledge of the legal obligations and problems involved in personnel management.

1.11.15   Knowledge of compensation, including wages, bonuses, incentive programs, and benefits.

1.11.16   Knowledge of methods for implementing a sales commission system.

1.11.17   Ability to describe the significance of a benefits program for staff and demonstrate an understanding in researching and selecting benefits.

1.11.18   Ability to write and implement thorough and legal job descriptions.

1.11.19   Knowledge of personnel time-management techniques.

1.11.20   Knowledge of administration, management, and development of a budget and of the financial aspects of a fitness center.

1.11.21   Knowledge of the principles of financial management.

1.11.22   Knowledge of basic accounting principles, such as accounts payable, accounts receivable, accrual, cash flow, assets, liabilities, and return on investment.

1.11.23   Ability to identify the various forms of a business enterprise, such as sole proprietorship, partnership, corporation, and S-corporation.

1.11.24   Knowledge of the procedures involved with developing, evaluating, revising, and updating capital and operating budgets.

1.11.25   Ability to manage expenses with the objective of maintaining a positive cash flow.

1.11.26   Ability to understand and analyze financial statements, including income statements, balance sheets, cash flows, budgets, and pro forma projections.

1.11.27   Knowledge of program-related break-even and cost/benefit analysis.

1.11.28   Knowledge of the importance of short-term and long-term planning.

1.11.29   Knowledge of the principles of marketing and sales.

1.11.30   Ability to identify the steps in the development, implementation, and evaluation of a marketing plan.

1.11.31   Knowledge of the components of a needs assessment/market analysis.

1.11.32   Knowledge of various sales techniques for prospective members.

1.11.33   Knowledge of techniques for advertising, marketing, promotion, and public relations.

1.11.34   Ability to describe the principles of developing and evaluating product and services, and establishing pricing.

1.11.35   Knowledge of the principles of day-to-day operation of a fitness center.

1.11.36   Knowledge of the principles of pricing and purchasing equipment and supplies.

1.11.37   Knowledge of facility layout and design.

1.11.38   Ability to establish and evaluate an equipment preventive maintenance and repair program.

1.11.39   Ability to describe a plan for implementing a housekeeping program.

1.11.40   Ability to identify and explain the operating policies for preventive exercise programs, including data analysis and reporting, confidentiality of records, relationships with healthcare providers, accident and injury reporting, and continuing education of participants.

1.11.41   Knowledge of the legal concepts of tort, negligence, liability, indemnification, standards of care, health regulations, consent, contract, confidentiality, malpractice, and the legal concerns regarding emergency procedures and informed consent.

1.11.42   Ability to implement capital improvements with minimal disruption of client or business needs.

1.11.43   Ability to coordinate the operations of various departments, including, but not limited to, the front desk, fitness, rehabilitation, maintenance and repair, day care, housekeeping, pool, and management.

1.11.44   Knowledge of management and principles of member service and communication.

1.11.45   Skills in effective techniques for communicating with staff, management, members, healthcare providers, potential customers, and vendors.

1.11.46   Knowledge of and ability to provide strong customer service.

1.11.47   Ability to develop and implement customer surveys.

1.11.48   Knowledge of the strategies for management conflict.

1.11.49   Knowledge of the principles of health promotion and ability to administer health-promotion programs.

1.11.50   Knowledge of health-promotion programs (e.g., nutrition and weight management, smoking cessation, stress management, back care, body mechanics, and substance abuse).

1.11.51   Knowledge of the specific and appropriate content and methods for creating a health-promotion program.

1.11.52   Knowledge of and ability to access resources for various programs and delivery systems.

1.11.53   Knowledge of the concepts of cost-effectiveness and cost-benefit as they relate to the evaluation of health-promotion programming.

1.11.54   Ability to describe the means and amounts by which health-promotion programs might increase productivity, reduce employee loss time, reduce healthcare costs, and improve profitability in the workplace.

Index

Note: Page numbers followed by *b*, *f*, or *t* indicate boxed, figures, or table material.